# 4th Edition
# CRASH COURSE

SERIES EDITOR
## Dan Horton-Szar
BSc(Hons), MBBS(Hons), MRCGP
Northgate Medical Practice
Canterbury
Kent, UK

FACULTY ADVISOR
## Sebastian Lucas
BA, BM BCh (Oxon), FRCP, FRCPath
Department of Histopathology
King's College London School of Medicine
London, UK

# Pathology

## Philip Xiu
MA MBBChir(Cantab) MRCP
CMT2, Royal Brompton Hospital, London, UK

MOSBY

ELSEVIER

Edinburgh London New York Oxford Philadelphia St Louis Sydney Toronto 2015

**ELSEVIER**
MOSBY

First edition 1999

Second edition 2002

Third edition 2007

Fourth edition 2012

Updated Fourth edition 2015

ISBN: 978-0-7234-3855-7

**British Library Cataloguing in Publication Data**
A catalogue record for this book is available from the British Library

**Library of Congress Cataloging in Publication Data**
A catalog record for this book is available from the Library of Congress

**Notices**
Knowledge and best practice in this field are constantly changing. As new research and experience broaden our understanding, changes in research methods, professional practices, or medical treatment may become necessary.

Practitioners and researchers must always rely on their own experience and knowledge in evaluating and using any information, methods, compounds, or experiments described herein. In using such information or methods they should be mindful of their own safety and the safety of others, including parties for whom they have a professional responsibility.

With respect to any drug or pharmaceutical products identified, readers are advised to check the most current information provided (i) on procedures featured or (ii) by the manufacturer of each product to be administered, to verify the recommended dose or formula, the method and duration of administration, and contraindications. It is the responsibility of practitioners, relying on their own experience and knowledge of their patients, to make diagnoses, to determine dosages and the best treatment for each individual patient, and to take all appropriate safety precautions.

To the fullest extent of the law, neither the Publisher nor the authors, contributors, or editors, assume any liability for any injury and/or damage to persons or property as a matter of products liability, negligence or otherwise, or from any use or operation of any methods, products, instructions, or ideas contained in the material herein.

**ELSEVIER** your source for books, journals and multimedia in the health sciences

**www.elsevierhealth.com**

  Working together to grow libraries in developing countries

**www.elsevier.com • www.bookaid.org**

The Publisher's policy is to use **paper manufactured from sustainable forests**

Printed in China

Last digit is the print line: 10  9  8  7  6  5  4  3  2  1

# Series editor foreword

The *Crash Course* series was first published in 1997 and now, 15 years on, we are still going strong. Medicine never stands still, and the work of keeping this series relevant for today's students is an ongoing process. These fourth editions build on the success of the previous titles and incorporate new and revised material, to keep the series up-to-date with current guidelines for best practice, and recent developments in medical research and pharmacology.

We always listen to feedback from our readers, through focus groups and student reviews of the *Crash Course* titles. For the fourth editions we have completely re-written our self-assessment material to keep up with today's 'single-best answer' and 'extended matching question' formats. The artwork and layout of the titles has also been largely re-worked to make it easier on the eye during long sessions of revision.

Despite fully revising the books with each edition, we hold fast to the principles on which we first developed the series. *Crash Course* will always bring you all the information you need to revise in compact, manageable volumes that integrate basic medical science and clinical practice. The books still maintain the balance between clarity and conciseness, and provide sufficient depth for those aiming at distinction. The authors are medical students and junior doctors who have recent experience of the exams you are now facing, and the accuracy of the material is checked by a team of faculty advisors from across the UK.

I wish you all the best for your future careers!

## Dr Dan Horton-Szar

# Prefaces

## Author

Pathology is the study of disease and is therefore central to all of medicine. Each chapter of this fourth edition has been updated to reflect the latest advances from a diverse range of research areas. Brand new clinical sketch boxes have been designed to integrate the understanding of pathology with clinical patient management for key diseases. Another new feature is extended matching questions (EMQs) and single best answers (SBAs) to add to the wide-ranging self-assessment offered by this edition, as well as the electronic edition. I hope this fourth edition proves a readily accessible but comprehensive tool throughout medical training, from lecture hall to hospital ward. Good luck with your studies!

**Philip Xiu**

## Faculty advisor

My predecessor, Prof Rosemary Walker did an excellent job in steering this incredibly comprehensive short text through several editions, providing a very good background to all aspects of pathology and their relevance to clinical medicine. Reflecting this Advisor's special interest, the text has been further revised and updated in several areas where there is progress, confusion and complexity: pregnancy-associated diseases, sickle cell disease, HIV and AIDS, leprosy, systemic sepsis, and infectious diseases in general. The classical areas of cancer and circulatory diseases have also been discretely amended to reflect current thinking where it matters. If all medical students knew most of what is in this text, with its appropriate organisation of knowledge, teachers could sleep more easily and the quality of diagnostic problem-solving among young doctors would be significantly improved. It will certainly help you in all aspects of your medical course. Special thanks and acknowledgement should also go to Philip Xiu for his work on the new edition.

**Sebastian Lucas**

# Acknowledgements

I would like to thank everyone who has helped during the writing of this book. I am grateful to the numerous friends who provided moral support and accepted having ideas thrown at them. Particular mentions must go to Kent Yip, Adam Young, Kevin McCarthy, Kari Schaitel, Oscar Bennett, Tom Clare, Saurabh Singh, Ben Pierce and Sarah Mason.

Finally I wish to thank the very helpful people involved in the production of this book, both in Edinburgh and Oxford.

## Figure Acknowledgements

Figs 3.3, 3.4, 3.6, 3.7, 6.21, 7.18, 11.2 and 13.23 and Fig. 5.15 are adapted with permission from General and Systematic Pathology, 5th Edition, edited by JCE Underwood. Churchill Livingstone, Edinburgh, 2009.

Figs 5.6 and 5.8 are adapted with permission from Anderson's Pathology, 10th edition, edited by I Damjanov and J Linder. Mosby, St.Louis, 1996.

Fig. 10.2 and Figs 5.11 and 7.8 are adapted with permission from medicshandbook. com, 2011.

Fig. 6.16 is adapted with permission from Robbins and Cotran, Pathologic Basis of Disease, 7th edition, edited by V Kumar, A Abbas, and N Fausto. Elsevier Saunders, Philadelphia, 2005.

Fig. 8.20 is adapted with permission from Clinical Medicine, 7th edition, edited by P Kumar and M Clark., Elsevier, London, 2009.

Fig. 8.37 is adapted with permission from Principles and Practice of Surgery, 3rd edition, edited by APM Forrest, DC Carter and IB Macleod. Churchill Livingstone, Edinburgh, 1995.

Fig. 8.40   is adapted with permission from Lecture Notes in General Surgery, 12th edn, by H Ellis, Wiley-Blackwell, 2010.

Fig. 11.14 is adapted with permission from Lecture Notes on Urology, 5th edition, by J Blandy. Blackwell Scientific, Oxford, 1998.

Fig. 13.4 is adapted with permission from Lecture Notes in Paediatrics, 8th Edition, by S Newell. Wiley-Blackwell, 2010.

Fig. 13.14 is adapted with permission from Essential Haematology, 5th edition, by AV Hoffbrand and JE Pettit. Wiley-Blackwell, Oxford, 2006.

Figs 13.30 and 13.31 are adapted with permission from Pathology Illustrated, 6th edition, by R Reid and F Roberts. Churchill Livingstone, Edinburgh, 2005.

# Dedication

For Helena – *In aeternum te amabo.*

**Phil**

# Contents

## Part I: Principles of pathology

## Part II: Systemic pathology

# Contents

# PART I
# PRINCIPLES OF
# PATHOLOGY

# Introduction to pathology

## DISEASES

A disease is an alteration from the normal function/structure of an organ or system, which manifests as a characteristic set of signs and symptoms.

## PATHOLOGY

Pathology is the scientific study of disease. It is concerned with the causes and effects of disease, and the functional and structural changes that occur. Changes at the molecular and cellular level correlate with the clinical manifestations of the disease.

Understanding the processes of disease assists in the accurate recognition, diagnosis and treatment of diseases.

### Divisions of pathology

Pathology is traditionally subdivided into five main clinical disciplines:

1. Histopathology—the study of histological abnormalities of diseased cells and tissues
2. Haematology—the study of primary diseases of the blood and the secondary effects of other diseases on the blood
3. Chemical pathology—the study of biochemical abnormalities associated with disease
4. Microbiology—the study of infectious diseases and the organisms that cause them
5. Immunopathology—the study of diseases through the analysis of immune function.

## Classification of disease

The causes of disease are numerous and diverse. For convenience, diseases are often classified as either congenital or acquired disorders. Congenital diseases are present from birth, whereas acquired disorders are incurred as a result of factors originating in the external environment.

### Congenital

Congenital causes can be either genetic (e.g. cystic fibrosis) or non-genetic (e.g. thalidomide anomalies).

### Acquired

Acquired causes can be any of the following:
- Trauma
- Infections
- Radiation injury
- Chemical injury
- Circulatory disturbances
- Immunological disturbances
- Degenerative disorders
- Nutritional deficiency diseases
- Endocrine disorders
- Psychosomatic factors
- Iatrogenic disease
- Idiopathic disease.

However, many, if not most, diseases are due to a combination of causes, and they are, therefore, said to have a multifactorial aetiology. Figure 1.1 illustrates the features of disease.

**Fig. 1.1** Characteristics of disease

| Characteristic | Explanation |
|---|---|
| Definition | A clear, concise and accurate description |
| Incidence | Number of new cases of disease occurring in a population of a defined size during a defined period |
| Prevalence | Number of cases of disease to be found in a defined population at a stated time |
| Aetiology | Cause of disease |
| Pathogenesis | Mechanism by which a disease is caused |
| Morphology | Form and structural changes |
| Complications and sequelae | Secondary consequences of disease |
| Treatment | Treatment regimens, effectiveness and side effects |
| Prognosis | Expected outcome of the disease |

**HINTS AND TIPS**

Autopsy room sessions can provide students with an excellent oppurtunity to correlate the gross histopathological features with the natural history of the disease.

## HOW PATHOLOGY IS COVERED IN THIS BOOK

### Part I: Principles of pathology

A limited number of tissue responses underlie all diseases. These responses are known as basic pathological responses. The first part of this book describes the principles of these in relation to our advancing knowledge of the molecular sciences.

### Part II: Systematic pathology

As well as an understanding of the basic pathological responses, it is also necessary to understand how they affect individual tissues and organs. The second part of this book describes the common pathology of the specific diseases as they affect individual organs or organ systems. This approach is termed systematic pathology, and it is illustrated by clinical examples of disease.

# Inflammation, repair and cell death

## ● Objectives

In this chapter, you will learn to:
- Describe the causes and mechanisms of acute and chronic inflammation.
- Describe the chemical mediators of inflammation.
- Understand the systemic effects of inflammation.
- Define the terms labile, stable and permanent tissue.
- Describe the mechanisms of wound healing.
- Describe necrosis and apoptosis as forms of cell death and understand the differences between them.

## INFLAMMATION

### Definition

Inflammation is the response of living tissues to cellular injury. It involves both innate and adaptive immune mechanisms.

### Purpose

The purpose of inflammation is to localize and eliminate the causative agent, limit tissue injury and restore tissue to normality.

Inflammation can be divided into two types: acute and chronic. The division of inflammation is based according to the time course and cellular components involved. These categories are not mutually exclusive, and some overlap exists (Fig. 2.1).

### Causes of acute inflammation

The causes of acute inflammation are:
- physical agents, e.g. trauma, heat, cold, ultraviolet light, radiation
- irritant and corrosive chemical substances, e.g. acids, alkalis
- microbial infections, e.g. pyogenic bacteria
- immune-mediated hypersensitivity reactions, e.g. immune-mediated vasculitis, seasonal allergic rhinitis (hay fever)
- tissue necrosis, e.g. ischaemia resulting in a myocardial infarction.

### Causes of chronic inflammation

Chronic inflammation usually develops as a primary response to:

- microorganisms resistant to phagocytosis or intracellular killing mechanisms, e.g. tuberculosis (TB), leprosy
- foreign bodies, which can be endogenous (e.g. bone, adipose tissue, uric acid crystals) or exogenous (e.g. silica, suture materials, implanted prostheses)
- some autoimmune diseases, e.g. Hashimoto's thyroiditis, rheumatoid arthritis, contact hypersensitivity reactions
- primary granulomatous diseases, e.g. Crohn's disease, sarcoidosis.

Inflammation becomes chronic when it occurs over a prolonged period of time with simultaneous tissue destruction and attempted repair. It may occur secondary to acute inflammation due to the persistence of the causative agent. Figure 2.2 shows the sequelae of inflammation.

## ACUTE INFLAMMATION

### Classic signs of acute inflammation

The classic signs of acute inflammation are:
- redness (rubor)
- heat (calor)
- swelling (tumour)
- pain (dolour)
- loss of function (functio laesa).

These classic signs are produced by a rapid vascular response and cellular events characteristic of acute inflammation.

The main function of these events is to bring elements of the immune system to the site of injury and prevent further tissue damage.

**Fig. 2.1** Comparison of acute and chronic inflammation

| | Acute inflammation | Chronic inflammation |
|---|---|---|
| Response | Immediate reaction of tissue to injury | Persisting reactions of tissue to injury |
| Onset | Rapid | Slow response |
| Immunity | Innate | Cell mediated |
| Predominant cell type | Neutrophil | Lymphocytes, plasma cells, macrophages |
| Duration | Hours to weeks | Weeks/months/years |
| Vascular response | Prominent | Less important |

*Note that the acute and chronic categories are not mutually exclusive.*

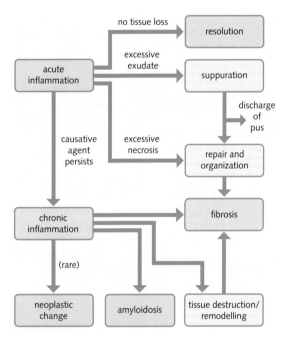

**Fig. 2.2** Sequelae of inflammation.

## Vascular response

### Vasodilatation

Blood flow to the capillary bed is normally limited by the precapillary sphincters. In acute inflammation, vasodilatation occurs when the arterioles and precapillary sphincters relax. This results in increased blood flow to the injured area.

### Increased vascular permeability

Endothelial intracellular proteins, contract under the influence of chemical inflammatory mediators, such as histamine, bradykinin, nitric oxide and leukotriene B4. Endothelial contraction results in:

- increased fenestrations between endothelial cells
- increased permeability of vessels to plasma proteins.

Proteins leak out of the plasma into the interstitial spaces, leading to a decrease in the plasma oncotic pressure. It includes circulating components such as immunoglobulins and coagulation factors.

### Inflammatory oedema

The combined increase in hydrostatic pressure and the decreased oncotic pressure (from leakage of proteins into interstitial spaces) causes net fluid movement from plasma into tissues; this is inflammatory oedema.

### Advantages of inflammatory oedema

- Fluid increase in the damaged tissue dilutes and modifies the action of toxins.
- Protein levels increase in the tissue—these include protective antibodies and fibrin.
- Non-specific antibodies act as opsonins for neutrophil-mediated phagocytosis and function to neutralize toxins.
- The formation of a fibrin net acts as a scaffold for inflammatory cells, preventing the spread of microorganisms.
- Circulation of the exudate into the lymphatic system assists in antigen presentation and helps mount a specific immune response.

## Cellular events

Neutrophil polymorphs pass between endothelial cell junctions and invade damaged tissue to combat the effects of injury. The movement of leucocytes out of the vessel lumen is termed extravasation, and is achieved in five stages (Fig. 2.3):

1. Margination to the plasmatic zone (Fig. 2.4). This is assisted by the slowing of the blood.
2. 'Rolling' of leucocytes due to the repeated formation and destruction of transient adhesions with the endothelium.
3. Adhesion ('pavementing')—leucocytes eventually firmly adhere to the vascular endothelium, due to the interaction of paired molecules on the leucocyte and endothelial cell surface, e.g. $\beta_2$-integrin and ICAM-1.
4. Transmigration (diapedesis)—leucocytes pass between the endothelial cell junctions, through the vessel wall into tissue spaces.
5. Chemotaxis—neutrophils migrate towards, and are possibly activated by, chemical substances (chemotaxins) released at sites of tissue injury. These chemotaxins are thought to be leukotrienes, complement components and bacterial products.

### HINTS AND TIPS

The predominant cell type of acute inflammation is the neutrophil. Lymphocytes, plasma cells and macrophages are the cells found in chronic inflammation.

## Phagocytosis and intracellular killing

Neutrophils and monocytes ingest debris and foreign particles at the site of injury (Fig. 2.5). Cellular pseudopodia engulf the foreign particle and fuse to produce a phagocytic vacuole or phagosome. Phagocytosis is assisted by opsonization with immunoglobulins and complement components.

Following phagocytosis, leucocytes attempt to destroy phagocytosed material by:

- discharge of lysosomal enzymes into the phagosome
- oxygen-dependent mechanisms, such as $H_2O_2$, $O_2^-$, $\bullet OH$
- oxygen-independent mechanisms, such as lactoferrin, lysozyme and hydrolases.

## CHEMICAL MEDIATORS OF INFLAMMATION

Several different inflammatory mediator systems interact to produce inflammation. No chemical mediator alone can be entirely responsible for any single feature of the inflammatory response.

Regulatory mechanisms exist in all mediator systems.

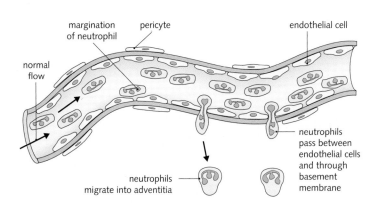

**Fig. 2.3** Cellular events in acute inflammation. Neutrophils are the predominant cell type of acute inflammation. They reach the injured tissues by margination, rolling, adhesion and transmigration.

margination of neutrophil · pericyte · endothelial cell · normal flow · neutrophils pass between endothelial cells and through basement membrane · neutrophils migrate into adventitia

---

**Fig. 2.4** Mechanism of margination of neutrophil polymorphs

Increased plasma viscosity → Decreased blood flow → White blood cells fall out of axial stream into plasmatic zone
(due to loss of intravascular (margination)
fluid)

**Fig. 2.5** Phagocytosis of foreign particle by leucocyte. (A) Attachment of foreign particle. (B) Pseudopodia engulfing particle. (C) and (D) Incorporation within the cell in a vacuole called a phagosome.

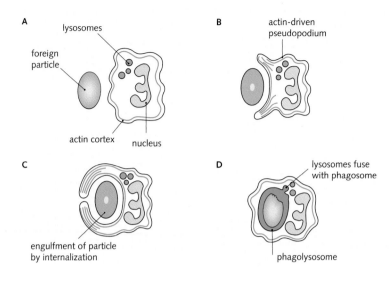

## The complement system

This cascading sequence of serum proteins is made up of more than 20 components; the activated product of one protein activates another (Fig. 2.6). The complement proteins have numerous functions (Fig. 2.7). The system can be activated in four ways during the acute inflammatory response:

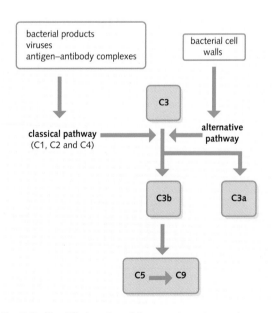

**Fig. 2.6** Simplified version of the complement cascade showing how the activated product of one protein activates another.

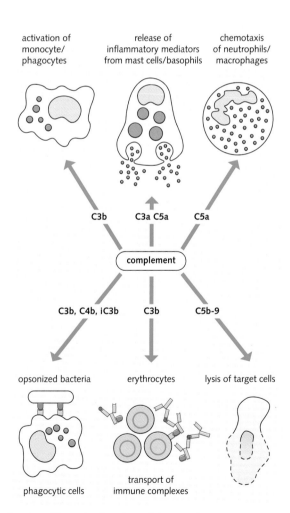

**Fig. 2.7** The major functions of the complement system.

1. Necrotic cells release enzymes that are capable of activating complement.
2. Antibody–antigen complexes activate complement through the classical pathway.
3. Gram-negative bacterial endotoxins activate complement through the alternative pathway.
4. Products of the kinin and fibrinolytic systems activate complement.

## Kinins

Kinins are small, vasoactive peptides and bradykinin is the most well known of all the kinins. It exerts its effects by increasing vascular permeability and producing pain. Both effects are cardinal features of acute inflammation.

The kinin system is stimulated by activated coagulation factor XII (the Hageman factor).

## Arachidonic acid, prostaglandins and leukotrienes

During acute inflammation, the membrane phospholipids of neutrophils and mast cells are metabolized to form prostaglandins and leukotrienes (Fig. 2.8).

The anti-inflammatory action of drugs (e.g. aspirin) is attributable to their ability to inhibit prostaglandin production.

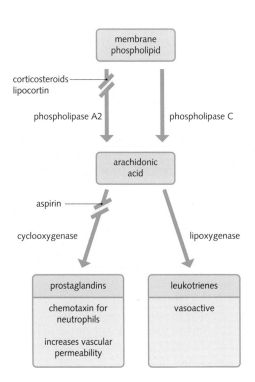

**Fig. 2.8** Formation of arachidonic acid and its metabolites.

**Clinical Note**

Corticosteroids (e.g. prednisolone) are very effective anti-inflammatory drugs but long-term use is associated with numerous side effects, including reduced bone density (osteoporosis), diabetes mellitus, increased blood pressure and cataracts. The prolonged use of corticosteroids is, therefore, carefully controlled, the lowest possible effective dose is prescribed.

## Platelet activation factors

Platelet activation factors are released from mast cells and neutrophils during degranulation. They have the following effects:

- Induce platelet aggregation and degranulation
- Increase vascular permeability
- Induce leucocyte adhesion to the endothelium
- Stimulate synthesis of arachidonic acid derivatives.

## Vasoactive amines

These are preformed inflammatory mediators and so can be rapidly released by inflammatory cells. The most notable example is histamine, which is released following the degranulation of mast cells.

## Cytokines

Cytokines are a family of chemical messengers that act over short distances by binding specific receptors on target cell surfaces. They include:

- interleukins—cytokines that act between leucocytes (more than 15 types)
- interferons—inhibit replication of viruses within cells and activate macrophages and natural killer (NK) cells
- growth factors
- tumour necrosis factors—kill tumour cells but also stimulate adipose and muscle catabolism leading to weight loss.

Tumour necrosis factor alpha (TNFα) and interleukin 1 (IL-1) are key cytokines in acute inflammation.

## Nitric oxide

Nitric oxide (NO) is a potent vasodilator that is released from endothelial cells and macrophages. NO acts as a regulator of inflammation, actively reducing the effect of other proinflammatory mediators.

## Acute-phase proteins

Proteins whose serum level dramatically increases during inflammation are called acute-phase proteins. These proteins are produced by the liver and induced by circulating levels of IL-1, e.g. the C-reactive protein.

### Clinical Note

C-reactive protein (CRP) can be measured in the serum as a non-specific marker of inflammation. Serial measurements can be used to monitor progress of an inflammatory disease.

## CHRONIC INFLAMMATION

### Mononuclear infiltration and granulation tissue

The site of chronic inflammation is dominated by:

- lymphocytes
- plasma cells (for antibody production)
- macrophages (for phagocytosis)—some macrophages fuse to form multinucleate giant cells.

Macrophages in inflamed tissue are formed from the transformation of blood monocytes (Fig. 2.9). The number of macrophages gradually increases during acute inflammation until they are the dominant cell type in chronic inflammation. These macrophages are activated by numerous stimuli, including interferon gamma (IFNy), which is produced by activated lymphocytes.

The macrophages gradually remove damaged tissue by phagocytosis and produce growth factors to aid repair through fibrosis. This results in the slow

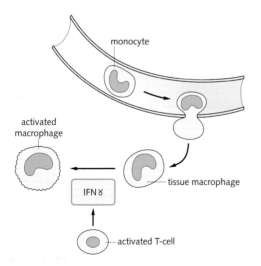

**Fig. 2.9** Monocytes and macrophages in chronic inflammation. Note that macrophages may be activated by stimuli other than interferon-gamma, including bacterial endotoxin and fibronectin.

replacement of damaged tissue with granulation tissue, which consists of new capillaries and new connective tissue formed from myofibroblasts and the collagen that they secrete.

The prolonged presence of activated macrophages in chronic inflammation leads to the overproduction of biologically active products and, therefore, tissue damage.

### HINTS AND TIPS

Chronic inflammation is a crucial process in many important diseases. Excellent examples are provided later in this book, including atherosclerosis (Chapter 6), tuberculosis (Chapter 7) and rheumatoid arthritis (Chapter 12).

### Wound healing

### Nature of cells

The regenerative capacity of tissue can be categorized in three main ways: labile, stable and permanent:

- Labile tissue is constantly dividing, usually through stem cell division. This allows the replacement of ageing tissue, such as the surface epithelia of the skin, gastrointestinal tract and uterus. Blood cells are derived from the labile cells of the bone marrow.
- Stable tissues are in a state of quiescence, meaning that the cells slowly replicate to maintain tissue size. However, such tissue may rapidly regenerate if stimulated.
- Permanent tissues consist of cells that have left the cell cycle and so are incapable of division. Neurons, cardiac and skeletal muscle cells are good examples.

### Clinical Note

A good example of stable tissue regeneration is the ability of the liver to regenerate after part of it is surgically removed (partial hepatectomy). In living-donor hepatic transplantations, one lobe of the donor's liver may be removed. Within weeks of the operation, the donor's liver returns to its original size by compensatory growth of the remaining lobes.

The ultimate consequence of tissue injury, therefore, depends on many factors. Although labile and stable cells may be capable of division, complex tissue architecture might not be replaced. The process of wound healing in the skin depends on the size of the injury; it occurs by two mechanisms:

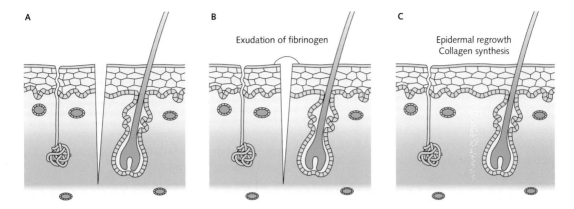

**Fig. 2.10** Skin incision healed by first intention. (A) Incision. (B) Weak fibrin join. (C) Strong collagen join.

## 1. Healing by first intention

Apposed wound margins are joined by fibrin deposition, which is subsequently replaced by collagen and covered by epidermal growth (Fig. 2.10), e.g. surgical incision wound.

## 2. Healing by second intention

Healing by second intention (Fig. 2.11) involves the following:

* Wound margins are unapposed due to extensive tissue damage
* Tissue defect fills with granulation tissue
* Epithelial regeneration to cover surface
* Granulation tissue eventually contracts resulting in scar formation.

**HINTS AND TIPS**

The type of healing process in the skin depends on the extent of tissue damage:
• Minimal tissue loss—involves healing by first intention.
• Extensive tissue loss—involves healing by second intention.

### Scar formation

Myofibroblasts within granulation tissue are attached to one another and to adjacent extracellular matrix. Their contraction draws together the surrounding matrix and thus reduces the size of the defect, but in doing so produces a scar.

## Patterns of inflammation

### Fibrinous inflammation

Fibrinous inflammation is the deposition of increased amounts of fibrin on a tissue surface, e.g. in acute pleurisy secondary to acute lobar pneumonia.

If the fibrin is eventually removed, resolution is said to have occurred. However, if the fibrin persists it may be converted to scar tissue (known as organization).

### Suppurative inflammation

Suppurative inflammation is characterized by the production of pus. It is usually caused by infection with pyogenic bacteria such as *Staphylococcus aureus* and *Streptococcus pyogenes*. Pus becomes surrounded by a 'pyogenic membrane' of sprouting capillaries, neutrophil polymorphs and fibroblasts.

**Fig. 2.11** Skin wound repaired by second intention. (A) Loss of tissue. (B) Granulation tissue. (C) Organization. (D) Early fibrous scar. (E) Scar contraction.

## Haemorrhagic inflammation

If damage is severe, blood vessels within the area may rupture, e.g. haemorrhagic pneumonia, meningococcal septicaemia.

## Granulomatous inflammation

Granulomatous inflammation is a form of chronic inflammation in which modified macrophages (termed epithelioid histiocytes) aggregate to form small clusters, or granulomas, surrounded by lymphoid cells. It usually occurs in response to indigestible particulate matter within macrophages. Causes of granulomatous inflammation include:

- microorganisms resistant to intracellular killing mechanisms, e.g. *Mycobacterium tuberculosis* and *Mycobacterium leprae*
- foreign bodies—endogenous (e.g. bone, adipose tissue, uric acid crystals) or exogenous (e.g. silica, suture materials, implanted prostheses)
- idiopathic, e.g. in Crohn's disease, sarcoidosis and Wegener's granulomatosis
- drugs, e.g. allopurinol and sulphonamides can cause hepatic granuloma.

Granulomas are aggregates of epithelioid histiocytes but commonly they fuse or divide without cytoplasmic separation to produce multinucleate giant cells. Examples include Langhans' giant cell (typical in tuberculosis) and foreign body giant cell (where indigestible foreign body is present).

> **HINTS AND TIPS**
>
> Commonly confused terms:
> - *A granuloma* is an aggregation of epithelioid histiocytes. It is a feature of some chronic inflammatory diseases.
> - *Granulation tissue* is a combination of capillary loops and myofibroblasts. It is a wound-healing phenomenon.

## Systemic effects of inflammation

Both acute and chronic inflammation can produce a number of systemic effects including:

- pyrexia—polymorphs and macrophages produce pyrogens (e.g. IL-1), which act on the hypothalamus
- constitutional symptoms—malaise, nausea and anorexia
- reactive hyperplasia of the mononuclear phagocyte system—enlargement of local and systemic lymph nodes

- haematological changes—increased erythrocyte sedimentation rate, leucocytosis and acute-phase protein release (e.g. C-reactive protein)
- weight loss—occurs in severe chronic inflammation, such as tuberculosis.

## CELL DEATH

Cells may be damaged either reversibly (sublethal damage) or irreversibly (lethal damage) (Fig. 2.12). The type of damage depends on the:

- nature and duration of injury
- type of cells affected
- regenerative ability of tissues.

There are two types of cell death: necrosis and apoptosis. Necrosis tends to occur after severe cellular injury and is always pathological. Apoptosis can be a physiological process that often follows DNA damage and cell-cycle arrest.

Note that there are no absolute ultrastructural criteria by which reversible and irreversible cellular injury can be distinguished, and that there is a continuum from a reversibly injured cell through to an irreversibly necrotically damaged cell.

## Mechanisms of cell death

The initiating mechanisms of cell death depend on the type of injury and are summarized in Fig. 2.13.

### Necrosis

Necrosis is the death of cells or tissues that are still part of the living organism. Necrosis is a pathological process following cellular injury, which results in an inflammatory response after the loss of plasma membrane integrity.

Regardless of the cause of cell injury, necrosis occurs with:

- depletion of intracellular energy systems
- disruption of cytoplasmic organelles
- liberation of intracellular enzymes
- production of oxygen free radicals
- disintegration of the nucleus
- alterations and failure of the plasma membrane
- alteration in ionic transport mechanisms
- increased permeability of membrane phospholipids
- physical disruption of the plasma membrane.

## Histological types of necrosis

### Coagulative necrosis

This is the most common form of necrosis. Dead tissue is initially swollen and firm, but later becomes soft as a result of digestion by macrophages. It usually evokes an

**Fig. 2.12** Relationships between sublethal and lethal cell damage. Sublethal damage can be repaired and the cell survives. Lethal cell damage is irreversible and results in cell death, which may occur by necrosis (as shown) or apoptosis. Types of cellular injury include mechanical trauma, loss of membrane integrity, inhibition of metabolic pathways, DNA damage and deficiency of essential metabolites.

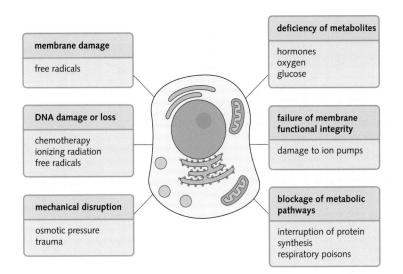

**Fig. 2.13** Mechanisms of cell death. Various cell and tissue types are differentially susceptible to various injurious agents, e.g. the cellular response to ischaemia.

inflammatory response; damaged tissue is removed by phagocytosis.

### Clinical Note

Coagulative necrosis is the classic pattern seen in myocardial tissue following a myocardial infarction (MI). It takes several hours to develop. However, the loss of plasma membrane integrity in necrosis allows the leaking of cardiac enzymes into the bloodstream very quickly, making them useful as biochemical markers. The levels of these enzymes (e.g. troponin T) in the blood are routinely used to aid the diagnosis of a MI.

## Liquefactive necrosis

This characteristically occurs in the central nervous system (e.g. a hypoxic stroke) due to minimal supporting stroma. Necrotic neural tissue undergoes total liquefaction and a glial reaction occurs around the periphery, with eventual cyst formation.

## Caseous necrosis (caseation)

This is commonly seen in tuberculosis. Histologically, the complete loss of normal tissue architecture is replaced by amorphous, granular and eosinophilic tissue. There are variable amounts of fat and an appearance reminiscent of cottage cheese, hence the term 'caseation'.

## Fibrinoid necrosis

This occurs in malignant hypertension, where increased arterial pressure results in necrosis of smooth muscle wall. Eosinophilic and fibrinous deposits are seen, although inflammation and actual necrosis are usually inconspicuous.

## Fat necrosis

This describes focal adipose tissue destruction, which may be due to:

- direct trauma—release of triglycerides following trauma elicits a rapid inflammatory response. Fat is phagocytosed by neutrophils and macrophages, which ultimately results in fibrosis
- enzymatic lipolysis—in acute pancreatitis, lipases liberated from damaged acini act on fat cells in the peritoneal cavity to release triglycerides.

## Apoptosis

Apoptosis is an energy-dependent mechanism of cell death for the deletion of unwanted individual cells; it is a form of 'programmed cell death'. Inhibition of

apoptosis results in cell accumulation, e.g. neoplasia (see Chapter 3). The rate of apoptosis must be matched by the rate of cellular division to maintain a stable tissue size. Increased apoptosis results in net cell loss, e.g. tissue atrophy.

Apoptosis can, therefore, be:

- physiological—such as in the maintenance of organ size, regulation of the immune system and the shedding of the endometrium at menstruation
- pathological—when cellular damage has occurred, often at the nuclear level (i.e. DNA damage). Apoptosis can, therefore, prevent the perpetuation of a genetically abnormal cell.

### HINTS AND TIPS

A key point: apoptosis is an energy-dependent process that does not result in an inflammatory response. This is in contrast to necrosis, an energy-independent process that can cause inflammation.

## Mechanisms of apoptosis

The execution of apoptosis is achieved by the activation of a cascade of proteases known as caspases. Caspase-3 is thought to be a crucial final enzyme in this caspase cascade, which can be initiated by two pathways (Fig. 2.14):

1. The extrinsic pathway—external 'death receptors' (e.g. TNF receptors) are activated by an appropriate ligand.
2. The intrinsic pathway—proapoptotic molecules are released from mitochondria after the breakdown of normal anti-apoptotic signalling (e.g. Bcl-2).

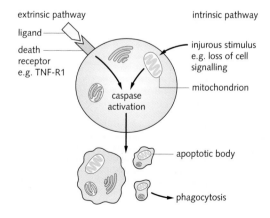

**Fig. 2.14** Initiation of apoptosis. The common caspase cascade may be triggered by the extrinsic ('death receptor') pathway or intrinsic (mitochondrial) pathway.

---

**Fig. 2.15** Comparison of cell death by necrosis and apoptosis

| Feature | Necrosis | Apoptosis |
|---|---|---|
| Induction | Pathological conditions | Pathological or physiological conditions |
| Number of cells | Groups of cells | Single cells |
| Plasma membrane | Loss of membrane integrity | Membrane remains intact |
| Morphology | Cell swelling and lysis | Cell shrinkage and fragmentation, formation of characteristic apoptotic bodies |
| Inflammation | Inflammatory response | No inflammatory response |
| Fate of cells | Phagocytosed by neutrophils and macrophages | Phagocytosed by neighbouring cells |
| Biochemical mechanism | Energy-independent Loss of ion homeostasis | Energy dependent Endonuclease activity |

Examples of where this occurs include the loss of cellular signalling and exposure to radiation or toxins.

The caspase cascade is the common result of both pathways. Morphologically, an apoptotic cell is characterized by:

- loss of cell surface markings
- cell shrinkage due to cytoskeletal breakdown
- nuclear chromatin condensation
- formation of apoptotic bodies with intact plasma membrane and organelles. These are eventually phagocytosed by adjacent cells.

A comparison of cell death by apoptosis and necrosis is given in Fig. 2.15.

# Cancer 3

## Objectives

In this chapter, you will learn to:
- Define tumour, dysplasia, metaplasia, hyperplasia and hypertrophy.
- Understand the differences between benign and malignant tumours.
- Briefly describe the epidemiology of cancer in the UK and worldwide.
- Describe the role of protooncogenes and tumour suppressor genes in the development of cancers.
- Understand the multistage model of tumour development.
- Describe the process of tumour growth and angiogenesis, invasion and metastasis.
- Describe the role of chemicals, radiation and viruses as carcinogenic agents.
- Describe the host defences against cancer.
- Understand the importance of tumour markers, grading and staging in clinical cancer pathology.

## DEFINITIONS AND NOMENCLATURE

## Definitions

### Tumour

A tumour can be defined as an abnormal mass of tissue resulting from autonomous disordered growth that persists after the initiating stimulus has been removed. A tumour results from genetic alteration and deregulated growth control mechanisms. There may be an inherited predisposition to tumour development (e.g. breast and ovarian cancer families), although this accounts for only a small proportion of total tumours. Tumours are:

- progressive—they are independent of normal growth control and continue to grow regardless of requirements and in the absence of any external stimuli
- purposeless—the abnormal mass serves no useful purpose
- parasitic—they are endogenous in origin but draw nourishment from the body while contributing nothing to its function.

All tumours have the suffix '—oma', which means a swelling.

Other related definitions are:

- neoplasm (i.e. new growth)—synonymous with tumour
- neoplasia—the process of tumour growth
- cancer—a malignant neoplasm
- anaplastic neoplasm—a very poorly differentiated neoplasm. Anaplastic specimens highlight the typical changes of a malignant neoplasm: pleomorphism (variation in shape and size) of cells and nuclei, numerous mitoses, abnormal nuclear morphology and cellular disorganization (i.e. loss of cellular polarity).

### Dysplasia

Dysplasia is the disordered development of cells resulting in an alteration in their size, shape and organization. It may be reversible but is also known to precede neoplasia. It is, therefore, referred to as a premalignant state in certain circumstances.

### Metaplasia

Metaplasia is the change from one type of differentiated tissue to another, usually in response to an irritating stimulus, e.g. a change from mucus-secreting epithelium to stratified squamous epithelium in the bronchial irritation associated with cigarette smoking. Metaplasia is reversible and often represents an adaptive response to environmental stress.

### Hyperplasia

This refers to an increase in the number of cells in a tissue or organ, which may result in an increase in the overall size. An example is the hyperplasia of breast tissue during pregnancy.

### Hypertrophy

Hypertrophy is an increase in tissue or organ size due to an increase in the size of cells. Crucially, there is no increase in the number of cells in the tissue. Cells that are permanent (e.g. myocardial fibres) cannot divide and so undergo hypertrophy to increase tissue size (e.g. left ventricular hypertrophy as a response to hypertension).

In general, tissues capable of division can undergo both hyperplasia and hypertrophy to increase tissue size.

## Benign versus malignant

Tumours are classified as either benign or malignant, according to their appearance and behaviour (Fig. 3.1). Benign tumours are usually well differentiated, localized cancers that do not invade the surrounding tissues or metastasize to other organs. Metastasis is the process whereby malignant cells spread from their site of origin (a primary tumour) to distant sites and grow into secondary tumours.

Malignant tumours are capable of invasion and spread to distant organs. This distinction is crucial in the clinic because metastatic disease is associated with significant morbidity and mortality. Malignant neoplasms can show a range of differentiations.

## Nomenclature of tumours

Tumour nomenclature (Fig. 3.2) is based on histological and behaviour patterns. Histology provides information about the type of cell from which the tumour has arisen, whereas behaviour provides information as to whether the cell is benign or malignant.

**Fig. 3.1** Characteristics of benign versus malignant tumours

| Benign | Malignant |
|---|---|
| Localized | Tumour spread |
| No invasion | Invasion |
| No metastases | Metastases |
| Slow growth rate | Rapid growth rate |
| Good differentiation | Poorly differentiated |
| Few mitoses | Many mitoses |
| Normal nuclear chromatin | Increased nuclear chromatin appearance |
| Uniform size cells | Cells and nuclei vary in size (pleomorphism) |
| Exophytic | Endophytic |
| Compression of normal tissue | Invasion and destruction of normal tissue |

Note that invasion is the only absolute distinguishing feature between benign and malignant neoplasms.

**Fig. 3.2** Important tumour nomenclature

| Histological type | Benign | Malignant |
|---|---|---|
| **Epithelial** | | |
| Glandular | Adenoma | Adenocarcinoma |
| Non-glandular | Papilloma | Carcinoma |
| **Connective tissue** | | |
| Adipose | Lipoma | Liposarcoma |
| Cartilage | Chondroma | Chondrosarcoma |
| Bone | Osteoma | Osteosarcoma |
| Smooth muscle | Leiomyoma | Leiomyosarcoma |
| Voluntary muscle | Rhabdomyoma | Rhabdomyosarcoma |
| Blood vessels | Angioma | Angiosarcoma |
| Nerve | Neurofibroma | Neurofibrosarcoma |
| Nerve sheath | Neurilemmoma | Neurilemmosarcoma |
| Glial cells | Glioma | Malignant glioma |
| **Others** | | |
| Haemopoietic | * | Leukaemia |
| Lymphoreticular | * | Lymphoma |
| Melanocytes | * | Malignant melanoma |
| Germinal cell | Benign teratoma | Malignant teratoma |

*Those tumours that are always malignant and do not have benign counterparts.

### HINTS AND TIPS

A few simple rules to follow:
- Carcinomas—malignant tumours of epithelial origin; prefixed by tissue of origin.
- '—oma' suffix for tumours, but there are some non-neoplastic '—omas', e.g. granuloma.
- '—sarcoma' suffix for malignant tumours of connective tissue origin.

## Classification of carcinomas

Carcinomas are malignant tumours of epithelial tissue. Carcinomas of non-glandular epithelium are prefixed by the name of the epithelial cell type. Malignant tumours of glandular epithelium are termed adenocarcinomas. Carcinomas can be further subclassified according to their ability to invade or not, and behavioural information can be gained from histological grading of cellular differentiation.

## Intraepithelial neoplasia

This covers the spectrum of changes short of invasive carcinoma:

- mild dysplasia
- moderate dysplasia
- severe dysplasia/carcinoma in situ.

> **Clinical Note**
>
> Cervical intraepithelial neoplasia (CIN) is a premalignant state that may exist for many years before cervical cancer develops. CIN is categorized according to the level of dysplasia seen in the squamous epithelium of the cervical transformation zone (the area examined on routine 'smear' screening). Three grades are observed:
> • CIN I—mildly dysplasic
> • CIN II—moderately dysplasic
> • CIN III—severely dysplasic (carcinoma in situ at high risk of invasion).

## Carcinoma in situ

This is an epithelial neoplasm with all the cellular features associated with malignancy but which has not yet invaded through the epithelial basement membrane.

The in-situ phase may not progress, or it may last for several years before invasion commences.

## Invasive carcinoma

This is an epithelial neoplasm that invades through the basement membrane. The tumour gains access to the vascular supply and lymphatics, and will often metastasize to distant tissues.

## Epidemiological aspects of cancer

### Cancer in the UK

As a cause of mortality in the UK, cancer is the second biggest killer (after cardiovascular disease). Its incidence (Fig. 3.3) is as follows:

- Almost 1 in 3 of the population will develop cancer during their lifetime.
- Almost 1 in 4 of the population will die of cancer.
- Incidence of cancer deaths increases with increasing age.
- Incidence of cancer varies between males and females.

### Cancer worldwide

The incidence of different cancers varies from country to country. This variation provides clues to the causes of the cancers. For example, in Japan, gastric carcinoma is 30 times more common than in the UK, whereas pancreatic cancer is much rarer. However, migration of a

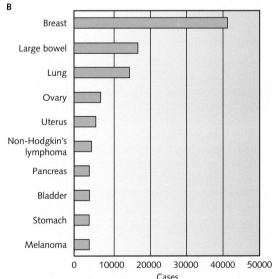

**Fig. 3.3** Incidence of the ten most common cancers of (A) men and (B) women in the UK. The data exclude non-melanoma skin cancers (e.g. basal cell carcinoma) because, although common, they are rarely fatal. Data from Cancer Research UK, 2003. (Adapted from Underwood, 2009.)

subset of the Japanese population to different geographical areas (e.g. USA, UK) alters the incidences of these diseases within that population. These findings suggest that environmental factors (such as diet and occupational, social and geographic effects) rather than genetic causes account for most of the observed differences between countries.

## MOLECULAR BASIS OF CANCER

### Oncogenes and tumour suppressor genes

Cell proliferation and division is usually tightly regulated by two sets of opposing functioning genes:

1. Growth-promoting genes, called protooncogenes
2. Negative cell-cycle regulators, called tumour suppressor genes (TSGs).

Abnormal activation of proto-oncogenes and loss of function of TSGs lead to the transformation of a normal cell into a cancer cell.

### Proto-oncogenes

Proto-oncogenes are genes that are expressed in normal cells. They code for oncoproteins, which positively regulate cell growth and differentiation (growth factors, transcription factors and receptor molecules). In healthy cells, the transcription of these genes is tightly controlled. Inappropriate expression of oncoproteins leads to abnormal cell growth and survival. Normally functioning proto-oncogenes can be activated into cancer-causing oncogenes in two ways:

- A mutation can produce an oncoprotein that is functionally altered and abnormally active. For example, intracellular signalling is affected by the hyperactive mutant *ras* protein.
- A normal oncoprotein can be produced in abnormally large quantities because of enhanced gene amplification (e.g. the *myc* oncogene in neuroblastomas) or enhanced transcription (formation of the Philadelphia chromosome from a translocation between chromosomes 9 and 22).

Oncogenes can be classified according to the function of their product. Oncogenes include genes that express:

- nuclear binding proteins, e.g. *c-myc*
- tyrosine kinase proteins, e.g. *src*
- growth factors, e.g. platelet-derived growth factor
- receptors for growth factors, e.g. *c-erb* B-2/HER-2, which is related to epidermal growth factor receptor
- GTP binding proteins, e.g. *ras*.

Expression of abnormal oncogene products corresponds to the behaviour and appearance of transformed cells. These include:

- independence from the requirement of extrinsic growth factors
- production of proteases that assist tissue invasion
- reduced cell cohesiveness, which assists metastasis
- ability to grow at higher cell densities
- abnormal cellular orientation
- increased plasma membrane and cellular motility.

### Tumour suppressor genes

Tumour suppressor genes (TSGs) (e.g. *p53* and *RB1*) encode proteins that prevent or suppress the growth of tumours. Inactivation of TSGs results in increased susceptibility to cancer formation. Genetically increased susceptibility to cancer formation was first proposed by Knudson, who studied the childhood retinal cancer retinoblastoma.

#### Clinical Note

Retinoblastoma is a rare malignant tumour of the retina. In familial cases (bilateral), a germline mutation in the *RB1* gene is present, meaning that only one further somatic mutation is required for tumour formation. Other cases of retinoblastoma are unilateral and sporadic, needing two somatic mutations on an initially fully functioning *RB1* gene. This requirement for separate mutations in both alleles of a TSG has been termed the 'two-hit' hypothesis of oncogenesis.

Examples of dysfunctional TSGs involved in human cancers are:

- *APC*—implicated in colorectal tumours and located on chromosome 5q
- *NF1*—implicated in neurofibrosarcoma and located on chromosome 17q
- *RB1*—implicated in retinoblastoma and located on chromosome 13q
- *BRCA1*—implicated in breast and ovarian cancer and located on chromosome 17q
- *p53*—implicated in many tumours and located on chromosome 17p.

Loss of function of TSGs or their protein products can result in uncontrolled neoplastic cell growth. TSGs can lose their normal function by a variety of mechanisms:

- Mutations (hereditary or acquired)
- Binding of normal TSG protein to proteins encoded by viral genes, e.g. human papilloma virus proteins E6/E7
- Complexing of normal TSG protein to mutant TSG protein in heterozygous cells.

TSGs function by maintaining the integrity of the genome through cell-cycle arrest in abnormally dividing cells and repair of DNA damage. They also function to promote cell suicide or apoptosis (see Chapter 2) in cells with sustained DNA damage.

One of the most studied TSGs is the *p53* gene, which is located at 17p; it is called 'the guardian of the genome'. *p53* is mutated or functionally altered in over 50% of all human cancers. In addition, a familial inherited mutation is found in Li-Fraumeni's syndrome, in which there is an increased predisposition to several tumour types.

*p53* can recognize damaged DNA and responds either through cell-cycle growth arrest at the $G_1$ check point or through the initiation of apoptosis. For example, the p53 protein product recognizes DNA damage caused by ultraviolet (UV) irradiation and activates apoptotic cell death pathways before the cell can divide and proliferate (Fig. 3.4).

Genes and proteins involved in the process of apoptosis include the death receptor and ligand families, cell-cycle-related genes, the *Bcl-2* family, the caspase family and the caspase substrates.

> ### HINTS AND TIPS
>
> Cellular proliferation is tightly regulated by two sets of opposing functioning genes. Proto-oncogenes are growth-promoting genes whereas tumour suppressor genes are growth-suppressing genes. Deregulated function of proto-oncogenes and tumour suppressor genes leads to cell transformation and tumourigenesis.

## Multistage model of tumour progression

Tumourigenesis is a multistage process that results from accumulated mutation. Tumours arise from single cells, which proliferate to form a clone of cells with identical abnormalities. As tumours develop, they undergo further somatic mutations, which cause abnormalities in other oncogenes and/or tumour suppressor genes. These additional mutations result in cells that are genetically different from each other but which are part of the same tumour: this is heterogeneity.

Fast-growing, less-differentiated cells take over and eliminate the slower-growing, better-differentiated cells.

Chemotherapy will kill the majority of tumour cells. However, tumour cells that are resistant to chemotherapy will survive and be selected for (because of ablation of competing, non-resistant cells), resulting in the regrowth of a tumour that is resistant to chemotherapy (Fig. 3.5). This highlights the concept of 'minimal residual disease', i.e. the small number of tumour cells that survive an intervention such as chemotherapy.

The progressive nature of tumourigenesis is clearly illustrated in Vogelstein's model of the development of colonic cancer. The accumulation over time of mutations in oncogenes such as *Ki-ras*, and loss of function mutations in tumour suppressor genes such as *APC*, results in the eventual formation of colon carcinoma (Fig. 3.6).

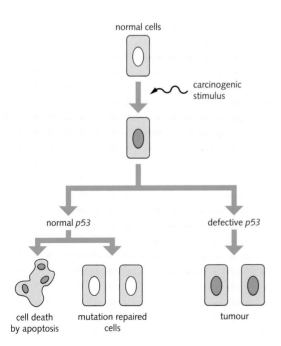

**Fig. 3.4** Role of p53 in cells with damaged DNA. Cells either undergo $G_1$ arrest and DNA repair, or cell death by apoptosis. (Adapted from Underwood, 2009.)

normal cells

carcinogenic stimulus

normal *p53*                    defective *p53*

cell death by apoptosis    mutation repaired cells    tumour

## TUMOUR GROWTH AND SPREAD

## Kinetics of tumour growth and angiogenesis

Angiogenesis is the formation of new blood vessels and is an important physiological process in normal embryogenesis, the female reproductive cycle and wound healing. However, pathological angiogenesis is a key player in many disorders, including cancer. This is because a solid tumour cannot grow beyond a few millimeters in diameter without a blood supply to maintain nutrient and oxygen provision and remove metabolic waste.

In normal cells, angiogenesis is a highly regulated mechanism. In contrast, tumour cells can release pro-angiogenic factors, which induce vascular proliferation.

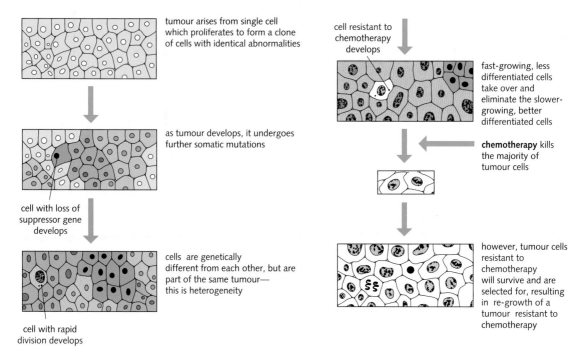

**Fig. 3.5** Tumour progression and genetic heterogeneity.

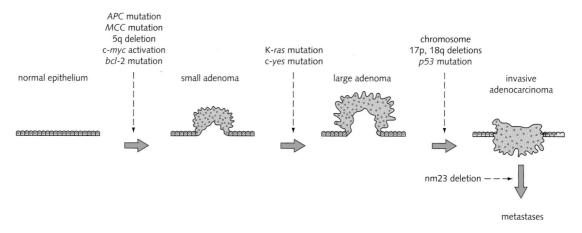

**Fig. 3.6** Multistep development of colonic cancer. The accumulation of genetic mutations corresponds to the altered behaviour of the tumour cells. (APC, adenomatous polyposis coli; MCC, mutated in colorectal cancer.) (Adapted from Underwood, 2009.)

This is sometimes called the angiogenic switch. The angiogenic switch results in the production of pro-angiogenic molecules such as vascular endothelial growth factor.

Eventually, the tumour outgrows its blood supply and areas of necrosis may appear, resulting in slower growth but a more malignant phenotype (Fig. 3.7). This is because only the strongest cells survive the hypoxic conditions.

## Mechanisms and pathways of invasion and metastasis

### Invasion

The ability to invade is the only absolute criterion for malignancy. Invading malignant cells have the following properties:

- Abnormal or increased cellular motility—due to loss of contact inhibition

**Fig. 3.7** Kinetics of tumour growth and angiogenesis. (A) Transformed cell. (B) Avascular tumour nodule. (C) Vascularized tumour. (D) Vascularized tumour with central necrosis. (TAF, tumour angiogenic factors.) (Adapted from Underwood, 2009.)

• Altered cellular adhesion—due to changes in surface adhesion molecules
• Increased secretion of proteolytic enzymes, e.g. metalloproteinases.

Metalloproteinases, such as collagenases and gelatinases, are the most important enzymes in neoplastic invasion. They digest the surrounding connective tissue, thus aiding invasion.

## Metastasis

In metastatic cancer, the total mass of secondary tumours usually exceeds that of the primary lesion. However, only a proportion of neoplastic cells in a malignant tumour are able to metastasize.

It can be impossible to find the primary lesion in some cancer patients who present with extensive secondary metastases.

To metastasize through vessels, neoplastic cells undergo the following sequence of events:

• Detachment of tumour cells from neighbouring cells
• Invasion of the tissue basement membrane and then surrounding connective tissue
• Intravasation into blood/lymphatic vessels
• Evasion of the host's defence mechanisms, often by forming a tumour cell embolus with platelets or host lymphoid cells
• Adherence to endothelium at a distant site

• Extravasation of cells from vessel lumen into surrounding tissue.

Following extravasation, the malignant cells proliferate and secrete more angiogenic growth factors for vascularization. Hence a new tumour is formed. However, not all cancer cells will grow at all distant sites. This is the seed and soil effect: conditions must be appropriate for cell proliferation.

## Main routes of metastasis

There are four main routes of metastasis (Fig. 3.8):

1. Local invasion—most common pattern of spread of malignant tumours is by direct growth into adjacent tissues.
2. Lymphatic spread—forms secondary tumours in lymph nodes.
3. Blood-borne (haematogenous) spread—cells enter the bloodstream and form secondary tumours in organs perfused by blood that has drained from a tumour.
4. Transcoelomic spread—in pleural, pericardial and peritoneal cavities.

### Clinical Note

It is clinically important to know the major tumours that spread to bone via the blood. These are cancers of the bronchus, breast, thyroid, kidney and prostate. Bone metastases can be evaluated using radionucleotide bone scanning, except in myeloma, where a skeletal survey is needed.

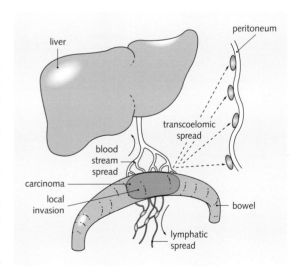

**Fig. 3.8** Routes of metastasis exemplified by a carcinoma of the bowel, i.e. via the bloodstream, via the lymphatic spread, through peritoneal cavities and via local invasion.

## CARCINOGENIC AGENTS

Carcinogens are substances known to cause an increased incidence of cancer.

Carcinogens can exert their effect either by genetic mechanisms (i.e. causing DNA alteration; this is the majority of carcinogens) or epigenetic mechanisms (i.e. acting on the protein product of growth-regulating genes).

## Chemical carcinogens

Most chemical carcinogens are procarcinogens and require metabolic conversion into an active form (ultimate carcinogens), usually by the cytochrome P450 system, which shows significant variability in activity (gene polymorphisms) between individuals. Some people are therefore inherently more susceptible to producing ultimate carcinogens.

Some carcinogens act directly to induce cellular damage. Examples of chemical carcinogens are given in Fig. 3.9.

| **Fig. 3.9** Examples of chemical carcinogens | |
|---|---|
| **Chemical compound** | **Cancer type** |
| **Indirect carcinogens** | |
| Polycyclic hydrocarbons | |
| • Soot [benzo(a)pyrene; dibenzanthracene] | Skin, colon |
| • Tobacco smoke | Lung, bladder, oral cavity, larynx, oesophagus |
| Aromatic amines | |
| • Benzidine, 2-naphthylamine | • Bladder |
| Nitrosamines | |
| • Chemotherapeutic agents | Oesophagus, stomach |
| • Cyclophosphamide, chlorambucil, thiotepa, busulphan | Leukaemias |
| Vinyl chloride | Liver (angiosarcoma) |
| Aflatoxins | Liver |
| **Unknown mechanisms** | |
| Heavy metals | |
| • Nickel, cadmium, chromium | Lung |
| • Arsenic | Skin |

## Stages of chemical carcinogenesis

The progressive model of carcinogenesis (Fig. 3.10) is based on observations of the effects of chemical carcinogens on laboratory animals. This model proposes three main stages of carcinogenesis:

1. Initiation—induction of a genetic alteration in an oncogene or TSG.
2. Promotion—a stimulus for proliferation of the initiated cell; this may be an external agent or a further random mutational genetic abnormality.
3. Persistence—when proliferation of tumour cells becomes autonomous, i.e. it no longer requires the presence of initiators or promoters.

## Radiation

Radiation can be:

• ionizing—natural radiation, therapeutic radiation and nuclear radiation
• non-ionizing—UV radiation.

### HINTS AND TIPS

The stages of chemical carcinogenesis are: initiation, promotion and persistence. The classic examples of initiation and promotion are the effects of methylcholanthrene and croton oil, discovered from experiments in mice. Remember that as humans are likely to be simultaneously exposed to initiators and promoters, chemical carcinogenesis is probably very complex.

Radiation can result in DNA damage in two ways:

1. Directly—causing strand breaks, base alterations and cross-linking of DNA.
2. Indirectly—ionization of $H_2O$ with formation of reactive oxygen free radicals, which interact with and damage DNA.

## Ultraviolet radiation

UV radiation is associated with many different kinds of skin cancer, particularly:

• Squamous cell carcinoma
• Basal cell carcinoma
• Malignant melanoma.

Skin cancer is the most common type of cancer in the UK and USA. It is more common in fair-skinned individuals.

UV light is thought to induce the formation of linkages between pyrimidine bases on the DNA molecule.

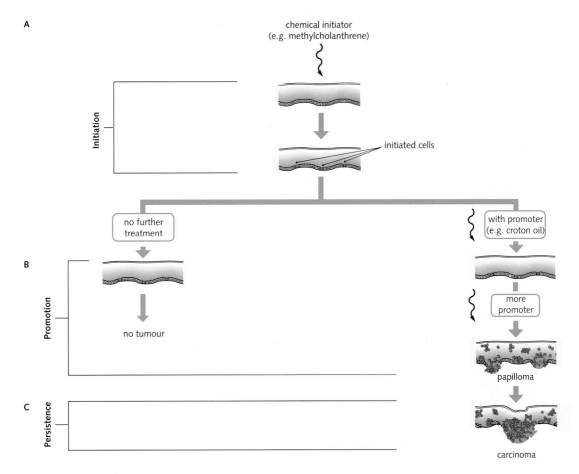

**Fig. 3.10** Stages of chemical carcinogenesis. (A) Initiation: induction of genetic changes in cells that result in neoplastic potential. (B) Promotion: induction of cellular proliferation in the initiated cell. (C) Persistence: proliferating tumour cells no longer require the presence of initiators or promoters. Tumour cells exhibit autonomous growth.

The risk is greatly increased in patients with xeroderma pigmentosum, a rare, autosomal recessive disease characterized by deficiency of DNA repair enzymes.

## Ionizing radiation

### X-ray radiation
Radiotherapy can cause cancer as well as curing it! It is associated with radiation-induced malignant neoplasms, often sarcomas. These tumours may occur months or years after radiation therapy, in the lungs, CNS, bones, kidneys and liver.

### Radioisotopes
Radioactive iodine, which is used to treat thyroid disease, is associated with an increased risk of cancer development as much as 15–25 years after treatment.

### Nuclear radiation
Survivors of the Hiroshima and Nagasaki atomic bombs, and of the accident at the Chernobyl nuclear power plant, have shown a greatly increased incidence of cancer, including leukaemia and carcinoma of the breast, lung and thyroid.

## DNA repair mechanisms and their failure

DNA is the cellular constituent most sensitive to radiation. Fortunately, cells have DNA repair genes (e.g. *MSH2*) that deal with DNA damage. Repair occurs rapidly in the vast majority of cases but damage is sometimes irreparable and major chromosomal and chromatid alterations occur. If such cells also evade cell-cycle arrest and apoptosis, a tumour may develop.

Repair of single-stranded breaks, particularly in rapidly dividing cells, is error prone and introduces single-base mutations.

Double-stranded cleavage leads to chromosome breakage. Attempts to repair multiple breaks result in inappropriate recombination events, e.g. translocation or interstitial deletion.

### Clinical Note

An excellent example of failed DNA repair mechanisms is the autosomal dominant condition hereditary non-polyposis colon cancer (HNPCC; discussed in Chapter 8). A DNA repair gene (e.g. *MSH2, MLH1)* is inactivated, resulting in failed mismatch repair and predisposition to multiple somatic mutations.

## Viruses

Certain DNA viruses and retroviruses (Fig. 3.11) can cause neoplasia, as follows:

- DNA viruses insert DNA directly into the host genome.
- Retroviruses have reverse transcriptase enzyme to produce a DNA copy of viral RNA. The DNA copy is then inserted into the host genome.

## Mechanism of viral carcinogenesis

Inserted viral genes may be viral oncogenes themselves *(v-onc)*, expression of which may lead to uncontrolled proliferation, or they may be activators or repressors of important cell-cycle regulating genes.

The mechanism of viral carcinogenesis is understood best in one of the most studied tumour viruses, the human papilloma virus. This double-stranded DNA virus has a tropism for squamous epithelium and subtypes 16 and 18 are implicated in cervical carcinoma. The viral genome incorporates into the host DNA and expresses the E6 oncoprotein, which inactivates the tumour suppressor protein p53. In addition expression of the E7 oncoprotein inactivates the tumour suppressor protein RB1. These oncoproteins, together with other factors, result in cervical intraepithelial neoplasia (CIN).

## HOST DEFENCES AGAINST CANCER

Some tumours are known to stimulate both innate (passive) and adaptive (active) immunological reactions in the host.

## Innate immunity

Activation of macrophages and natural killer cells can prevent growth of some tumours in vitro. Some tumours activate complement via the alternative pathway.

## Adaptive immunity

### Humoral

Antibodies may have a protective role, through complement activation or opsonization of tumour cells for cell-mediated destruction. They are more likely to be effective against free cells (e.g. leukaemia or metastasizing tumours) than those in solid lumps.

### Cell-mediated immunity

Cell-mediated immunity is involved in recognition and monitoring of cells progressing towards malignancy. Therefore, cells that become significantly different to

**Fig. 3.11** Examples of oncogenic human viruses

| Type | Virus | Tumour type |
|---|---|---|
| Retroviruses | Human T cell leukaemia virus (HTLV) | T cell leukaemia |
| | Human immunodeficiency virus (HIV) | AIDS-related lymphomas |
| DNA viruses | Human papillomavirus | Skin papilloma (common wart) |
| | | Cervical carcinoma |
| | Epstein–Barr virus | Carcinoma of the nasopharynx |
| | | Burkitt's lymphoma |
| | Hepatitis B virus | Hepatocellular carcinoma |

be recognized as 'foreign' may be eliminated by the immune system. This is particularly true of those tumours with a suspected viral aetiology.

The importance of immune surveillance in the prevention of cancer is clearly illustrated in immuno-compromized patients. For example, lymphomas associated with Epstein–Barr virus can present 4–7 years post-immunosuppressive therapy following organ transplant.

Cytotoxic T cells are thought to play a role in tumour regression, particularly in virus-associated neoplasms. Infiltration of some tumours by lymphocytes and macrophages is associated with better prognosis.

Although many immune mechanisms are known to be active against tumour cells, most tumours are not distinguishable from normal host cells and so are not easily detected by the immune system. Additionally, tumour cells develop mechanisms to evade the immune system. These are thought to include reducing the expression of the surface major histocompatibility complex (MHC), antigen masking and actually suppressing the host immune system through cytokine release or apoptosis stimulation.

## CLINICAL CANCER PATHOLOGY

Tumour markers are increasingly being used for prognostic and management decision processes. These are products derived from the tumour that can be found in the blood and used for diagnosis, assessing response to treatment and detecting recurrence. Examples include the CA125 ovarian tumour marker, the prostate-specific antigen (PSA) marker in prostate carcinoma and the α-fetoprotein in hepatocellular carcinoma and testicular teratoma.

Pathology reports of resected tumours contain macroscopic and microscopic descriptions that give information about the size and type of a cancer, local invasion and lymph node metastasis.

The grade of a tumour is based on morphological study (proliferation, differentiation, pleomorphism) and indicates tumour differentiation. Staging is used to determine how advanced a tumour is. For example, colorectal tumours can be staged by the Dukes classification (A–C/D). The TNM (tumour size, lymph node spread, metastasis formation) system is used to stage many tumours.

# Infectious disease

## Objectives

In this chapter, you will learn to:
- Define infection, colonization, pathogen, commensals, pathogenicity and virulence.
- Understand the principles of Koch's postulates of disease.
- Outline the categories of infectious agents, their key features and main differences.
- Describe host defences against infection and how microorganisms attempt to evade them.
- Describe the mechanisms of viral and bacterial pathogenicity, and the immune responses of the host.
- Understand how bacterial antibiotic resistance develops and spreads.
- Understand the importance of hospital-acquired infection and the pathogens responsible.
- Describe the inflammatory responses to infection.

## GENERAL PRINCIPLES OF INFECTION

### Infection and colonization

Infectious diseases are a common cause of morbidity and mortality. The prevalence of infectious diseases varies considerably between developed and developing nations. The burden of specific diseases depends on the quality of the drinking water, sanitation, healthcare system and the prevailing social and climatic conditions.

Infection is the invasion and proliferation of microorganisms in the tissues of the body. This usually follows the successful breach of host barriers and immune defence mechanisms.

Transmission of infectious agents can be:
- human to human spread (horizontal and vertical transmission)
- animal to human (zoonoses)
- environment to human (airborne, water, fomites)
- medical institution to patient (nosocomial).

Following invasion, infective organisms can spread to distant tissue sites by:
- local spread
- lymphatic spread
- haematogenous spread
- dissemination in the tissue fluid
- neural spread.

Colonization is the inhabitation of the external body surfaces—the skin, gastrointestinal (GI) tract, external genitalia and vagina—usually by harmless microorganisms. This generally occurs soon after birth.

## Pathogens and commensals

Pathogens are microorganisms that are normally absent from the body but which have mechanisms to invade and cause infection. Commensals are those microorganisms that constitute the normal flora of a healthy body. They do not normally cause disease and they are often advantageous to the host by the production of nutrients, such as vitamin $B_{12}$, and by the exclusion of harmful bacteria. For example, the normal commensal flora of the skin prevents colonization by pathogenic bacteria.

### HINTS AND TIPS

The distinction between commensals and pathogens is not absolute. Many commensals are potential pathogens, i.e. they are harmless only so long as they are kept at bay by the host's defence mechanisms.

## Other characteristics of microorganisms

### Pathogenicity

Pathogenicity is the capacity of a particular microorganism to cause disease.

### Virulence

Virulence is a measure of the pathogenicity of a microorganism, which can be said to be highly virulent if a small number of microbes can cause severe disease.

## Opportunistic infection

Opportunistic infection is an infection by organisms of low pathogenicity, usually due to impaired immune responses. Opportunistic infections are common in immunocompromized patients, such as those with a primary or second immunodeficiency. Examples include:

- children with severe combined immunodeficiency (SCID), a rare group of inherited syndromes (often X-linked) that require bone marrow transplantation to prevent death in early infancy
- patients infected with human immunodeficiency virus (HIV), which results in the destruction of CD4+T cells
- transplant patients using immunosuppressive drugs.

### Clinical Note

Deficiency of specific immune defences predisposes individuals to characteristic patterns of infection. For example the T-cell-deficient disease, DiGeorge syndrome, results in chronic viral, fungal and intracellular bacterial infections. This syndrome occurs due to the lack of development of the thymus and parathyroid glands.

## CATEGORIES OF INFECTIOUS AGENT

There are numerous different categories of infectious agent. The classification of the major pathogens is shown in Fig. 4.1.

nucleocapsid

nucleic acid    capsid

envelope

derived from host cell membrane
(surface, internal, nuclear)
with inserted glycoproteins

**Fig. 4.2**   Structure of an enveloped virus.

## Viruses

Viruses carry nucleic acids but lack synthetic machinery. They can therefore replicate only within the host cell, i.e. they are obligate intracellular parasites (Fig. 4.2).

Viruses have the following characteristics:

- They consist of a nucleic acid core and protein coat (capsid), which together constitute the nucleocapsid.
- Some, but not all, viruses are enveloped by a membrane of host-cell origin.
- Morphology is icosahedral, helical or complex.
- Classification is usually based on type of nucleic acid (Fig. 4.3).

**Fig. 4.1** Classification of major pathogens

|  | Viruses | Bacteria | Fungi | Protozoa | Helminths and ectoparasites |
|---|---|---|---|---|---|
| Size | 20–300 nm | 0.1–5 µm | 2–10 µm | 2–100 µm | 0.5–35 cm |
| Pro- or eukaryote | Neither | Prokaryote | Eukaryote | Eukaryote | Eukaryote |
| Nucleic acid | DNA or RNA | DNA + RNA | DNA + RNA | DNA + RNA | DNA + RNA |
| Replication | Intracellular | Intra- and/or extracellular | Intra- and/or extracellular | Intra- and/or extracellular | Extracellular |
| External cell wall | No | Yes (usually): peptidoglycan | Yes: rigid chitin | No | No |
| Reproduction | Assembly | Binary fission | Binary fission and sexually | Binary fission and sexually | Sexually |

**Fig. 4.3** Classification of viruses based on nucleic acid type

| Virus type | Mode of replication | Examples |
|---|---|---|
| DNA viruses | Utilize host cell polymerases for mRNA synthesis<br>Can remain in infected cell and establish<br>persistent infections (latent, immortalizing viruses) | Herpes simplex virus<br>Varicella-zoster virus<br>Adenovirus<br>Papillomavirus |
| RNA viruses | Encode their own replicative enzymes for formation of more mRNA<br>(Host enzymes cannot replicate RNA) | Measles virus<br>Mumps virus<br>Influenza virus<br>Rabies virus<br>Poliovirus |
| Retroviruses<br>(RNA) | Contain 'reverse transcriptase' enzyme for production of viral mRNA<br>Viral DNA is inserted into host genome | HIV I and II<br>HTLV I and II |

## Pathogenesis of cell injury

Viruses produce tissue injury by:

- direct cytopathic effect—viral replication within cells leads to degenerative changes, including cell lysis, e.g. respiratory epithelial cells infected with influenza virus
- induction of an immune response—stimulated by viral proteins on the surface of host cells
- incorporation of viral genes into the host genome—often inducing cellular death by apoptosis, e.g. HIV
- cellular transformation—some viruses can cause cellular proliferation and transformation to produce cancers, e.g. Epstein–Barr virus, human papillomavirus (see Chapter 3).

Therefore, the harmful effects of viral infections include cell death, acute and chronic tissue damage, triggering of an autoimmune response and transformation of cells to form tumours.

Viral infections can be detected by a variety of methods:

- Direct detection of the virus by electron microscopy
- Observed specific cellular cytopathic effects
- Detection of viral proteins by immunofluorescence techniques
- Detection of host-produced antiviral antibodies by enzyme-linked immunosorbent assay (ELISA)
- Detection of viral nucleic acid by polymerase chain reaction (PCR).

## Bacteria

Bacteria are prokaryotes with a single circular DNA chromosome. Bacteria are divided into two broad groups—Gram-positive and Gram-negative—based on their reaction to the Gram stain (a staining procedure used with light microscopy).

> **HINTS AND TIPS**
>
> Gram staining is a key microbiological test. Crystal violet and iodine are used to stain the bacterial cell wall. Gram-positive bacteria (lots of cell wall peptidoglycan) retain these components on challenge with acetone, and so stain purple. Gram-negative bacteria (little peptidoglycan) lose the iodine and crystal violet colouring with the addition of acetone, instead staining pink from the use of safranin counterstain.

Not all bacteria stain using the Gram method, e.g. *Mycobacterium tuberculosis* requires a special staining technique known as Ziehl–Neelsen.

Further classification is based on practical characteristics, i.e. size, shape, respiration and reproduction. Biochemical and immunological measures can provide further information. For example, Gram-positive cocci can be distinguished by testing for the production of the catalase enzyme; *Staphylococcus* species produce catalase whereas *Streptococcus* species do not.

A generalized structure of a bacterium is shown in Figure 4.4 and an example of the characteristics used to classify bacteria is shown in Figure 4.5.

The pathogenic effects of bacteria are the results of the release of endotoxins and exotoxins. These produce acute and chronic inflammation and tissue damage.

Bacterial infections can be diagnosed from a number of different samples obtained from the patient. These include blood, faeces, urine, cerebral spinal fluid and swabs taken from infected wounds. Samples will

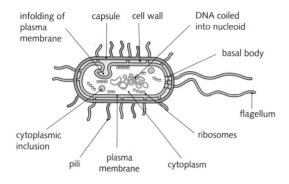

infolding of plasma membrane
capsule
cell wall
DNA coiled into nucleoid
basal body
flagellum
ribosomes
cytoplasm
plasma membrane
pili
cytoplasmic inclusion

**Fig. 4.4** Generalized structure of a bacterium.

generally be cultured to determine the species of bacteria and their sensitivity to different antibiotics.

## Fungi

Fungi are unicellular, multicellular or multinucleate organisms (Fig. 4.6). They are eukaryotes and contain ergosterol instead of cholesterol in their plasma membranes.

Fungi have a well-defined cell wall composed of polysaccharides and chitin; they can be moulds, yeasts or dimorphic.

Fungal infections are either superficial (e.g. involving the skin, hair, nails and mucous membranes) or systemic (e.g. involving the lungs, brain or heart); the latter are usually found only in the immunocompromized. Such opportunistic fungi include *Aspergillus, Candida* and *Cryptococcus*.

**Clinical Note**

Some fungi produce toxins termed mycotoxins. For example, *Aspergillus flavus* proliferates on food stored in humid conditions and produces aflatoxins, which are highly carcinogenic mycotoxins. Ingestion of food contaminated with aflatoxins causes an increased risk of hepatocellular carcinoma in humans, particularly where there is underlying hepatitis B infection.

## Protozoa

Protozoa are unicellular eukaryotes that may develop into cysts in harsh environmental conditions. The main divisions of protozoa are shown in Figure 4.7. Protozoa species may be capable of replicating intracellularly or extracellularly. The most important protozoal disease worldwide is malaria, which is caused by the *Plasmodium* species.

Identification of protozoa often occurs by microscopy of patient specimens. Specimens include faeces, blood and tissue. Culture methods are not routinely applied for identification purposes.

## Helminths and ectoparasites

Helminths are a group of parasitic worms, as shown in Figure 4.8. Ectoparasites (e.g. bed bugs, crab louse, fleas, etc.) are parasites that live on the outer surfaces of the host.

Microscopy of patient specimens (faeces, blood, tissue) allows the identification of most helminths and ectoparasites.

| staining | shape | respiration | shape/reproduction | genus | species |
|---|---|---|---|---|---|
| Gram-positive | cocci (spherical) | aerobic | clusters | Staphylococcus | S. aureus |
| | | | chains/pairs | Streptococcus | S. pyogenes |
| | | anaerobic | | Peptococcus | P. magnus |
| | bacilli (rod-shaped) | aerobic | sporing | Bacillus | B. anthracis |
| | | | non-sporing | Listeria | L. monocytogenes |
| | | anaerobic | sporing | Clostridium | C. tetani |
| | | | non-sporing | Propionibacterium | P. acnes |

**Fig. 4.5** The characteristics used to classify bacteria, using Gram-positive bacteria as an example.

**Fig. 4.6 Classification of fungi**

| Yeast-like form | Hyphal form | Dimorphic form |
|---|---|---|
| | | |
| single, rounded cells<br><br>multiply by budding,<br><br>e.g. *Candida albicans*, *Cryptococcus neoformans* | branching filaments interlaced to make mycelium or mould<br><br>produce spores<br><br>hyphae may be several hundred mm in length,<br><br>e.g. *Aspergillus fumigatus*, dermatophytes | can assume either yeast or hyphal form depending on environment,<br><br>e.g. *Histoplasma capsulatum*, *Blastomyces dermatitidis* |

**Fig. 4.7 Main divisions of protozoa**

| Sporozoa | Flagellates | Amoebae | Ciliates |
|---|---|---|---|
| | | | |
| all are intracellular parasites, e.g. Plasmodium in red blood cells | move by beating one or more flagella, e.g. Trypanosoma | move by extending pseudopodia; they have no fixed shape, e.g. Entamoeba | move by beating many cilia, e.g. Balantidium |

## Chlamydiae, Rickettsiae and Mycoplasmas

*Chlamydiae* and *Rickettsiae* are obligate intracellular organisms. *Chlamydia* replicates within vacuoles formed inside epithelial cells. *Chlamydia trachomatis* is an important cause of female infertility (scarring of fallopian tubes) and preventable blindness (corneal scarring and opacification).

*Rickettsiae* are transmitted by arthropod vectors (e.g. lice, ticks, mites) and replicate in the cytoplasm of epithelial cells to produce injury (usually a haemorrhagic vasculitis).

*Mycoplasma* lack cell walls and are the smallest free-living organisms known to man (typically 125–300 nm). They can be transmitted between people by aerosol to produce an atypical pneumonia.

**Fig. 4.8  Main groups of helminths (parasitic worms)**

| Nematodes (roundworms) | Cestodes (tapeworms) | Trematodes (flukes) |
|---|---|---|
| | | |
| resistant cuticle; longitudinal muscles; complete digestive system; separate sexed reproductive system, e.g. *Ascaris lumbricoides*, *Strongyloides stercoralis* | cellular epithelium; no digestive system; all hermaphrodites, e.g. *Taenia solium*, *Echinococcus granulosus* | cellular epithelium; circular and longitudinal muscles; incomplete digestive system; mostly hermaphrodites, e.g. *Schistosoma* |

## Prions

Prions are an abnormal isoform of a normal host protein (the prion protein; PrP). Prions are not microorganisms but are infectious proteins that are highly resistant to decontamination methods, such as standard autoclaving or disinfectants. Humans express normal prion proteins but their function is unknown. Inoculation of an abnormal prion protein into a normal host induces conformational changes in the normal host prions, resulting in their conversion to abnormal host prions. Disease occurs when the abnormal prion protein is resistant to protease breakdown where the original protein was protease sensitive.

Thus, the original inoculated prion protein is able to catalyse a chain reaction in which host proteins become conformationally abnormal.

The net result is the formation of amyloid plaques of prion protein in the CNS. These plaques result in vacuolar spongiform degeneration of neuronal processes with neuronal loss and glial proliferation.

In humans, several forms of prion protein disease exist—including kuru and Creutzfeldt–Jakob disease (CJD), both of which are always fatal, usually within 6 months. Since the 1990s, an emerging variant (vCJD) has occured in people under the age of 50. The consumption of offal contaminated with bovine spongiform encephalopathy (BSE) prions has been proven in its aetiology.

### HINTS AND TIPS

Infective agents include bacteria, viruses, fungi, parasites and prions. Remember, prions are not infective organisms.

## MECHANISMS OF PATHOGENICITY

## Host defences and routes of entry

The majority of infectious agents encountered by an individual are prevented from entering the body by a variety of biochemical and physical barriers (Fig. 4.9). For example, anatomical barriers such as the skin, mucous membranes, GI tract and genitourinary tract provide a physical environment of unfavourable growth conditions for bacteria.

Further host defence is provided by the innate and adaptive immune mechanisms. Innate immunity consists of non-specific mechanisms that contribute to resistance and recovery from infection. Innate immunity includes soluble proteins (complement, acute-phase proteins), immune cells [macrophages, neutrophils, natural killer (NK) cells] and receptors (Toll-like receptors). Adaptive immunity is specific and includes cellular immunity (cytotoxic and helper T cells) and humoral immunity (B cells). Adaptive immunity is characterized by antigen specificity and clonal proliferation. In addition, the generation of immunological memory initiates a heightened response to subsequent antigen exposure.

However, despite these defences, pathogenic microorganisms possess efficient mechanisms for attaching to, and often penetrating, the body surfaces where they proliferate and disseminate. If they are to be transmitted to a fresh host, the microorganisms must also exit from the body.

The different routes of entry and exit of microorganisms are outlined in Figure 4.10.

packaged together with the RNA into new virus particles and released.

## Release of new virus particles

### Cell lysis (cytolysis)
Non-enveloped viruses (e.g. adenoviruses) are released directly into the extracellular environment by lysis of the host cell; their mode of release results in the death of the cell.

### Budding
Enveloped viruses (e.g. HIV and herpesvirus) are released by 'budding' from the host cell membrane:

- Nucleocapsid proteins are inserted into the host cell membrane.
- A modified area of host cell membrane extends out from the cell surface and is pinched off (i.e. budded) from the host cell enclosing the new viral particle.

This mechanism does not cause the death of the cell, and so viral replication can continue.

## Immune reaction to virally infected cells

Cytotoxic T cells kill virally infected cells as follows:

- Virally infected cells express viral peptides bound to major histocompatibility complex (MHC) class I on their cell surfaces.
- Cytotoxic T cells ($T_C$) recognize viral antigen via the T-cell receptor.
- $T_C$ cells secrete cytolysins, which results in the lysis of the virally infected cells.

NK cells can do the same, but less effectively. The activity of these cells is enhanced by interferons produced by $T_C$ and helper T cells ($T_H$). Interferons also prevent adjacent cells from becoming infected by intercellular viral transport.

It is worth noting that as well as spreading infection, immune responses can lead to tissue injury. For example, the liver damage following hepatitis B infection is largely mediated by the strong immune response of $T_C$ cells towards infected hepatocytes.

## Bacterial infections

### Adherence

Certain bacteria are able to adhere specifically to epithelial cells by means of pili (also called fimbriae), which are slender filamentous processes on the surfaces of some bacteria. Pili are coated with recognition molecules called adhesins. Specific interactions between adhesins of pili and molecules on the surface epithelial cells enable the bacterium to adhere to the host cell membranes. Polymorphisms in host cell-surface glycoproteins may

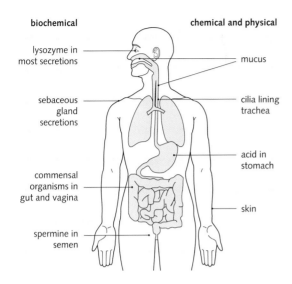

**biochemical**                    **chemical and physical**

lysozyme in most secretions

mucus

sebaceous gland secretions

cilia lining trachea

acid in stomach

commensal organisms in gut and vagina

skin

spermine in semen

**Fig. 4.9**  Exterior host defences.

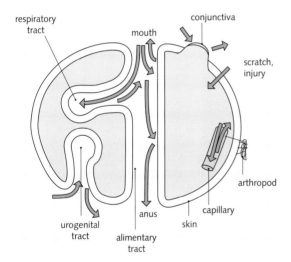

respiratory tract

conjunctiva

mouth

scratch, injury

arthropod

urogenital tract

anus        skin

capillary

alimentary tract

**Fig. 4.10**  Routes of entry and exit of microorganisms.

## Virus infections

### Viral replication cycles
Figure 4.11 outlines two types of viral replication cycle:

1. DNA viruses have their own DNA and use the host's cellular machinery to make more DNA, protein and glycoprotein. These are then reassembled into new virus particles prior to release from the cell.
2. RNA retroviruses first make viral DNA using the viral reverse transcriptase enzyme. Viral DNA is then inserted into the host genome prior to its transcription to form messenger RNA (mRNA). Viral RNA is in turn translated into viral protein, which is

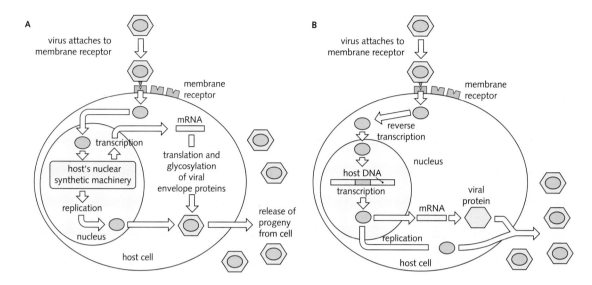

**Fig. 4.11** Viral replication cycles. (A) DNA virus: DNA viruses have their own DNA. The viruses use the host's cellular machinery to make more DNA, protein and glycoprotein. These are then reassembled into new virus particles prior to release from the cell. (B) RNA retrovirus: RNA retroviruses first make viral DNA using viral 'reverse transcriptase'. Viral DNA is then inserted into the host genome prior to its transcription to form mRNA. Viral RNA is in turn translated into viral protein, which is packaged together with the RNA into new virus particles and released.

make an individual more susceptible to binding by certain types of bacterial adhesins.

Pili are more common in Gram-negative bacteria, although a few Gram-positive bacteria also possess them. Lipoteichoic acids (Gram-positive bacteria only) can function in a similar manner to pili by binding to fibronectin and epithelial cells.

## Exotoxins and endotoxins

Toxins are responsible for many of the local and distant effects of bacterial infection.

### Exotoxins

Exotoxins are proteins secreted by bacteria which are highly toxic to the host. The modes of action of some exotoxins are considered below:

- Enzymatic lysis—α-toxin (phospholipase C) of *Clostridium perfringens* breaks down host cell membranes
- Pore forming—α-toxin of *Staphylococcus aureus* disrupts host cell membrane by pore formation
- Inhibiting protein synthesis, e.g. diphtheria toxin
- G protein hyperactivation, e.g. cholera toxin
- Affecting synaptic transmission at neuromuscular junctions, e.g. tetanus and botulinum toxins.

Treating exotoxin with formaldehyde or high temperatures can denature the toxin to form toxoids, which can be useful for vaccination.

### Endotoxins

Endotoxins are integral parts of bacterial cell walls, normally released only when the bacterium dies. They are typically lipopolysaccharides contained within the cell walls of Gram-negative bacteria. (But note that an exception is the 'superantigen' endotoxin TSST1, which is produced by the Gram-positive *Staphylococcus aureus* and causes toxic shock syndrome.)

These endotoxins are not in themselves toxic but can induce toxic effects by their potent activation of:

- the complement cascade, causing inflammatory damage
- the coagulation cascade, potentially causing disseminated intravascular coagulation
- cytokines, notably tumour necrosis factor and interleukin-1 released from leucocytes, causing fever.

In overwhelming infections, the patient is said to suffer from endotoxic shock with fever, hypotension and cardiac and renal failure.

## Aggressins

Aggressins are bacterially produced enzymes that act predominantly in the local tissue environment. They include enzymes such as coagulase, streptokinase and collagenases. Aggressins facilitate the growth and proliferation of the bacteria.

## Avoiding death by phagocytosis

Successful microorganisms have evolved numerous ingenious antiphagocytic devices:

- Phagocyte killing, e.g. via exotoxin release.
- Prevention of opsonization—the microbe produces protein that prevents interaction between opsonizing antibody and phagocyte.
- Preventing phagocyte contact—some bacteria have an external capsule of polysaccharide, which gives a slimy surface and provides protection against phagocytosis, e.g. *Streptococcus pneumoniae*.
- Protection against intracellular death—this allows the microorganism to survive within the phagocyte by, for example, inhibition of phagosome and lysosome fusion (*Mycobacterium tuberculosis*) or escaping from the phagolysosome into cytoplasm (*Listeria monocytogenes*).

## Antibiotic resistance and plasmids

Many bacteria are resistant to antibiotics. Resistance is conferred by genes that encode bacterial enzymes that block the effect of an antibiotic. These genes are not usually contained within the bacterial genome, but rather within extrachromosomal DNA termed 'plasmids'. These plasmids are capable of self-replication and can be transferred from bacterium to bacterium.

Antibiotic-susceptible bacteria (those lacking plasmids conferring antibiotic resistance) can acquire plasmids from resistant bacteria and so gain antibiotic resistance. These newly resistant forms are then differentially selected under antibiotic treatment, with the non-resistant bacteria being deleted from the population.

**HINTS AND TIPS**

Resistance to antibiotics can be transferred between bacteria by any of the methods of bacterial genetic recombination i.e. conjugation, transduction and transformation.

## Hospital-acquired infection

Hospital-acquired infection (nosocomial infection) occurs in up to 10% of uninfected admitted patients. It is thought to be the direct cause of 5000 deaths per year in the UK and it contributes to a further 15 000 deaths. Common pathogens include *Streptococcus pyogenes*, *Staphylococcus aureus*, *Escherichia coli* and *Pseudomonas aeruginosa*. Common sites of nosocomial infections include the:

- urinary tract
- surgical wounds
- lower respiratory tract
- skin
- blood (bacteraemia)—either by direct introduction such as through a venous catheter (primary), or by spread from another site such as a urinary tract infection (secondary).

Such infections can delay recovery, increase complication rates and ultimately result in the death of a patient. Of particular concern is the emergence of multi-drug-resistant infections that do not respond to traditional broad-spectrum antibiotics. Important examples include methicillin-resistant *Staphylococcus aureus* (MRSA) and vancomycin-resistant enterococci (VRE).

Although measures should be put in place to reduce levels of nosocomial infection, it is important to remember that many hospital patients are at inherently high risk of developing an infection in hospital regardless of these measures.

**Clinical Note**

Important measures to reduce levels of hospital acquired infection include hand-washing (staff and visitors), minimizing the length of preoperative hospital stays, careful use of prophylactic antibodies before certain procedures, isolating infected patients in side-rooms and using barrier-nursing techniques.

## SEPSIS

Sepsis is defined as the association of systemic inflammatory responses with evidence of a microbial origin. In the absence of infection this is known as systemic inflammatory response syndrome (SIRS). There are abnormal clinical physiological variables such as pulse rate, body temperature, hypotension, abnormal leucocyte count, and – critically – response to restorative measures and fluid administration. The source of the infection may be organ-specific (e.g. lung in pneumonia, or abdomen in peritonitis), but often there is only blood stream infection – bacteraemia. The diagnosis is often presumptive because blood and other site microbiological cultures may be negative, partly from previous antibiotic administration.

A key concept in sepsis is the host response with production of cytokines (see Chapter 2). Some patients over-react to a standard infection stress and may suffer severe sepsis.

Early antibiotic treatment and supportive care are the mainstays of management. In the example of meningococcal sepsis (*Neisseeria meningitidis*), the moment it is suspected from the clinical status of the patient and the haemorrhagic skin rash, antibiotics are given and the microbiological investigations follow later.

## INFLAMMATORY RESPONSES TO INFECTION

### Suppurative polymorphonuclear inflammation

This is characterized by the production of pus, such as in a boil or abscess, which is usually caused by infection with pyogenic bacteria (e.g. *Staphylococcus aureus, Streptococcus pyogenes*).

### Chronic inflammation and scarring

This is caused by persisting reactions of tissue to injury and it occurs over weeks, months or even years. The cell-mediated immune response is characterized by lymphocytes, plasma cells and macrophages.

Examples include hepatitis B viral infection, which may lead to liver cirrhosis.

### Granulomatous mononuclear inflammation

This is a form of chronic inflammation in which modified macrophages—epithelioid cells—aggregate to form small clusters or granulomas surrounded by lymphoid cells. It occurs in response to the presence of microorganisms within macrophages that are resistant to intracellular cell killing (e.g. *Mycobacterium tuberculosis*).

### Necrotizing inflammation

#### Gangrene

In gangrene, necrotic tissue is invaded by putrefactive organisms, notably clostridia. Tissue appears green or black because of the breakdown of haemoglobin.

# PART II
# SYSTEMIC PATHOLOGY

# Pathology of the nervous system

## Objectives

In this chapter, you will learn to:
- Describe common pathological presentations in the central nervous system (CNS).
- Describe congenital malformations, developmental diseases and perinatal injury of the CNS.
- Recall traumatic injuries to the CNS and describe their effects.
- Understand cerebrovascular disease.
- Describe the infections of the CNS.
- Understand demyelinating and degenerative diseases of the CNS.
- Briefly describe the effect of metabolic disorders and toxins on the CNS.
- Recall the neoplasms that affect the central and peripheral nervous systems, briefly describing them.
- Give examples of peripheral neuropathies of hereditary, traumatic, inflammatory, infectious, metabolic and toxic origin.
- Describe disorders of the sympathetic and parasympathetic nervous system.

## DISORDERS OF THE CENTRAL NERVOUS SYSTEM

### Common pathological features

#### Intracranial herniation

Intracranial herniation is the movement of part of the brain from one space to another with resultant damage. It usually occurs following a critical increase in intracranial pressure caused by an expanding lesion, e.g. tumour or haematoma. However, it may be inadvertently precipitated by withdrawing cerebrospinal fluid (CSF) at lumbar puncture.

Figure 5.1 shows a diagrammatical representation of the sites of intracranial herniation.

#### Cerebral oedema

This is an abnormal accumulation of fluid in the cerebral parenchyma. It may be the result of breakdown of the blood–brain barrier (vasogenic oedema), parenchymal cell membrane injury (cytotoxic oedema) or a combination of the two. Possible causes include:
- ischaemia, e.g. from infarction
- trauma, e.g. from head injury
- inflammation, e.g. encephalitis or meningitis
- cerebral tumours (primary or secondary)
- metabolic disturbances, e.g. hyponatraemia or hypoglycaemia.

The condition is associated with raised intracranial pressure and may result in herniation.

### Hydrocephalus

Hydrocephalus is an increase in the volume of CSF within the brain resulting in the expansion of the cerebral ventricles and eventual increase in intracranial pressure. It can occur by one of three mechanisms:

1. Obstruction to flow of CSF (the most common form)
2. Impaired absorption of CSF at arachnoid villi (rare)
3. Overproduction of CSF by choroid plexus neoplasms (very rare).

Hydrocephalus can be classified into non-communicating and communicating forms.

#### Non-communicating (obstructive hydrocephalus)

This can be congenital or acquired.

Congenital hydrocephalus occurs in 1 per 1000 births, due to Arnold–Chiari and Dandy–Walker malformations (see page 39) and cerebral aqueduct stenosis.

Acquired obstructive hydrocephalus can result from any lesion that obstructs the CSF within the ventricles preventing flow into the subarachnoid space, such as:

- tumours—especially of the posterior fossa, as the fourth ventricle aqueducts are easily obstructed
- haemorrhage—intraventricular or in the posterior fossa.

#### Communicating hydrocephalus

Caused by an impairment outside the ventricular system in the absence of any CSF flow obstruction, e.g. meningitis or subarachnoid haemorrhage. Normal pressure

**Fig. 5.1** Sites of intracranial herniation. (A) Subfalcine herniation. (B) Transtentorial herniation. (C) Tonsillar herniation. (D) Herniation of swollen brain through any defect in the dura and skull.

lateral ventricle

falx cerebri

A herniation of cingulate gyrus beneath falx cerebri

skull

D herniation of swollen brain through any defect in dura and skull

expanding lesion

dura

collapse of ventricle

midbrain

tentorium cerebelli

B herniation of medial part of temporal lobe over tentorium cerebelli

pons

cerebellum

medulla

C herniation of lower part of cerebellum through foramen magnum

hydrocephalus (intermittent pressure hydrocephalus) is a particular form of communicating hydrocephalus. This is a rare condition of progressive dementia associated with ventricular dilatation. Random sampling shows normal CSF pressure, but continuous monitoring reveals intermittent increases.

### Secondary or compensatory hydrocephalus

In this special type of hydrocephalus, an increase in CSF occurs as a compensatory measure following loss of brain tissue, e.g. due to infarction or atrophy. There is no associated increase in CSF pressure.

### Clinical Note

Congenital hydrocephalus may be diagnosed antenatally via ultrasound (if severe) or present as a considerably enlarged head at birth. In acquired hydrocephalus, enlargement of the head is prevented by the inability of skull expansion (sutures are fused), resulting in increased intracranial pressure. Associated features include dementia, gait disturbances and incontinence. Treatment involves insertion of a ventricular shunt to drain CSF into the peritoneum, attempting to prevent irreversible brain damage.

## Malformations, developmental disease and perinatal injury

### Neural tube defects and posterior fossa abnormalities

The aetiology of central nervous system (CNS) malformations includes genetic factors, maternal infections, toxicity, metabolic factors and irradiation in utero.

Neural tube defects are the most common congenital abnormalities of the CNS and are caused by defective closure of the midline structures over the neural tube. The most common forms in the newborn affect the spinal cord (e.g. spina bifida). Screening for neural tube defects can be performed with ultrasound or by measurement of a-fetoprotein in the maternal serum or amniotic fluid (raised in 90% of cases).

Posterior fossa abnormalities are the second most common development abnormality of the CNS. Figure 5.2 illustrates the types of congenital abnormalities.

### Syringomyelia and hydromyelia

Syringomyelia is a rare condition in which a cyst (syrinx) develops within the spinal cord, usually posterior to the central canal (Fig. 5.3). The cavity is lined with astrocytes by the process of gliosis. It is most common in the cervical spinal cord, but it may extend into the medulla (syringobulbia).

| Fig. 5.2 Types of congenital abnormality | |
| --- | --- |
| Condition | Features |
| **Neural tube defects with cranial involvement** | |
| Anencephaly | Absence of the cranial vault and failure in the development of the cerebral hemispheres |
| Encephalocele | Ossification defects in the bones of the skull result in herniation of the brain and meninges. Most common form is occipital |
| **Neural tube defects with spinal involvement** | |
| Spina bifida occulta | Abnormal development of the vertebral arches but the cord and meninges are normal. Usually asymptomatic |
| Spina bifida cystica | Abnormal development of the vertebral arches results in cystic outpouching. Presents either with protrusion of CNS tissue through a vertebral column defect (meningomyelocele: 90% of cases) or protrusion of only the meninges (meningocele: 10% of cases) |
| **Posterior fossa abnormalities** | |
| Arnold–Chiari malformation | Prolongation of the cerebellum downwards through the foramen magnum often resulting in obstructive hydrocephalus |
| Dandy–Walker malformation | Obstruction of the foramina of Luschka and Magendie (exit of the fourth ventricle) results in the formation of a cyst-like structure between the cerebellar hemispheres |

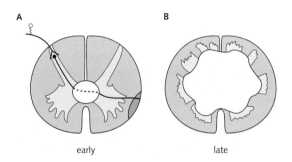

**Fig. 5.3** Syringomyelia. (A) Early effects: damage to the decussating sensory fibres, with loss of temperature and touch in local segments. (B) Late effects: destruction of grey matter and gradual affection of long tracts with loss of local reflexes, severe sensory loss and spastic paralysis.

Hydromyelia is the term used when the ependyma-lined central canal of the spinal cord (containing CSF) is dilatated.

These conditions are usually acquired due to trauma, ischaemia or associated spinal cord tumours. Rarely, they occur because of congenital abnormalities such as the Arnold–Chiari malformation.

Syringomyelia may produce muscle weakness and atrophy in the upper limbs due to compression of the anterior horn cells. There is loss of the sensations of pain and temperature, but preservation of those of position and vibration, due to damage of nerve fibres crossing the cord in the lateral spinothalamic tracts.

## Perinatal injury

This term refers to any brain injury sustained in the period shortly before and after birth. It is an important cause of childhood disability.

### Cerebral palsy

Cerebral palsy describes brain malformation or damage affecting motor areas of the brain. It is the leading cause of handicap in children, affecting 2 per 1000 live births. The different presentations of cerebral palsy are outlined in Figure 5.4.

> **HINTS AND TIPS**
>
> Note that cerebral palsy is a general term covering any non-progressive motor deficit caused by perinatal injury. Possible presentations include spasticity (increased muscle tone), dystonia (disordered muscle tone), ataxia (disordered muscle coordination) and paresis (incomplete paralysis).

| Fig. 5.4 Types of cerebral palsy and their associated characteristics | |
|---|---|
| **Type** | **Characteristics** |
| Spastic cerebral palsy (70%) | Hypertonia, ankle clonus and extensor plantar response |
| Dystonic (athetoid) cerebral palsy (10%) | Irregular, involuntary muscle movements |
| Ataxic cerebral palsy (10%) | Hypotonia, weakness, uncoordinated movements and intentiontremor |
| Mixed cerebral palsy (10%) | — |

### Ischaemia and hypoxia

Ischaemia and hypoxia are major causes of severe peri-natal brain damage. Perinatal hypoxia is usually due to asphyxiation associated with the trauma of birth, whereas perinatal ischaemia is commonly caused by intracranial haemorrhages.

Premature infants are highly susceptible to develop-ing intracranial haemorrhages because of disturbances in the cerebral circulation, possibly caused by in-utero hypoxia/ischaemia. Mortality is high; one-third of survivors develop cerebral palsy, epilepsy or mental retardation.

In full-term infants, intracranial haemorrhages with the formation of small haematomas may occur during difficult deliveries, although this is less common with modern obstetric care.

## Traumatic injuries to the central nervous system

The common types of CNS trauma are summarized in Figure 5.5 and discussed in more detail below.

| Fig. 5.5 Examples of common central nervous system trauma | |
|---|---|
| **Level of injury** | **Pathology** |
| Skull | Fracture |
| Parenchymal tissue | Concussion Contusions and lacerations Diffuse axonal injury |
| Vascular system | Extradural (epidural) haemorrhage Subdural haemorrhage Subarachnoid haemorrhage Intracerebral haemorrhage |
| Spinal cord | Open injuries Closed injuries |

## Skull fractures

Skull fractures occur in approximately 80% of fatal cases of head injuries. The most common are linear fractures of the vault of the skull; such fractures may extend into the base of the skull causing cranial nerve laceration.

The other types of skull fracture are:

- penetrating—increased risk of infection due to tear-ing of the dura
- compound—increased risk of infection due to lacer-ation of the scalp and tearing of the dura
- depressed—increased incidence of epilepsy
- comminuted (fragmented)—increased incidence of massive brain damage.

## Parenchymal damage

### Concussion

This is an abrupt transient loss of consciousness due to temporal neuronal dysfunction following a relatively slight impact. It is caused by an enormous, but short-lived, increase in pressure within the cranium at time of impact. Full recovery usually ensues, although amnesia for the event often persists.

### Contusions and lacerations

A contusion is a bruise with extravasation of blood but with the pia-arachnoid intact. A laceration is where the pia-arachnoid is torn. Both are focal types of brain dam-age occurring at the moment of injury, caused by strik-ing the brain against adjacent bone. They are most common at the frontal and occipital poles and mainly affect the crests of gyri. Both lesions are characteristically haemorrhagic.

Types of contusion:

- Fracture contusion—occurs at the site of fracture.
- Coup contusion—occurs at point of impact in absence of fracture.
- Contrecoup contusion—occurs diametrically oppo-site to the site of impact.
- Herniation contusion—e.g. when the cerebellar ton-sils are impacted and bruised by the foramen magnum.
- Gliding contusion—occurs at the superior margins of the cerebral hemispheres; usually caused by inter-ference of the dura with a rotational movement of the brain.

### Diffuse axonal injury

This condition is produced as a result of rotational movements of the brain within the skull during angular acceleration or deceleration. It often occurs in the ab-sence of any skull fracture or cerebral contusions. There are two main features:

1. Small haemorrhagic lesions in the corpus callosum and the dorsolateral quadrant of the brainstem (macroscopic)
2. Widespread tearing of axons, usually at the nodes of Ranvier (microscopic).

Diffuse axonal injuries occur in up to 50% of patients who develop coma shortly after trauma. It is associated with head injuries involving vehicular accidents.

## Traumatic vascular injury

Bleeding from craniocerebral trauma is often associated with high mortality. It can occur in one or more of the potential spaces surrounding the brain, e.g. extradural and subdural.

### Extradural (epidural) haemorrhage

This type occurs in 2% of all head injuries and in 15% of fatal cases. Haemorrhage occurs into the potential space between the skull and dura, gradually stripping dura from bone to form a large, saucer-shaped haematoma.

This injury is almost always the result of skull fracture, usually of the temporal bone, with laceration of the middle meningeal artery that runs through it (a branch of the maxillary artery).

It is associated with a post-traumatic lucid interval of several hours followed by a rapid increase in intracranial pressure.

### Subdural haemorrhage

Haemorrhage occurs into the potential space between the dura and the outer surface of the arachnoid membrane. Usually caused by a rupture of the small bridging veins or the venous sinuses within the subdural space. The resulting haematoma is often extensive because of the loose attachment of the dura and arachnoid membranes.

Subdural haemorrhage can occur following acute severe head injury or chronically, over days and weeks. Chronic subdural haemorrhage is more common in:

• the elderly—even with minimal trauma, due to brain atrophy and the subsequent stretching of bridging veins
• infants—because the bridging veins have thin walls.

Subdural haemorrhage may present with focal signs relating to compression of a particular brain area. Personality change, memory loss and confusion are commonly detected.

### Subarachnoid haemorrhage

Arterial rupture into the subarachnoid space is usually secondary to superficial contusions or lacerations of the brain. Small amounts of blood can be disposed of by arachnoid granulations. Larger haemorrhages cause arachnoid fibrosis leading to meningeal irritation and raised intracranial pressure. It can also occur as a result of hypertension, aneurysms, embolisms or infarction.

### Intracerebral haemorrhage

This is caused by direct rupture of the intrinsic cerebral vessels at the time of injury.

Resulting haematomas are classified into three types:

1. Solitary—occur in association with cortical contusions; common in temporal and frontal poles
2. Multiple—associated with severe contrecoup lesions; often fatal
3. Burst lobe—intracerebral or intracerebellar haematoma in continuity with subdural haematoma; most common in temporal and frontal lobes; rapidly fatal.

## Spinal cord injuries

Most spinal injuries occur in males aged under 40 years. Road traffic accidents account for more than 80% of such injuries.

There are two types of spinal cord injury: open and closed.

### Open injuries

These are rare. They are a result of direct trauma to the spinal cord and nerve roots and can be either perforating (i.e. with extensive disruption and haemorrhage) or penetrating (i.e. with incomplete cord transection—Brown–Séquard syndrome).

### Closed injuries

These are in the majority and are associated with fracture or dislocation of the spinal column causing compression of the cord by distortion of the spinal canal.

The consequences depend mainly on the site and severity of the lesion. Cervical lesions may result in tetraplegia; lower thoracic lesions may result in paraplegia.

> **HINTS AND TIPS**
>
> Remember that with limited CNS repair mechanisms, the site of trauma is more important than the size of lesion. For example, a small lesion of the frontal lobe may be clinically silent, but would cause tetraplegia if located in the cervical spinal cord, and death if in the brainstem.

## Cerebrovascular disease

Cerebrovascular disease is the third leading cause of death in the UK.

Stroke is a common outcome of cerebrovascular disease and it is defined as a sudden event in which neurological deficit develops over minutes or hours and lasts for longer than 24 hours.

If CNS disturbance lasts for less than 24 hours the condition is termed a transient ischaemic attack (TIA).

The incidence of stroke is 2 or 3 per 1000 per year, but is much higher than this in the elderly, affecting males more than females. Causes are:

- cerebral infarction (80%)
- intracerebral haemorrhage (10%)
- subarachnoid haemorrhage (10%).

Pathological effects occur because of extensive hypoxic neuronal damage. The area of brain affected can be readily localized since the blood supply of the brain has a fairly constant anatomic distribution. Figure 5.6 shows the territories of the major arteries.

Clinical features of stroke depend on localization and the nature of the lesion. Risk factors are atherosclerosis, ischaemic heart disease, hypertension and diabetes mellitus.

## Hypoxia, ischaemia and infarction

Cerebral infarction is the process whereby a focal area of necrosis is produced in the brain in response to a decreased supply of oxygen (and glucose) in the territory of a cerebral arterial branch. There are two main causes of infarction:

1. Hypoxia—the reduction of oxygen supply to tissues despite an adequate blood supply, e.g. following respiratory arrest.
2. Ischaemia—blood supply to tissues is absent, or severely reduced, usually as a result of constriction or obstruction of a blood vessel.

Ischaemia accounts for the majority of cases of cerebral infarction.

### Mechanisms of ischaemia

Ischaemia may be caused by:

- vascular disease, e.g. thrombosis, embolic occlusion or vasculitis

**Fig. 5.6** Territories of the major arteries. (1) Main cerebral arteries forming circle of Willis. (2) Their territories: (A) Lateral view. (B) Inferior view. (C) Medial view. (Reproduced with permission from Anderson's Pathology, Damjanou, ed., Mosby.)

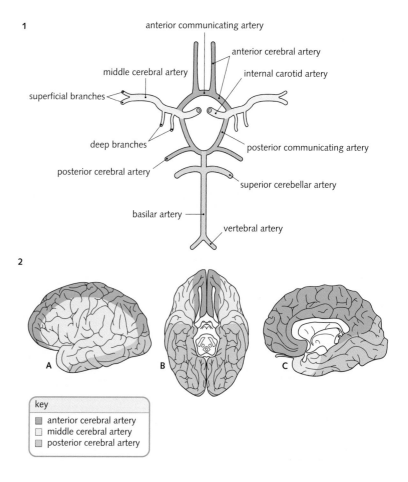

1

anterior communicating artery
anterior cerebral artery
middle cerebral artery
internal carotid artery
superficial branches
deep branches
posterior communicating artery
posterior cerebral artery
superior cerebellar artery
basilar artery
vertebral artery

2

A
B
C

key
anterior cerebral artery
middle cerebral artery
posterior cerebral artery

- cardiac disease, e.g. prolonged hypotension (producing global cerebral ischaemia) or cardiac embolism
- trauma—head injury leading to vascular occlusion, dissection or rupture.

Infarcted tissue becomes swollen and soft with the loss of definition between grey and white matter. It undergoes liquefactive (colliquative) necrosis and shows microglial macrophage infiltration. Eventually, the necrotic tissue is completely phagocytosed to leave a fluid-filled cystic cavity with a gliotic wall.

In global cerebral ischaemia, the peripheral cortical ribbon of brain undergoes infarction, starting at the watershed areas where cerebral artery territories appose.

Figure 5.7 shows the macroscopic and microscopic pathological features of cerebral infarction.

## Atraumatic haemorrhage

### Intracerebral haemorrhage
The majority of intracerebral haemorrhages are thought to arise from Charcot–Bouchard microaneurysms associated with hypertension and diabetic vascular disease. These haemorrhages occur most frequently in the basal ganglia.

The resulting haematoma acts as a space-occupying lesion leading to increased intracranial pressure and herniation.

### Subarachnoid haemorrhage
This can occur at any age, but it is an important cause of death and disability in the 20–40-year age group. The majority of subarachnoid haemorrhages are caused by saccular (berry) aneurysms, which develop at proximal branch points in the major cerebral vessels on the circle of Willis (Fig. 5.8).

These aneurysms occur in 1–2% of the population, but they are more common in the elderly and those with hypertension.

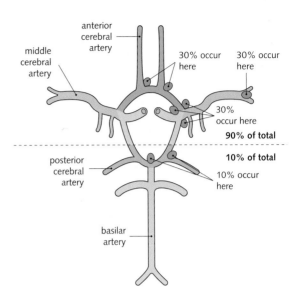

**Fig. 5.8** Berry aneurysms: approximate frequency and distribution. The dotted line separates anterior from posterior circulation. (Redrawn with permission from Anderson's Pathology, Damjanou, ed., Mosby.)

## Hypertensive cerebrovascular disease

Systemic hypertension can affect the CNS, resulting in neurological dysfunction:

- Atheroma of the larger cerebral vessels leads to a loss of autoregulation of cerebral blood flow. It may also allow small cavitary (lacunar) infarcts to develop, particularly in the lenticular nucleus and thalamus.
- Aneurysms—both saccular (berry) and microaneurysms—may cause spontaneous intracerebral haemorrhage.
- Encephalopathy—pathogenesis is uncertain but damage to the blood–brain barrier leads to forced cerebral hyperperfusion.

**Fig. 5.7** Pathological features of cerebral infarction

| Time | Macroscopic | Microscopic |
| --- | --- | --- |
| Before 24 hours | No naked eye abnormalities | Some neuronal damage |
| After 24 hours | Softening and swelling (oedema) of affected tissue | Line of demarcation between normal and abnormal myelin in white matter |
| After a few days | Necrotic tissue | Infiltrating macrophages Proliferating astrocytes and capillaries |
| After weeks/months | Fluid-filled cystic cavity with gliotic wall | Necrotic tissue removed Thickened capillary walls Only astrocytes remain |

Chronic hypertension may lead to multiple infarct events, often producing a syndrome of dementia and neurological deficit (multi-infarct dementia).

# Infections of the central nervous system

Meningitis refers to inflammation of the meninges; specifically, the leptomeninges and CSF within the subarachnoid space. Pachymeningitis refers to inflammation centred on the dura, whereas meningoencephalitis is inflammation of the meninges and brain parenchyma.

## Aseptic (viral) meningitis

This is the most common cause of meningitis, usually caused by viral infection. The term 'aseptic' is confusing, referring to an absence of recognizable (bacterial) organisms. It is a benign and self-limiting illness, usually less severe than bacterial meningitis.

### Common causative organisms

The common causative organisms are enteroviruses (e.g. echoviruses, Coxsackie viruses, polioviruses) and mumps virus. It may occur as a complication of viral infection, e.g. mumps or measles.

Affected individuals present with headache, irritability and rapid development of meningeal irritation.

## Acute pyogenic (bacterial) meningitis

Organisms that typically cause this condition vary between age groups (Fig. 5.9).

The clinical features are headache, photophobia, drowsiness and neck stiffness. These indicators of meningeal irritation usually occur with systemic signs of infection (e.g. fever) and the development of a petechial rash.

Treatment is with vigorous intravenous antibiotic therapy.

Important complications include:

- intracerebral abscess (see below)
- cerebral infarction due to an obliterative endarteritis of local arteries
- hydrocephalus due to subarachnoid adhesions blocking CSF flow
- epilepsy
- disseminated intravascular coagulation (DIC)
- adrenal haemorrhage (Waterhouse–Friderichsen syndrome).

Mortality varies by bacteria, but may be as high as 60% with *Streptococcus pneumoniae*, particularly affecting the very young and the elderly (see Figure 5.5).

## Brain abscess

A brain abscess is a severe focal infection of the brain and is typically 1–2 cm across. It starts as an area of cerebritis—inflammation of the brain parenchyma—and develops into a pus-filled cavity walled off by gliosis and surrounded by cerebral oedema. Multiple abscesses may develop, particularly with haematogenous spread of the causative organism. It often results in raised intracranial pressure.

The aetiology of brain abscesses is as follows:

- Middle ear infection (60%)—temporal lobe and cerebellar abscesses
- Frontal sinusitis (20%)—frontal lobe abscesses
- Bacteraemia/septicaemia (10%)—usually frontal lobe abscesses
- Penetrating skull trauma
- Secondary to meningitis
- Unknown causes.

Common causative organisms are *Streptococcus vividans*, *Staphylococcus aureus* and *Klebsiella* species, but it can also be caused by fungal infection.

Treatment involves antibiotic therapy at an early stage, with surgical aspiration or excision of the capsule.

| Fig. 5.9 Typical meningitis-causing bacteria by age-group | | | |
|---|---|---|---|
| **Neonates** | **Infants** | **Young adults** | **Elderly** |
| Escherichia coli<br>Group B<br>streptococci | Neisseria meningitidis<br>Streptococcus<br>pneumoniae | Neisseria meningitidis<br>Streptococcus<br>pneumoniae | Streptococcus pneumoniae<br>Neisseria meningitidis<br>Listeria monocytogenes |

Anticonvulsant medication may be required as epilepsy frequently develops.

Overall mortality is between 10 and 20%, often because of a delay in diagnosis.

## Subdural empyema

This is a collection of pus in the subdural space and it is relatively uncommon. In adults, it usually results from frontal sinusitis, whereas in infants it is usually secondary to meningitis.

Clinically, patients with subdural empyema are usually very ill. The pus spreads rapidly on the surface of a hemisphere, producing hemiparesis, raised intracranial pressure, fits and meningism.

## Chronic meningoencephalitis

### Tuberculous meningitis

This is meningitis due to infection by *Mycobacterium tuberculosis*. It is rare in the UK but a major problem in developing countries.

The disorder is almost always secondary to tuberculosis elsewhere in the body; infection usually reaches the CNS via the bloodstream.

*Pathogenesis*—granulomatous inflammation affects the basal meninges, large arteries and cranial nerves, covering the brain in a gelatinous, greenish exudate.

It presents clinically with slow-onset, subacute meningitis. It may be accompanied by isolated cranial nerve palsies.

Hydrocephalus may result from impaired reabsorption of CSF or obstruction of CSF outflow from arachnoid fibrosis.

CSF shows an initial increase in mononuclear cells and polymorphs (Fig. 5.10). Untreated, the disease is usually fatal. Intensive treatment with antituberculous drugs lowers mortality to 15–20%.

### Neurosyphilis

This is caused by invasion of the CNS by the micro-organism *Treponema pallidum*. It can occur weeks, months or years after initial infection (tertiary-stage syphilis).

Meningitic illness occurs in only approximately 10% of cases of untreated syphilis. It is usually mild or even asymptomatic, but it may be severe with transient cranial nerve palsies and convulsions.

## Lyme disease

This disorder is caused by the tick-borne spirochete *Borrelia burgdorferi*. It is a systemic illness characterized by skin lesions and neurological features.

## Viral encephalitis

This is a virally induced diffuse inflammation of the brain, which is usually concomitant with meningo-encephalitis. It is a common complication of many viral illnesses. Common causative viruses are:

- arboviruses
- herpes simplex virus I and II
- measles
- cytomegalovirus
- polio and enteroviruses
- rabies
- human immunodeficiency virus (HIV).

Most cases are mild and self-limiting. However, some cases (e.g. those involving herpes simplex virus type I and rabies) result in extensive tissue destruction and may be fatal.

Mortality for the more severe type is 50%, and the majority of survivors have severe, permanent brain damage.

## Fungal infections

These are relatively rare and occur mainly in the immunosuppressed (e.g. associated with chemotherapy, steroid treatment, acquired immune deficiency syndrome; AIDS), but some organisms, e.g. *Cryptococcus neoformans*, can produce disease in the absence of immunosuppression.

**Fig. 5.10** Typical CSF results from lumbar puncture. (Redrawn with permission from (Medicshandbook.com)

| Type | Pyogenic | Tuberculosis | Viral-aspetic |
|---|---|---|---|
| Appearance | Turbid | Fibrin webs | Usually clear |
| Predominant cell | Neutrophils | Lymphocytes | Lymphocytes |
| Cell count/mm$^3$ | 90–1000+ | 10–1000 | 50–1000 |
| Glucose | <0.5 plasma | <0.5 plasma | >0.5 plasma |
| Proteins (g/L) | >1.5 | 1–5 | <1 |
| Organisms | On stain and culture | On Ziehl-Neelsen stain | Not seen |

The spread can be haematogenous (e.g. from the lungs, which is the most common) or direct (e.g. from the nose and paranasal sinuses, which is rare).

The most common causative organisms are *Cryptococcus neoformans* and *Candida albicans* (causes fungal abscesses).

## Protozoal infection toxoplasmosis

This is caused by infection with *Toxoplasma gondii*. It may be acquired by eating poorly cooked infected meat or food contaminated with feline faeces. It has two forms: congenital and acquired.

In the congenital form, the organism is transmitted to the fetus through the placenta during maternal infection, potentially leading to:

- abortion or stillbirth
- severe brain damage leading to early death
- moderate brain damage and chorioretinitis, compatible with life but with permanent disability.

Acquired toxoplasmosis is the most common opportunistic infection of the CNS in adults with AIDS. It results in:

- necrotizing cerebritis
- chronic abscesses
- meningoencephalitis.

However, in healthy subjects, it rarely causes cerebral symptoms.

Other protozoan organisms that may cause infection of the CNS are:

- free-living amoebae
- *Plasmodium falciparum*
- trypanosomes.

## Progressive multifocal leucoencephalopathy

Multifocal destruction of oligodendrocytes results in demyelination with minimal inflammation and damage to axons. It is caused by the DNA JC polyomavirus, and it occurs in association with underlying diseases such as AIDS, chronic lymphocytic leucaemia, carcinoma and systemic lupus erythematosus (SLE).

Patients present with progressive dementia. The disease is progressive and death usually occurs within a few months.

## Subacute sclerosing panencephalopathy

This subacute encephalitis occurring in children is due to persistent measles infection. It presents with progressive neurological dementia, and death usually occurs within 2 years of onset. It is now rare due to immunization with the MMR vaccine.

## Spongiform encephalitis (Creutzfeldt–Jakob disease)

This presents as rapidly progressive dementia, ataxia and myoclonus; it is rare in the UK (1 per million people per year). Spongiform changes include the formation of intracellular vacuoles in neurons and glia. The infectious agent is a prion protein (PrP; see page 32). The condition has an incubation period of up to 30 years, but it is always fatal, usually within 6 months. The disease typically affects people over 70 years old.

Variant Creutzfeldt–Jakob disease (vCJD) is a human disease associated with bovine spongiform encephalopathy that shows the potential for prion transmission between species. Descriptions of the disease are relatively recent but it appears to affect younger individuals than does classic CJD. Neurological decline seems to be slower, but fatal progression is—so far—universal. A genetic predisposition may increase susceptibility to vCJD from eating infected beef. Recent estimates have suggested that the disease might be responsible for hundreds or thousands of cases.

## Demyelinating diseases

This group of diseases has a common factor of primary damage to myelin of nerves while the axons and nerve cells remain relatively intact.

## Multiple sclerosis

Multiple sclerosis (MS) is the most common demyelinating disorder of the CNS, affecting 50 per 100 000 in the UK. Peak incidence is between 20 and 40 years, with a slight female predominance.

MS is characterized by relapsing and remitting episodes of immunologically mediated demyelination within the CNS. Recovery from each episode of demyelination is usually incomplete, leading to progressive deterioration. There is an association between the disease and certain human leucocyte antigens (HLA, e.g. A3, B7, DR2 and DQ1). The incidence also increases with distance from the equator, suggesting a possible environmental trigger.

*Pathogenesis*—activated T lymphocytes cross the blood–brain barrier, reacting to self-antigens against myelin that are presented by microglia. A strong inflammatory reaction follows, enhanced by the release of proinflammatory cytokines. Acute demyelination occurs in the central white matter in discrete areas known as plaques.

Abnormalities are confined to the CNS; the peripheral nervous system (PNS) is usually spared. Common sites are the optic nerve, brainstem, cerebellum, periventricular regions and cervical spinal cord.

**Fig. 5.11** Clinical manifestations of MS and their causes

| Manifestations | Causes |
|---|---|
| **Early clinical symptoms** | |
| Blurring of vision | Optic nerve disease |
| Incoordination | Cerebellar peduncle disease |
| Abnormal sensation | Disease of long ascending sensory tracts |
| **Late stages** | |
| Blindness, paraplegia and incontinence | Spinal tract involvement |
| Ataxia | Spinal and cerebellar involvement |
| Intellectual dysfunction | Loss of hemispheric white matter |

Figure 5.11 lists the clinical manifestations of MS and their causes.

**Clinical Note**

MS diagnosis involves identification of abnormal CNS areas (e.g. by MRI scanning) in the absence of another explanation. The CSF may show increased lymphoid cells and oligoclonal bands of IgG. There is no specific treatment, but high-dose intravenous corticosteroids may accelerate remission in relapse. Beta-interferon has also been used to some success. Most follow a relapsing-remitting course with variable disability, but a minority (5%) suffer rapidly progressive (fulminant) disease, which is fatal within 5 years.

# Degenerative disorders

These diseases primarily affect the grey matter, with progressive neuronal loss. A common feature of this group is the development of protein aggregates (cellular inclusions) that are resistant to degradation.

## Cortical Alzheimer's disease

This is the most common cause of dementia in Western countries.

Dementia is defined as the progressive loss of cognitive function, independent of the state of attention, and occurs due to degeneration of the cerebral cortex. Alzheimer's disease affects 5% of people over 65 years, and 15% of people over 80 years in the UK; females more than males. Also of significance is the subgroup of early-onset patients (40–60 years).

Genetic studies have shown that there is an increase in incidence of sporadic cases in individuals with ApoEe4 genotype on chromosome 19. The amyloid precursor protein *(APP)* gene on chromosome 21 has been implicated in the familial cases.

The aetiology and pathogenesis are unknown; some cases (5%) are familial, but most (95%) are sporadic.

Macroscopically, there is marked cortical atrophy, especially of the frontal lobes; the brain is reduced in weight to 1000 g or less (normal average 1400 g). There is a loss of cortical grey and white matter.

Histological hallmarks are as follows:

- Senile (neuritic) plaques—composed of an extracellular core of amyloid protein (10–150 nm diameter) surrounded by dystrophic neurites; occur most frequently in the hippocampus, cerebral cortex and deep grey matter. The main component of the core is Aβ, a readily aggregating peptide that is thought to be central in the pathogenesis of dementia.
- Neurofibrillary tangles—abnormal tangles of insoluble cytoskeletal-like proteins (tau proteins – paired helical filaments) that form within the cytoplasm of neurons.
- Neuropil threads—distorted, twisted and dilated dendritic processes and axons of cerebral cortex found around amyloid plaques.

Clinically, there is failure of memory and disturbance of emotions. There tends to be progressive physical decline with poor food intake and inability to walk. Death is commonly due to the development of pneumonia.

# Basal ganglia

## Parkinsonism

This term is used to refer to patients whose clinical presentation typically consists of:

- akinetic rigidity
- stooped posture with slow voluntary movements
- diminished facial expression
- festinating gait (progressively shortened, accelerated steps)
- resting ('pill-rolling') tremor.

The causes include:

- Parkinson's disease
- postencephalitic parkinsonism (very rare)
- neuroleptic drugs
- cerebral anoxia.

## Parkinson's disease

This is characterized by rest tremor, slowness of voluntary movement and rigidity. It occurs in 1 per 1000 adults, but 1 per 200 over the age of 65. The aetiology is unknown.

*Pathogenesis:*

- The disorder shows degeneration of pigmented dopaminergic neurons of the substantia nigra, the locus caeruleus and several other brainstem nuclei.
- Degeneration of these cells causes disease by reducing the amount of dopamine in the corpus striatum.
- Surviving cells in the substantia nigra contain eosinophilic spherical inclusions (Lewy bodies), which contain cytoskeletal filaments.

The disease can be symptomatically treated with drugs, such as L-Dopa, that correct neurotransmitter imbalance. Eventually, there is failure of response to treatment and patients die from wasting and poor nutritional intake. Several genes have been implicated in the development of Parkinson's disease, including those encoding the proteins $\alpha$-synuclein and parkin.

## Motor neurons

### Motor neuron disease (amyotrophic lateral sclerosis)
This progressive, neurodegenerative disease is characterized by the selective loss of both upper and lower motor neurons from the spinal cord, brainstem and motor cortex. Its prevalence is 5 per 100 000 of the population, with male incidence greater than female.

The majority of cases are sporadic but 5% of cases are familial—due to mutation of the superoxide dismutase gene.

It eventually progresses to severe paralysis with loss of swallowing and respiration, leading to death in 2–3 years.

Other degenerative disorders are considered in Figure 5.12.

## Metabolic disorders and toxins

### Vitamin deficiencies

#### Vitamin B$_1$ (thiamine) deficiency
This is common in chronic alcoholics, resulting in:

- Wernicke's encephalopathy—memory impairment, ataxia, visual disturbances and peripheral neuropathy
- Korsakoff's psychosis—confused state, memory loss and confabulation.

If both occur, it is known as Wernicke–Korsakoff syndrome.

#### Vitamin B$_{12}$ (cyanocobalamin) deficiency
This produces weakness and paraesthesia in the lower limbs with loss of vibration and proprioception resulting from subacute combined degeneration of the spinal cord (Fig. 5.13). Replacement therapy at an early stage reverses the degenerative process, but long-standing cases show irreversible axonal damage with reactive gliosis.

#### Iodine deficiency
Severe iodine deficiency causes hypothyroidism; it is the most important endocrine disorder to affect the CNS in children. In the fetus, severe iodine deficiency causes cretinism characterized by dwarfism, mental defect and spastic diplegia. This can be prevented by iodine supplements during pregnancy.

### Toxins

#### Carbon monoxide
Carbon monoxide (CO) binds irreversibly to haemoglobin, rendering erythrocytes incapable of oxygen transport. CO poisoning therefore results in brain damage due to hypoxia. This poisoning may be accidental or associated with attempted suicide.

The amounts of carbon-monoxide-bound haemoglobin (HbCO) with corresponding clinical symptoms are as follows:

- > 20%—dyspnoea and slight headache
- 30%—severe headache, fatigue and impaired judgement

**Fig. 5.12** Additional types of degenerative disease

| Degenerative disorder | Features |
| --- | --- |
| Pick's disease | Progressive dementia with severe memory and speech loss. Atrophy of cortex in areas of the frontal and temporal lobes. Surviving neurons contain Pick's bodies |
| Huntington's disease | Autosomal dominant disorder (trinucleotide repeat, chromosome 4) characterized by chorea and progressive dementia. Cerebral atrophy in the caudate nucleus and putamen |
| Friedreich's ataxia | Autosomal recessive spinocerebellar disease<br>Degeneration of the posterior columns, corticospinal and spinocerebellar tracts |

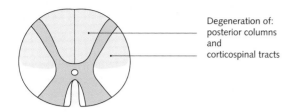

Degeneration of:
posterior columns
and
corticospinal tracts

**Fig. 5.13**  Subacute combined degeneration of the spinal cord. Degeneration of posterior columns leads to sensory loss (vibration and proprioception) causing ataxia. Degeneration of corticospinal tracts leads to upper motor neuron damage causing spastic paralysis.

- 60–70%—loss of consciousness
- > 70%—rapidly fatal.

Hypoxia results in neuronal necrosis with a predilection for globus pallidus. Other selectively vulnerable regions are the hippocampus and the cerebral and cerebellar cortices.

### Methanol

Methanol is highly toxic to the CNS, particularly to the retina. It is lipid soluble, so readily diffuses into the CSF and aqueous humour in concentrations higher than in plasma.

Methanol is metabolized into formic acid and formaldehyde. It is the formaldehyde that is thought to be the mediator of toxic effects. There are two types of methanol poisoning:

1. Acute—sudden death with multiple haemorrhagic lesions in the cerebral hemispheres
2. Chronic—atrophy of retinal ganglion cells with secondary degeneration of the optic nerve.

### Ethanol

The consequences of excessive ethanol intake on the CNS are manifold (Fig. 5.14).

## Neoplasms of the CNS

### Gliomas

Gliomas are tumours that arise from glial supportive tissue of brain. They are the most common primary brain tumours, accounting for 50% of all CNS tumours.

> **HINTS AND TIPS**
>
> Note that glial cells are the support cells of the CNS. The group includes astrocytes (throughout the CNS), oligodendrocytes (form myelin sheaths), ependymal cells (line the ventricular system) and microglia (act as CNS macrophages).

### Astrocytoma

This is a glioma derived from astrocytes. It is more common in children, usually occurring in the cerebellum. It accounts for 10% of all primary tumours in adults, usually in the cerebral hemispheres. Common types of astrocytomas and their corresponding tumour grading include:

- pilocytic astrocytoma (grade I)—relatively benign, often affecting children
- well-differentiated fibrillary astrocytoma (grade II)—small increase in glial cell nuclei
- anaplastic astrocytoma (grade III)—densely cellular with nuclear pleomorphism

**Fig. 5.14** Consequences of excess ethanol intake on the central nervous system

| Disease | Features | Mechanism |
| --- | --- | --- |
| Fetal alcohol syndrome | Cerebral malformations<br>Facial and somatic malformations<br>Growth retardation | Direct toxicity |
| Acute intoxication | Cerebral oedema<br>Petechial haemorrhages | Direct toxicity |
| Cerebral and cerebellar atrophy | Neuronal loss | Direct toxicity |
| Nutritional disorders | Wernicke's encephalopathy<br>Korsakoff's syndrome | Deficiency of vitamin $B_1$ |
| Hepatocerebral syndromes | Hepatic encephalopathy<br>Chronic hepatocerebral degeneration | Hepatic toxicity with secondary effects on CNS |
| Demyelinating disorders | Central pontine myelinolysis | Electrolyte disturbances |

*(Adapted from Underwood, 2009.)*

- glioblastoma (grade IV)—the most common and most malignant of primary brain tumours, relatively poorly differentiated. Areas of necrosis and haemhorrage surrounded by a 'pseudopalisade' arrangement of tumour cells.

## Oligodendrogliomas

These ill-defined, slow-growing tumours arise from oligodendrocytes in the white matter of the cerebral hemispheres, especially the temporal lobe. They account for 5% of all primary CNS neoplasms in adults. They are characterized by large nuclei cells with perinuclear halo, the so-called 'fried egg' appearance.

## Ependymoma

These tumours arise from the ependymal cells lining the ventricle and central canal of the spinal cord. Ependymoma is the most common tumour of the spinal cord, accounting for 5% of all primary CNS neoplasms. It is common in children and young adults.

## Medulloblastoma

This highly malignant tumour of primitive neuroepithelial cells arises in the cerebellum of children. It is the most common tumours of childhood CNS. The tumour is highly radiosensitive, but without treatment it is rapidly fatal.

## Other tumours

### Metastatic tumours

These tumours are more common than any primary intracranial neoplasms. The cerebellum is the preferred site but they can affect any part of the brain as well as other intracranial structures, especially meninges (malignant meningitis). Metastases often occur at the boundary between grey and white matter, surrounded by oedema.

The most common neoplasms to metastasize to the CNS are:

- breast carcinomas
- bronchus carcinomas
- kidney carcinomas
- colon carcinomas
- malignant melanoma.

### Meningiomas

These account for approximately 15% of adult intracranial tumours and are the second most common primary intracranial neoplasms. Tumours arise from the arachnoid mater. They are usually benign and external to the brain. They are characterized by laminated calcified psammoma bodies.

# DISORDERS OF THE PERIPHERAL NERVOUS SYSTEM

Disorders of peripheral nerves are termed neuropathies. They can be predominantly sensory, predominantly motor or mixed, depending on which nerves are affected.

> **HINTS AND TIPS**
>
> Note that:
> - Disorders affecting many peripheral nerves are termed polyneuropathies, and they usually cause symmetrical deficits.
> - Disorders affecting only one (mononeuropathy) or a few (multiple mononeuropathies) peripheral nerves typically cause asymmetrical deficits.
> - Radiculopathies are disorders of nerve roots.

## Hereditary neuropathies

### Hereditary motor and sensory neuropathies (HMSN)

#### Peroneal muscular atrophy (HMSN I+II; Charcot–Marie–Tooth disease)

This disorder is characterized by pronounced atrophy of the calf muscles with associated sensory deficits as a result of slowly progressive symmetric neuropathy. It is the commonest of the hereditary neuropathies, and it is usually autosomal dominant. It impedes ambulation and causes foot deformities (pes cavus), but it does not shorten the lifespan.

Figure 5.15 provides a table of the different types of peroneal muscular atrophy and their characteristics.

### Hereditary sensory and autonomic neuropathies (HSAN)

This group of autosomal inherited diseases produces mainly sensory and autonomic neuropathies. There are three major types, as described in Figure 5.16.

## Traumatic neuropathies

### Laceration

This is a jagged tear of the peripheral nerve in which there is partial or complete loss of continuity of the nerve. It occurs most commonly from cutting injuries, misplaced intramuscular injections or fragments of fractured bone.

**Fig. 5.15** Different types of peroneal muscular atrophy and their characteristics

|  | HMSN I | HMSN II |
| --- | --- | --- |
| Type of neuropathy | Demyelinating neuropathy | Axonal neuropathy |
| Relative occurrence | 75% | 25% |
| Type of axonal loss | Large calibre axons | Large and small calibre axons |
| Nerve conduction velocity | Impaired (< 30 m/s) | Normal (> 45 m/s) |
| Time of onset | Early (first decade) | Later (second decade) |
| Effects | Severe distal wasting in legs | Weakness and wasting less marked |

HMSN, hereditary motor and sensory neuropathy.

**Fig. 5.16** Types of hereditary sensory and autonomic neuropathies

|  | HSAN I | HSAN II | HSAN III |
| --- | --- | --- | --- |
| Clinical syndrome | Ulcerative acropathy due to numbness | Congenital sensory neuropathy | Familial dysautonomia |
| Eponym | Morvan's | Ciacci's | Riley–Day |
| Inheritance | Autosomal dominant | Autosomal recessive | Autosomal recessive |
| Affected neurons | Degeneration of large myelinated fibres of both peripheral nerves and posterior columns of spinal cord | Degeneration of large and small myelinated fibres | Degeneration of non-myelinated fibres with preservation of myelinated fibres. Loss of neurons of autonomic ganglia |

HSAN, hereditary sensory and autonomic neuropathies

## Avulsion

This is the tearing of nerve fibres from the surface of the spinal cord or from a muscle. It may be partial or complete depending on whether all or only some of the nerve rootlets are involved.

Nerve roots may be avulsed from the spinal cord in two ways:

1. Tensile stresses from cervical plexus transmitted centrally can stretch and finally avulse the nerve roots.
2. A spinal cord injury, such that displacement of the cord acts directly on the nerve roots between their attachment to the cord and their entry into the intravertebral foramen.

Both laceration and avulsion injuries cause the severed ends of the damaged nerve to retract and then to undergo Wallerian degeneration to form a traumatic neuroma (a type of benign tumour). Subsequently, the proximal portion of the nerve develops neuritic sprouts which, if sited in proximity to the severed distal nerve, may reinnervate by slow regrowth along the nerve sheath.

If continuity of the nerve is completely interrupted, basal laminae sheaths no longer form continuous tubes to guide regeneration sprouts and so the potential for recovery is limited.

## Compression/entrapment neuropathy

Compressed nerves undergo segmental demyelination with decreased nerve conduction velocity. If compression is prolonged or severe, axonal degeneration may occur. Symptoms of nerve compression are paraesthesia, anaesthesia and loss of muscle strength.

### Clinical Note

Common sites of nerve compression are:
- nerve roots in the intervertebral foramina by prolapsed intervertebral discs or osteophytes due to osteoarthritis of the spine
- median nerve in the carpal tunnel at the wrist
- ulnar nerve in flexor carpal tunnel at the medial epicondyle of humerus
- common peroneal nerve at the neck of the fibula.

### Carpal tunnel syndrome

This is a disorder in which the size of the carpal tunnel is significantly reduced, causing compression of the median nerve. Causes include inflammation of the flexor retinaculum and arthritic changes.

## Inflammatory neuropathies

### Guillain–Barré syndrome (acute inflammatory demyelinating polyradiculopathy)

This is the most common form of acute neuropathy caused by immune-mediated demyelination of peripheral nerves, usually occurring 2–4 weeks after viral illnesses such as Epstein–Barr infection. The pathogenesis is unclear, but it appears that virus infection triggers a T-cell-mediated autoimmune-like response against peripheral nerves.

Affected patients develop motor neuropathy that rises from the peripheral limbs ('ascending paralysis'), with lesser sensory changes due to widespread demyelination of the peripheral nerves. Recovery (i.e. remyelination) occurs over 3–4 months and is usually complete.

## Infectious neuropathies

### Leprosy (Hansen's disease)

A chronic granulomatous disease caused by *Mycobacterium leprae*. It is the most common cause of peripheral neuritis worldwide, affecting about 10 million patients in total.

The clinicopathological features of leprosy are dependent on the host's response to infection, with a spectrum of disease ranging from tuberculoid to lepromatous form (see Fig. 5.17).

### Varicella-zoster virus

An invasion of cutaneous sensory nerves during primary infection with varicella-zoster virus (VZV, the virus that causes chickenpox) leads to infection of the dorsal root ganglia where the virus enters a latent state. Reactivation of VZV may occur years later causing shingles—painful, vesicular skin eruptions in the distribution of sensory dermatomes, usually thoracic or trigeminal. The reason for reactivation is unknown but there is increased incidence in immunocompromised individuals.

## Metabolic and toxic neuropathies

### Peripheral neuropathy of diabetes mellitus

This occurs in both type I and II diabetes mellitus with a prevalence of 10–60% clinically, but up to 100% when evaluated by nerve conduction studies. There is increased prevalence with increased duration of the disease.

#### Pathogenesis

Vascular occlusion of the blood vessels supplying the nerves results in neuronal atrophy. There are four types:

1. Symmetrical and predominantly sensory polyneuropathy
2. Autonomic neuropathy
3. Proximal painful motor neuropathy
4. Cranial mononeuritis (mainly CN III, IV and VI).

**Fig. 5.17** Comparison of peripheral nerve damage by lepromatous and tuberculoid forms of leprosy

|  | Lepromatous | Tuberculoid |
|---|---|---|
| Immune mechanism | Minimal immune response (occurs in patients with low cellular immunity) | Vigorous T-cell mediated (delayed) hypersensitivity |
| Spread of organisms | Bacteraemia occurs in peripheral sites | Bacteraemia rare |
| Distribution in nerves | Widely disseminated diffuse nerve involvement | One or a few sites (asymmetrical) |
| Nerve enlargement and damage | Intense infiltration of nerves by vacuolated macrophages | Hallmark of nerve involvement is discrete, well-formed granulomas |
| Neurological deficit | Sensory and motor involvement Patchy loss of sensation | Sensory, motor and autonomic involvement Peripheral nerve palsies Anaesthetic areas prone to injury and secondary infection |
| Prognosis | Progressive and lethal | Progression slow, but immune response produces extensive destruction of tissue resulting in severe disfigurement Eventually heals spontaneously |

## Metabolic and nutritional causes

### Uraemic neuropathy in renal failure
Approximately 60% of patients with chronic renal failure have symptoms of uraemic neuropathy at onset of dialysis. It is typically distal and symmetrical, producing pain and paraesthesia with the lower extremities preferentially involved. Dialysis usually improves symptoms.

## Toxic neuropathies
Many toxins cause damage to peripheral nerves. The most common toxins are:

- drugs—e.g. isoniazides, sulphonamides, vinca alkaloids, dapsone and chloroquine
- alcohol—in cases of chronic abuse
- industrial toxins—e.g. acrylamide, hexane, organophosphates, lead, arsenic, mercury.

Most toxins produce a 'dying back' pattern of axonal damage resulting in a distal symmetric pattern of sensorimotor involvement. There is a 'stocking glove' distribution at onset but continued exposure to the toxin extends the deficit to the lower calves and forearms.

## Neuropathies associated with malignancy (metastatic neuropathy)
Cancer patients frequently have mononeuropathies caused by direct infiltration of individual nerves or plexuses, e.g. brachial plexopathy due to apical lung cancer.

## Neoplasms of peripheral nerves
Peripheral nervous system tumours are illustrated in Figure 5.18.

## DISORDERS OF THE AUTONOMIC NERVOUS SYSTEM

## Disorders of the sympathetic nervous system

### Horner's syndrome
An uncommon condition caused by loss of sympathetic innervation to the eye. It is characterized by:

- pupillary constriction (miosis) due to unopposed action of the pupillary constrictor
- partial ptosis (drooping) of the upper eyelid due to paralysis of smooth muscle fibres contained in the levator muscle of the upper eyelid
- enophthalmos (eye sunken into socket)
- anhidrosis (loss of sweating) on affected side of the face.

**HINTS AND TIPS**

Lesions affecting any part of the sympathetic pathway (Fig. 5.19) may produce Horner's syndrome:
- brainstem—tumours, vascular lesions, or syringobulbia
- cervical cord—tumours or syringomyelia
- cervical sympathetic chain—pancoast tumours (apical tumours of the lung) frequently invade adjacent sites; invasion of the superior cervical sympathetic ganglion often results in Horner's syndrome.

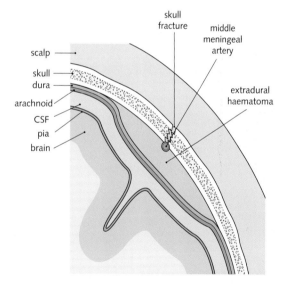

**Fig. 5.19** Sympathetic innervation to the eye and face showing the relationship of the sympathetic trunk to the apex of the lungs.

| Fig. 5.18 Peripheral nervous system tumours | |
|---|---|
| **Tumour** | **Features** |
| Schwannoma | Benign tumour of schwann cells of the nerve sheaths. Most common site is the vestibular branch of CN VIII |
| Neurofibroma | A tumour of the neural crest cells derived from the epineurium and endoneurium |

## Trauma/surgical section of the sympathetic trunk

Surgical sympathectomies are sometimes performed for the relief of such conditions as:

- Raynaud's phenomenon—pallor, pain and numbness of the fingers caused by vasospastic constriction of the digital arteries; sympathectomy is occasionally performed to improve limb perfusion
- causalgia—severe burning pain that occurs following injury to the major peripheral nerves of the limbs (e.g. median, ulnar, sciatic) presumed to be due to disturbances of sympathetic reflexes
- hyperhidrosis—excessive sweating.

The consequences of either traumatic or surgical section of the sympathetic chain depend on the level of the section, but may cause:

- loss of blood pressure control → syncope (fainting)
- impairment of sweating → hyperpyrexia
- impairment of bladder and bowel functions
- interruption of pathway to erectile tissue → impotence.

## Phaeochromocytoma

This is a rare tumour arising from chromaffin cells of the adrenal medulla, occurring in 1 in 1000 cases of hypertension. The majority are sporadic but about 10% are familial. Most are benign but about 5% are malignant.

The effects are those of hypersecretion of catecholamines, i.e. hypertension, hypermetabolism and hyperglycaemia. There is also pallor, headaches, sweating and nervousness.

It may be associated with other endocrine neoplasias, namely:

- multiple endocrine neoplasia syndrome (especially MEN2 syndromes)
- von Recklinghausen's disease—associated with neurofibromatosis
- von Hippel–Lindau syndrome—associated with renal cell carcinomas and multiple hemangiomas.

It is diagnosed by increased amounts of urinary excretion of catecholamines and their metabolites, such as vanillylmandelic acid (VMA).

Surgical removal of the tumour relieves hypertension and other effects.

# Diseases of the parasympathetic nervous system

## Effects of ablation of parasympathetic innervation

The most common site of parasympathetic ablation is the vagus nerve (vagotomy) for treatment of duodenal ulcers. This is less common now because of increasing awareness of the bacterial aetiology (Helicobacter pylori) of intestinal ulcers.

# Pathology of the cardiovascular system (6)

## Objectives

In this chapter, you will learn to:
- Understand the fetal circulation and how alterations produce congenital abnormalities of the heart.
- Describe the key processes of atherosclerosis, hypertension and thrombosis (arterial and venous).
- Describe the spectrum of ischaemic heart disease and the commonly resulting heart failure.
- Understand the disorders of heart valves, including infective endocarditis.
- Recall the diseases of the myocardium itself.
- Describe the diseases of the pericardium—effusions and pericarditis.
- Understand the development of aneurysms, particularly affecting the aorta.
- Briefly describe the inflammatory and neoplastic diseases of the vasculature.
- Briefly describe other diseases of the veins and lymphatics.

## CONGENITAL ABNORMALITIES OF THE HEART

### Epidemiology

Congenital heart abnormalities are relatively common, affecting nearly 1% of live births. The incidence is higher in premature babies.

### Causes

#### Sporadic

These are the majority of cases and no teratogenic factors can be identified.

#### Maternal factors

There is an increased incidence associated with certain maternal factors including:

- maternal infection, especially with rubella
- maternal alcohol abuse (causes fetal alcohol syndrome)
- intrauterine radiation
- maternal use of teratogenic drugs, e.g. phenytoin, thalidomide.

These factors are of greatest importance between the fourth and ninth week after conception.

#### Genetic or chromosomal abnormalities

These are associated with an increased incidence of congenital heart malformations (e.g. Down's syndrome).

### Clinical features

Most cardiac abnormalities become apparent at or shortly after birth, usually by some manifestation of heart failure such as cyanosis, breathlessness, feeding difficulties, or a failure to thrive. However, it is possible for some conditions to be undetected until adulthood.

### Classification

Congenital heart defects may be divided into two main groups depending on whether the lesions cause:

1. abnormal shunting of blood between the two sides of the heart. A shunt is defined as an abnormal communication between heart chambers or blood vessels. In congenital heart disease there may be either left-to-right (more common) or right-to-left shunts
2. obstruction to blood flow by narrowing of chambers, valves or blood vessels. Complete obstruction is termed an atresia.

### Fetal circulation

As the fetus does not breathe in the uterus, blood flow is controlled by three unique mechanisms (Fig. 6.1):

- Foramen ovale—connection from the right atrium to the left atrium allows oxygenated maternal blood from the umbilical vein to bypass the lungs and directly enter the left side of the heart.
- Ductus arteriosus—connection between the pulmonary artery and aorta allows blood entering the pulmonary circulation to be diverted away from the lungs and to the body. This blood is generally less oxygenated, having entered the heart from the

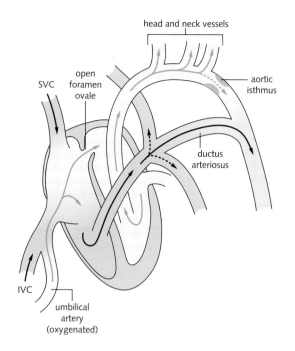

**Fig. 6.1** Schematic representation of the fetal circulation. Note the role of the foramen ovale and ductus arteriosus in diverting blood away from the immature lungs. The aortic isthmus ensures that highly oxygenated blood is delivered to the crucial head and neck structures, with less oxygenated blood supplying the immature organ systems. (IVC, inferior vena cava; SVC, superior vena cava.)

| **Fig. 6.2** Prevalence of left-to-right shunts | |
|---|---|
| **Type** | **% of all CHD abnormalities** |
| Ventricular septal defect | 25–30 |
| Atrial septal defect | 10–15 |
| Patent ductus arteriosus | 10 |
| Atrioventricular septal defect | 5 |
| *CHD, congenital heart disease.* | |

## Ventricular septal defect

This defect of the interventricular septum is the most common cardiac abnormality, accounting for 25–30% of all cases of congenital heart disease (Fig. 6.3). The interventricular septum can be divided into a membranous (fibrous) portion and a muscular portion.

Most congenital defects are perimembranous, i.e. occurring at the junction of the membranous and muscular portions.

There are small and large defects:

- Small defects—often confined to the tiny membranous area, many of which spontaneously close
- Larger defects—also involve the muscular wall of the septum.

superior vena cava, so avoiding diversion through the foramen ovale. The high resistance of the immature lungs aids flow through this low-resistance pathway.

- Aortic isthmus—this constriction in the fetal aorta after the origin of the head and neck arteries ensures that relatively low oxygenated blood from the ductus arteriosus supplies the immature organ systems of the body, rather than crucial head and neck structures.

After birth, pulmonary vascular resistance drops, allowing the foramen ovale and ductus arteriosus to close. The aortic isthmus also expands shortly after birth.

## Left-to-right shunts

These are malformations that result in the shunting of blood from the left side of the heart to the right because of the higher pressures in the left side of the heart; they are the most common group of congenital heart abnormalities. These defects clinically are acyanotic as the blood does not bypass the lungs.

Figure 6.2 lists the prevalence of left-to-right shunts.

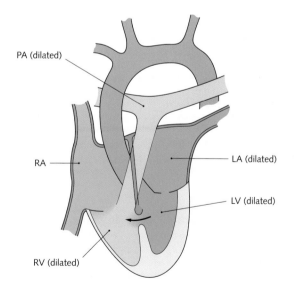

**Fig. 6.3** Ventricular septal defect. Larger defects involve the septal muscle but smaller defects may be confined to the maladie de Roger (tiny membranous region). (LA, left atrium; LV, left ventricle; PA, pulmonary artery; RA, right atrium; RV, right ventricle).

The size and site of the defect determines the extent of shunting of the blood from left to right. Defects may present as cardiac failure in infants, or as a murmur in older children or adults.

### Clinical Note

The clinical presentation of a ventricular septal defect includes:

- pansystolic murmur, caused by flow from the high-pressure left ventricle to the low-pressure right ventricle during systole. The smallest defects generally produce the loudest murmurs
- tachypnoea
- indrawing of the lower ribs on inspiration
- right and left ventricular hypertrophy.

   Small defects need no treatment; larger ones require surgical repair to prevent cardiac failure.

## Atrial septal defect

This is a common congenital heart defect, affecting females more than males by 2:1. Blood flows from left to right due to the high compliance of the right ventricle. The defect may be of two types (Fig. 6.4):

1. Ostium primum—defect is at the level of the atrioventricular septum and is associated with an abnormal mitral valve (split anterior leaflet).

2. Ostium secundum—the foramen ovale fails to close, remaining patent as the fossa ovalis. This is the most common form of atrial septal defect.

Most children are asymptomatic, however some children present with dyspnoea, chest infections, cardiac failure or arrhythmias (e.g. atrial fibrillation).

The characteristic physical signs are a systolic flow murmur over the pulmonary valve and wide splitting of the second heart sound.

Atrial septal defects should be closed surgically to prevent shunt reversal (see below). If performed before this develops, the prognosis after surgery is excellent.

## Patent (persistent) ductus arteriosus

This persistence of the embryological connection between the aorta and the pulmonary is shown in Figure 6.5. Patent (open) ductus arteriosus occurs in about 10% of all cases of congenital heart disease, affecting females more than males. There is a recognized association with maternal rubella.

A continuous 'machinery-like' murmur is classically detected, as high volumes of oxygenated blood are shunted from the high-pressure aorta back into the lungs. This can dramatically increase the work of the heart in a large defect, leading to eventual cardiac failure without early surgical correction.

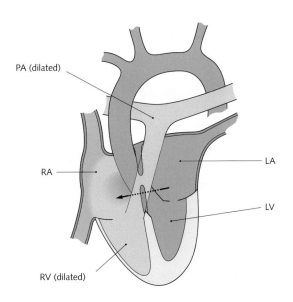

**Fig. 6.4**   Atrial septal defect. The defect is usually located at the level of the fossa ovalis. (LA, left atrium; LV, left ventricle; PA, pulmonary artery; RA, right atrium; RV, right ventricle).

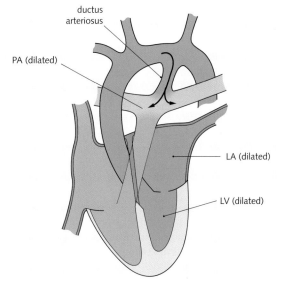

**Fig. 6.5**   Patent ductus arteriosus. Persistence of the duct is more common in females, and it is associated with maternal rubella.

## Eisenmenger's syndrome

All the left-to-right shunts described above have the potential to result in pulmonary hypertension, partly due to the obliteration of small vessels in the lungs and the increase in flow. Eventually, this increase in pulmonary resistance can be so great that reversal to a right-to-left shunt occurs, producing marked cyanosis as deoxygenated blood is pumped around the body (Eisenmenger's syndrome).

The condition is irreversible and usually prevents surgery to correct the original congenital defect.

## Right-to-left shunts

These are less common than left-to-right shunts. The result of a right-to-left shunt is that deoxygenated blood bypasses the lungs to enter the systemic circulation. Cyanosis may, therefore, develop in the early postnatal period with any of these conditions.

### HINTS AND TIPS

Understanding the embryonic development of the heart assists in the understanding of congenital abnormalities, for example, the involvement of the embryonic foramen ovale in the development of atrial septal defects, and the congenital abnormality created by a persistent ductus arteriosus.

## Tetralogy of Fallot

This is the most common cause of cyanotic congenital heart disease, occurring in about 1 in 2000 live births. The abnormality consists of four defects (Fig. 6.6):

1. Ventricular septal defect
2. Over-riding aorta sitting astride the ventricular septal defect
3. Pulmonary stenosis (causing systolic murmur)
4. Right ventricular hypertrophy.

Aetiopathogenesis—defects are caused by the abnormal embryological development of the bulbar septum, which normally separates the ascending aorta from the pulmonary artery (and should fuse with the interventricular septum).

Pulmonary stenosis leads to inadequate perfusion of the lungs and the over-riding aorta receives blood from both the right and left ventricles. The net result is that the systemic circulation contains deoxygenated blood, causing cyanosis in affected individuals.

Clinical features are:

- cyanosis—especially after a crying attack. This is termed a 'Fallot's spell', as adrenergic stimulation exacerbates the right ventricular outflow obstruction,

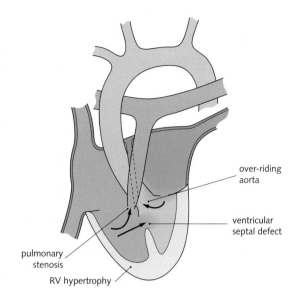

**Fig. 6.6** Fallot's tetralogy is an important cause of right-to-left shunting.

so increasing the amount of blood shunted. Squatting after exertion can relieve these symptoms by increasing the afterload of the left heart
- loud ejection systolic murmur—either from the ventricular septal defect or pulmonary stenosis.

Most cases are now surgically corrected, with a good prognosis if performed in early childhood. Complications include endocarditis and consequent cerebral infarction or brain abscess.

## Transposition of the great arteries

Connections between the right and left ventricle, aorta, and pulmonary artery are disordered—the aorta emanating from the right ventricle and the pulmonary artery arising from the left (Fig. 6.7).

Postnatal survival is possible only if one or more of the following shunts exists:

- atrial septal defect—this is often surgically enlarged in early life to ensure adequate oxygenated blood mixes into the systemic circulation
- ventricular septal defect
- patent ductus arteriosus.

Surgical correction is possible, at which point all shunts are closed.

## Persistent truncus arteriosus

Both the aorta and pulmonary artery develop from a single tube: the truncus arteriosus. Persistence of the truncus results in a single great artery that receives

**Fig. 6.7** Transposition of the great vessels. Survival is possible only if other shunts are present at either the atrial (A), ventricular (B) or ductus (C) level.

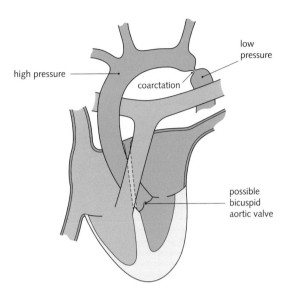

**Fig. 6.8** Coarctation of the aorta. Signs and symptoms depend largely on the size of the narrowing.

blood from both ventricles. A ventricular septal defect is also present.

Cyanosis occurs due to the mixing of blood from the right and left ventricles.

## Obstructive congenital defects

### Coarctation of the aorta

This is a stenotic narrowing of the aorta, usually located in the region where the ductus arteriosus joins the aorta, i.e. the fetal aortic isthmus (Fig. 6.8). About 50% of affected individuals have an associated bicuspid aortic valve. 'Berry' aneurysms of the cerebral circulation are also more common in these individuals.

This defect accounts for up to 5% of all forms of congenital heart disease, and it affects 1 in 4000 live births, male incidence being greater than female by 2:1.

*Clinical features*—stricture produces:

- hypertension proximal to the stenosis, leading to symptoms such as headache and dizziness
- hypotension distal to the stenosis, leading to generalized weakness and poor peripheral circulation.

Characteristically, the blood pressure is raised in the upper body but is normal or low in the legs:

- Upper body—abnormally large arterial pulsations may be seen in the neck, and severe hypertension leads to the development of collateral circulations, which may be visible or present on imaging in older children and adults, e.g. pericapsular and intercostal arteries.

- Lower body—femoral pulses are weak and delayed when compared to the radial pulse.

A systolic murmur may sometimes be heard posteriorly over the coarctation.

*Pathological complications*—in untreated severe cases death may occur in several ways:

- Left ventricular failure, following prolonged hypertension
- Dissection of the aorta, particularly in patients with associated bicuspid aortic valves
- Bacterial endocarditis, usually at the site of aortic constriction
- Cerebral haemorrhage.

### Pulmonary artery stenosis or atresia with intact ventricular septum

This presents as a narrowing (stenosis) or fusion (atresia) of the trunk of the pulmonary artery. In atretic cases, the patent foramen ovale forms the only outlet for blood from the right side of the heart. The ductus arteriosus is always patent and represents the only access route to the pulmonary circulation.

### Aortic stenosis and atresia

Semilunar aortic valves may be stenosed or atretic. If fusion is complete, the aorta, left ventricle and left atrium are markedly underdeveloped. This is usually

**Fig. 6.9** Summary of congenital cardiac malformations

**Left-to-right shunts**

- Ventricular septal defect
- Atrial septal defect
- Patent ductus arteriosus
- Atrioventricular septal defects

**Right-to-left shunts**

- Tetralogy of Fallot
- Transposition of the great arteries
- Persistent truncus arteriosus
- Total anomalous venous connection

**Obstructive congenital defects**

- Coarctation of the aorta
- Pulmonary artery stenosis/atresia
- Aortic stenosis/atresia

accompanied by an open ductus arteriosus which delivers blood into the aorta. The condition is associated with severe cyanosis.

Figure 6.9 gives a summary of congenital cardiac malformations.

# ATHEROSCLEROSIS, HYPERTENSION AND THROMBOSIS

## Definitions and concepts

### Arteriosclerosis

This is an imprecise term meaning thickening and loss of elasticity of the arteries caused by any condition. Three patterns of arteriosclerosis exist:

1. Atherosclerosis—the most common form. A degenerative disease involving the intima of large- and medium-sized arteries. Atherosclerotic lesions are termed atheromas. This is discussed in greater detail below.
2. Mönckeberg's medial calcific sclerosis—this degenerative disease of older individuals involves the deposition of calcium in the media of medium-sized muscular arteries. These deposits do not reduce the size of the vessel lumen.
3. Arteriolosclerosis—the thickening of small artery and arteriole vessel walls, with subsequent reduction in lumen size. This is associated with systemic hypertension and diabetes mellitus, and particularly affects vessels in the kidney, pancreas, gall bladder, small intestine, adrenals and retina.

**HINTS AND TIPS**

The terms 'arteriosclerosis' and 'atherosclerosis' are often confused. They are not synonymous and they should not be used interchangeably. Arteriosclerosis is hardening or loss of elasticity of the arteries from any cause, whereas atherosclerosis implies hardening or loss of elasticity due to atheroma.

## Consequences of arteriosclerosis

The consequences particularly of atherosclerosis and arteriolosclerosis are:

- vessel thickening $\rightarrow$ narrowing of lumen $\rightarrow$ poor tissue perfusion
- inelasticity of vessels $\rightarrow$ predisposition to vessel rupture and haemorrhage
- alterations in vascular endothelium $\rightarrow$ increased predisposition to thrombosis.

Arteriosclerosis contributes to the high frequency of cardiac (myocardial infarction, angina pectoris), cerebral (stroke, transient ischaemic attack), colonic (malabsorption, ischaemic colitis) and peripheral (intermittent claudication, rest pain) diseases in the elderly population.

Certain diseases are known to accelerate and aggravate arteriosclerosis, e.g. hypertension and diabetes.

## Atherosclerosis

A degenerative, progressive and inflammatory disease of large- and medium-sized arteries (but not veins), this is characterized by the focal accumulation of lipid-rich material in the intima of arteries and associated cellular reactions. Although essentially a disease of the vessel intima, atherosclerosis also has an impact on the structure and function of the underlying media.

Atherosclerotic lesions are found to some extent in virtually every adult over the age of 40 as well as in many younger individuals. The consequences of atherosclerosis account for half of all deaths in the Western world.

Commonly affected arteries are:

- aorta (especially the abdominal aorta)
- coronary arteries
- cerebral arteries
- common iliac/femoral arteries.

Atherosclerosis is rare in the arteries of the upper limb and in the pulmonary arteries.

Epidemiological studies have identified risk factors associated with atheroma development. These can be broadly classified into:

- fixed (constitutional) risk factors, i.e. inherent to an individual

- modifiable risk factors, i.e. those that may be controlled (although often to a very limited extent).

  Fixed risk factors are:

- age—atherosclerotic lesions increase in number with increasing age
- gender—females have half the incidence of males up to the age of 55, due to the protective effect of oestrogens; over 55 years, the male to female ratio is equal
- familial traits—familial increase in predisposition is often associated with familial hyperlipidaemia
- race—wide interracial variations exist in the incidence of atheroma, but this may be due to dietary differences. The condition is relatively uncommon in China, Japan and Africa.

Modifiable risk factors lead to an increased severity of atherosclerosis. Such factors are multiplicative rather than additive—this means that combinations of risk factors massively increase the risk of atherosclerosis. Examples are:

- hypercholesterolaemia [increased serum levels of cholesterol or low-density lipoprotein (LDL)]—usually dependent on diet, but may also occur as a result of some forms of familial hypercholesterolaemia
- hypertension—increased blood pressure, both the systolic and diastolic levels
- diabetes mellitus—probably because it results in hypercholesterolaemia
- cigarette smoking—there is a strong link between smoking and deaths from coronary artery disease; the mechanism is unclear
- sedentary lifestyle—exercise decreases the incidence of sudden death from ischaemic heart disease but it is not clear whether it directly reduces atherosclerosis formation
- obesity—particularly central or truncal obesity, probably a reflection of poor diet and resultant hyperlipidaemia.

Following development of atherosclerosis, factors such as stress, personality traits and coagulation disorders may alter the risk of a related event (e.g. stroke or ischaemic heart disease).

### Clinical Note

The clinical management of atherosclerosis is based on minimizing risk factors:

- antihypertensive medication, e.g. diuretics, β-blockers
- HMG CoA reductase inhibitors (statins)—lower cholesterol by inhibiting hepatic synthesis
- anticoagulants—75 mg aspirin (low-dose aspirin) daily to minimize thrombotic risk
- lifestyle advice, e.g. stopping smoking, healthier diet and increased exercise.

## Pathogenesis

The pathogenesis of the characteristic lipid plaques of atherosclerosis is described by the response to injury hypothesis. This states that atherosclerosis is a chronic inflammatory response of the arterial wall to endothelial injury.

Atherosclerosis begins early in life; the first signs of the disorder are termed fatty streaks, which usually occur in areas of altered arterial stress (e.g. bifurcations and sites of endothelial injury). Endothelial dysfunction may also have a role in the early pathogenesis of plaque formation.

Low-grade endothelial injury may be induced by:

- cigarette smoking
- altered haemodynamics—the damaging effect of turbulent blood flow (e.g. at major arterial bifurcations) may be further worsened by hypertension
- homocysteine—this amino acid may directly damage the arterial wall. Individuals with the rare genetic disorder homocystinuria, which results in raised blood homocysteine levels, develop premature vascular disease
- hyperlipidaemia—possibly causing direct endothelial damage and promotion of platelet attachment
- others—viruses, other infectious agents and inflammatory cytokines have all been suggested as potential inducers of endothelial injury.

### Stages of development in atherosclerosis

The key stages in the development of atherosclerotic plaques (atheromas) are as follows:

1. Chronic endothelial injury results in endothelial dysfunction, causing an increased permeability of the vessel wall, and the expression of receptors for leucocyte adhesion.
2. Plasma proteins (including LDL) diffuse into the arterial intima.
3. Monocytes bind newly expressed receptors and migrate into the intima, differentiating into macrophages. These macrophages take up oxidized LDL to form foam cells. When they die, release of the cellular contents of these cells forms extracellular lipid pools.
4. Adhesion of platelets to the endothelium.
5. Release of cytokines and growth factors (e.g. platelet-derived growth factor) by platelets and activated macrophages results in the migration of smooth muscle cells from the media to the intima (myointimal cells). These muscle cells change from a contractile to repair phenotype, producing collagens in an attempt to stabilize the growing lesion.

The above scheme outlines the formation of a stable atherosclerotic plaque (see Fig. 6.10, parts A–C). Such a plaque can remain asymptomatic for many years, slowly growing to the point where it may significantly obstruct blood flow.

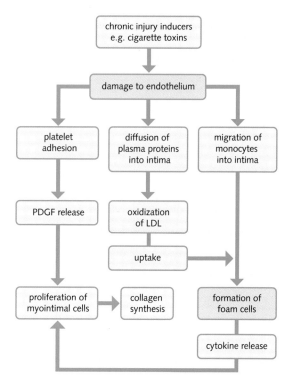

**Fig. 6.11** Summary of events involved in pathogenesis of atherosclerosis.

The maintenance of a stable atherosclerotic plaque depends on the balance between inflammation (macrophage mediated) and repair (smooth muscle mediated). If activated macrophages start producing additional cytokines (e.g. interleukin-1, matrix metalloproteinases), the muscle cells forming the protective fibrous cap may become senescent, resulting in an unstable plaque. Thinning of the cap follows, with potential for erosion, rupture (releasing prothrombotic material) or ulceration (see Fig. 6.8, part D).

Figure 6.11 provides a summary of the events involved in the pathogenesis of atherosclerosis.

**Fig. 6.10** Atheroma formation. (A) Endothelial injury: allows entry of cholesterol-rich, low-density lipoproteins (LDLs) into the intima. (B) 'Fatty streaks': barely visible pale bulges form as a result of phagocytosis and accumulation of lipid by intimal macrophages. (C) Stable plaques: raised, yellow lesions within the intima consisting of free lipid released by macrophages and collagen deposited by myointimal cells (repair phenotype). (D) Unstable plaque with ulceration: allowing platelet aggregation and thrombosis with the potential for embolism to a distant site. Note that pressure atrophy of the underlying media and elastic lamina results in weakening of the arterial wall.

### Arterial remodelling

The migration of smooth muscle cells away from the arterial media produces the complex effect of remodelling. Two types have been proposed:

1. Negative remodelling—some arterial segments affected by atherosclerosis constrict, increasing the likelihood of occluding the lumen.
2. Positive remodelling—affected arterial segments dilate, potentially compensating for the plaque and maintaining the size of the lumen.

Thinning of the muscular arterial media predisposes an artery to aneurysm.

# Hypertension

Elevated blood pressure is an important and treatable cause of cardiac failure. It is a major risk factor for atherosclerosis and cerebral haemorrhage. Any increase in blood pressure is associated with an increased risk of disease.

## Functional or operational definition

Hypertension is increasingly being defined by the level at which intervention (e.g. antihypertensive medication) is of proven benefit. Sustained systemic blood pressure above 140 mmHg systolic and/or above 85 mmHg diastolic should be treated to reduce cardiovascular events such as strokes. Target levels for those with diabetes and renal disease are lower.

## Aetiological classification

Hypertension can be classified into two main types according to its aetiology (Fig. 6.12):

1. Primary (essential or idiopathic) hypertension—a complex, multifactorial disease in which blood pressure is elevated with age, but with no apparent cause. This accounts for 90% of all cases and probably has a strong genetic determinant.
2. Secondary hypertension—elevated blood pressure due to an identifiable cause. It accounts for 10% of hypertension. Examples include renal hypertension, endocrine causes and coarctation of the aorta.

## Pathological classification

Hypertension can also be classified according to the clinical course of disease:

- Benign hypertension—stable elevation of blood pressure over many years
- Malignant (accelerated) hypertension—a rare condition characterized by a dramatic elevation of blood pressure over a short period of time.

### Benign hypertension
Here, vessel changes develop gradually in response to a persistent elevated blood pressure; males are affected more than females. Histologically, it is characterized by:

- hypertrophy and thickening of muscular media
- thickening of elastic lamina

**Fig. 6.12** Causes of hypertension

| Primary hypertension: unknown aetiology but probably multifactorial involving : | |
| --- | --- |
| Genetic predisposition | Strong familial association |
| Socioeconomic factors | Related to social deprivation |
| Dietary factors | Obesity, high salt intake, high alcohol, caffeine intake |
| Hormonal factors | Abnormalities in renin–angiotensin–aldosterone system |
| Neurological factors | Excessive sympathetic nervous system activity |
| **Secondary hypertension: secondary to :** | |
| Renal disease | Parenchymal disease, e.g. chronic pyelonephritis, glomerulonephritis, polycystic kidneys, amyloidosis<br>Vascular disease, e.g. stenosis of renal artery |
| Adrenal disorders | Pheochromocytoma, Cushing's syndrome, Conn's syndrome (primary hyperaldosteronism), congenital adrenal hyperplasia |
| Other endocrine disorders | Thyrotoxicosis, hypothyroidism, acromegaly, hyperparathyroidism, diabetes with renal involvement |
| Cardiovascular disorders | Coarctation of the aorta, arteriovenous fistulae and shunts |
| Drugs | e.g. Oral contraceptives, anabolic steroids, corticosteroids, epinephrine (adrenaline) and related sympathomimetic drugs |
| Pregnancy | ±Pre-eclampsia |

- fibroelastic thickening of intima
- hyaline deposition in arteriole walls (hyaline arteriolosclerosis).

The effects are:

- reduced size of vessel lumen leads to tissue ischaemia
- increased rigidity leads to limited capacity for expansion and constriction
- increased fragility of vessels leads to an increased risk of haemorrhage (especially cerebral).

After many years of benign progression, 5% of such patients enter an accelerated malignant phase.

### Malignant hypertension

Acute, destructive changes occur in the walls of small arteries when blood pressure rises suddenly and markedly. This results in necrosis of the vessel wall and infiltration of the necrotic media by fibrin (i.e. fibrinoid necrosis of vessels).

The destructive changes result in a cessation of blood flow through small vessels with multiple foci of tissue necrosis, often with intravascular thrombosis. Areas typically affected include the retina (high-grade retinopathy) and the kidneys (glomerular disease).

Figure 6.13 lists the features of malignant and benign hypertension.

## Complications and effects of hypertension

### Vascular effects

Hypertension accelerates atherosclerosis, which causes thickening of the media of muscular arteries, particularly the smaller arteries and arterioles. Structural changes perpetuate further rises in blood pressure, causing a progressively worsening clinical picture.

The normal flow of protein into the vessel wall is increased resulting in intramural protein deposition termed hyaline in benign hypertension, and fibrinoid in malignant hypertension:

- Hyaline deposition—a common feature of ageing small arteries ($<1$ mm diameter); refers to the homogeneous appearance of vessel walls due to infiltration by plasma proteins
- Fibrinoid deposition—a combination of fibrin infiltration with necrosis of the vessel wall.

### Heart

The left ventricle undergoes hypertrophy resulting from the increased workload, causing increased susceptibility to spontaneous arrhythmias. Ischaemic heart disease due to accelerated atherosclerosis is a common complication of hypertension.

### Brain

Intracerebral haemorrhage is a frequent cause of death in hypertension. Small-vessel damage within the cerebral hemispheres results in the development

**Fig. 6.13** Features of benign and malignant hypertension

|  | Benign | Malignant |
|---|---|---|
| Incidence | Very common (at least 5% of UK population) | Rare |
| Age | Begins at < 45 years but prolonged into 6th and 7th decades | Young adults (25–35 years) |
| Sex | Females > males | Females = males |
| Aetiology | Majority of cases due to primary hypertension | Majority of cases secondary to renal disease (few cases arise out of benign essential hypertension) |
| Disease progression | Very slow (many years) | Rapid (months to 1–2 years) |
| Blood pressure | Very slow rise Diastolic = 90–120 mmHg | Rapid rise Diastolic $\geq$ 120 mmHg |
| Arterial changes | Potentiates atheroma → accelerated arteriosclerosis | Intimal fibrous thickening → accelerated arteriosclerosis |
| Arteriole changes | Hyaline thickening with narrowed lumen | Fibrinoid necrosis of vessel wall Lumen occluded by thrombus Affects mainly kidney and abdominal viscera |

of micro-infarcts, which form hypertensive lacunae, i.e. small areas of destroyed brain filled with fluid.

### Kidneys

Arteriolosclerosis leads to progressive ischaemia of the nephrons and chronic renal failure. This is termed benign hypertensive nephrosclerosis, and it is a common cause of chronic renal failure in the middle-aged and elderly population.

### Retina

Hypertension may produce retinal ischaemia and infarction, visible on fundoscopic examination.

Figure 6.14 outlines the complications and effects of hypertension.

## Pulmonary hypertension

### Definition and causes

This is defined as pulmonary arterial pressure in excess of 30 mmHg. Figure 6.15 lists the causes of pulmonary hypertension.

### Effects of pulmonary hypertension

With acute onset, there is a massive transudation of fluid from the pulmonary capillaries into the alveoli (pulmonary oedema), leading to shortness of breath and expectoration of bloodstained, watery fluid. Chronic onset has three effects:

1. Hyperplastic arteriosclerosis—muscular hypertrophy, intimal fibrosis and dilatation of the pulmonary arteries
2. Necrotizing arteriolitis—increased pressure within the pulmonary arteries causes weakening of the vessel wall with repeated episodes of haemorrhage into the alveolar spaces, which contain haemosiderin-laden macrophages
3. Cor pulmonale—right ventricular hypertrophy and dysfunction as a result of increased workload.

## Effects of diabetes mellitus on the vessels

Individuals with diabetes suffer from an increased severity of atherosclerosis and capillary microangiopathy in which thickening of the small-vessel walls is attributed to hyaline arteriolosclerosis and marked expansion of the basement membrane.

Vessel damage is complex and is probably due to the increased plasma levels of cholesterol and triglycerides. Biochemically there is abnormal glycosylation of protein within the vessel wall. Clinical sequelae of diabetic vessel damage are described in detail in Chapter 10; they include diabetic retinopathy, diabetic nephropathy and peripheral neuropathy.

**Fig. 6.14** Complications and effects of hypertension

|  | Benign | Malignant |
|---|---|---|
| Vessels | Hyaline deposition due to infiltration by plasma proteins | Fibrinoid deposition due to combination of fibrin deposition and necrosis of vessel wall |
| Heart | Hypertrophy of left ventricle → ↑susceptibility to spontaneous arrhythmias Heart failure in 60% of cases Ischaemic heart disease | Hypertrophy of left ventricle → ↑susceptibility to spontaneous arrhythmias Focal myocardial necrosis Acute heart failure Ischaemic heart disease |
| Brain | Cerebral haemorrhage | Encephalopathy (fits and loss of consciousness) due to cerebral oedema Cerebral haemorrhage |
| Kidney | Nephrosclerosis, but not usually serious | Severe renal damage; death in uraemia |
| Retina | Ischaemia and infarction ('cotton wool' exudates) Association with central retinal vein thrombosis | Ischaemia and infarction ('cotton wool' exudates) Association with central retinal vein thrombosis |
| Other organs | No significant damage | Focal necrosis, e.g. perforation of gut |

| **Fig. 6.15** Causes of pulmonary hypertension | |
| --- | --- |
| **Mechanism** | |
| **Precapillary causes** | |
| Increased pulmonary blood flow | Left-to-right shunts, e.g. atrial septal defects, ventricular septal defects |
| **Capillary causes** | |
| Destruction of lung capillary bed | Emphysema<br>Interstitial fibrosis of lungs |
| Mechanical arterial occlusion | Recurrent pulmonary emboli |
| Alveolar hypoxia causing pulmonary vasoconstriction | High altitude<br>Obesity<br>Chronic obstructive airways disease |
| **Postcapillary causes** | |
| Pulmonary venous congestion | Mitral valve disease, e.g. stenosis<br>Chronic left ventricular failure |
| **Idiopathic causes** | |
| Primary pulmonary hypertension | Rare disease of young women due to increased tone in pulmonary vessels → progressive vascular changes and death |

## Thrombosis

Thrombosis is the formation of a solid mass of blood constituents—thrombus—within the vascular system. It is not to be confused with a clot, which occurs in non-flowing blood.

Thrombosis can affect both arteries and veins.

**HINTS AND TIPS**

A thrombus is different from a clot! A clot is defined as blood coagulated outside the vascular system or within the vascular system after death.

### Arterial thrombosis

This is most commonly superimposed on an atheroma. As the plaque enlarges, it causes turbulent blood flow, which results in the loss of intimal cells. The exposure of vessel collagen predisposes to platelet activation. Turbulence itself will predispose to fibrin deposition and platelet clumping.

The greatest degree of turbulence occurs at the downstream side of the forming thrombus; thrombi, therefore, grow in the direction of the blood flow (propagation). An arterial thrombosis may result in tissue infarction and ischaemia either directly or through embolization.

### Venous thrombosis

Many venous thrombi begin at damaged valves that produce turbulence. Furthermore, blood stasis during surgery or due to immobilization may result in the formation of a deep vein thrombosis (risking pulmonary embolism). However, some thrombi form at sites with no known predisposing factors. Often thrombi grow by successive deposition of alternating bands of platelets and red blood cells. These patterns are known as the lines of Zahn.

A thrombosed vein may cause an inflammatory response (thrombophlebitis) or a vein that is inflamed may thrombose (phlebothrombosis). A histological differentiation between the two types is in most cases impossible.

#### Affected sites
The most commonly affected sites are:

- deep leg veins (90% of cases), particularly the lower leg
- skull and dural sinuses
- portal venous tributaries
- pelvic veins.

## Outcomes

Outcomes of venous thrombosis include:

- lysis—dissolution of the thrombus by activated fibrinolytic system
- propagation—spread of the thrombus proximally in the veins
- organization—reparative process with ingrowth of fibroblasts
- recanalization—usually incomplete re-establishment of blood flow
- embolism—thrombus migrates to a distant site.

## Complications

The most serious acute complication is embolism of the thrombus to the pulmonary arteries, causing a pulmonary embolism (PE). These are divided into massive, major and minor events and are discussed in detail on page 109.

Chronic complications are aching pains due to varicose veins, venous congestion, oedema, venous eczema and ulceration.

### Clinical Note

Deep vein thrombosis (DVT) is a key clinical topic, as a resulting pulmonary embolus may be life-threatening. High-risk patients should be identified and offered prophylaxis. DVTs typically present as a painful unilaterally swollen calf, which is warm to the touch. Diagnosis is aided by radiographic venograms and non-invasive ultrasound (large veins only). Immediate treatment involves heparin and prolonged warfarin, the latter being used continuously in those with repeated DVTs.

## Virchow's triad

Factors that predispose any blood vessel to thrombosis can be classified into three main groups, collectively known as Virchow's triad (Fig. 6.16):

- Changes in the blood constituents—forming a hypercoaguable state
- Changes in the blood vessel endothelium—usually at the point of injury
- Changes in the pattern of blood flow—stasis or turbulence.

## Hypercoagulability

### Primary (hereditary)

Hereditary defects of hypercoagulability lead to a life-long tendency to thrombosis (thrombophilia). They usually affect the venous system:

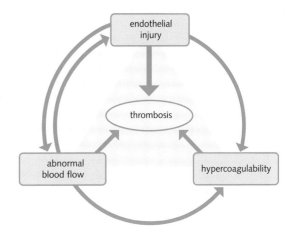

**Fig. 6.16** Virchow's triad in thrombosis. Endothelial integrity is the single most important factor: injury can affect local blood flow and/or coagulability. Abnormal blood flow (turbulence or stasis) can, in turn, cause endothelial injury. The elements of the triad may act independently or combine to cause thrombus formation. (Redrawn with permission from Robbins and Cotran, Pathologic Basis of Disease, 7th edition, V Kumar, A Abbas, and N Fausto, Elsevier Saunders, 2005).

- Antithrombin III deficiency—autosomal dominant condition characterized by recurrent venous thromboses usually starting in early adult life. Primary defect is a deficiency of antithrombin III, which usually neutralizes thrombin and other activated clotting factors.
- Protein C deficiency—autosomal dominant condition resulting in failure of neutralization of activated factors V and VIII. Protein S is a cofactor for protein C. Therefore, protein S deficiencies produce a similar pathology.
- Factor V Leiden—point mutation in the factor V gene, which results in factor V protein that is resistant to neutralization by protein C. This is very common, affecting up to 5% of Caucasians.
- Prothrombin G20210A—this prothrombin gene polymorphism occurs in 2% of the population and is associated with increased levels of prothrombin and venous thromboembolism.

### Secondary (acquired)

Defects are as follows:

- Malignancy—patients with carcinoma of the breast, lung, prostate, pancreas or bowel have an increased risk of venous thrombosis.
- Blood disorders, e.g. increased viscosity (especially polycythaemia rubra vera) and thrombocytosis lead to an increased risk of venous thrombosis.
- Oestrogens—associated with raised plasma levels of various clotting factors leading to an increased risk of venous thrombosis.

- Antiphospholipid antibody syndrome—leads to the interaction of antibodies (lupus anticoagulant and anticardiolipin antibodies) with phospholipid-bound proteins involved in coagulation. This causes prolongation of clotting times in vitro, with a paradoxical increased risk of venous and arterial thrombosis. Often found in patients with autoimmune disease, especially systemic lupus erythematosus (SLE).
- Cholesterol—partly genetic, partly acquired (diet/lifestyle), leads to an increased risk of arterial thrombosis.
- Smoking—has been implicated as a predisposing risk factor for thrombosis, possibly by causing a hypercoagulable state.

### Endothelial injury

Direct injury to the endothelium as seen in trauma (including intravenous cannulation) and inflammation may lead to thrombosis. Damage to the endothelium also occurs in association with atheroma.

### Alterations to blood flow

Alterations are:

- stasis—allows platelets to come in contact with endothelium. Slow flow prevents blood from diluting activated coagulation components, e.g. prolonged immobilization.
- turbulence—may cause physical trauma to endothelial cells. Loss of laminar flow may bring platelets into contact with endothelium.

## ISCHAEMIC HEART DISEASE AND HEART FAILURE

Ischaemic heart disease (IHD) is a condition caused by a reduction or cessation of the blood supply to the myocardium (myocardial ischaemia). This is usually as a result of atherosclerosis, although in rare cases it may be caused by coronary embolism, arteritis or ostial obstruction. The left ventricle is more prone to ischaemia because of its greater bulk and work requirement, and its higher oxygen demand.

IHD is the most common type of cardiac disease and a leading cause of death in the Western world, accounting for about one-third of all male deaths and one-quarter of all female deaths. Risk factors for the development of ischaemic heart disease are the same as those for the development of atherosclerosis.

## Classification

IHD results in four main syndromes:

1. Stable angina (chronic manifestation) or unstable angina (acute manifestation)

2. Myocardial infarction (acute manifestation)
3. Sudden cardiac death (acute manifestation)
4. Congestive cardiac failure (chronic manifestation).

The acute manifestations of cardiac ischaemia form the continuous spectrum of disease termed the acute coronary syndromes (ACS).

## Angina pectoris

Angina pectoris is episodic chest pain caused by ischaemia of the myocardium following exercise. Ischaemia is usually the result of stenosis of one or more of the coronary arteries resulting in reduced blood flow to the myocardium.

Stenosis of the coronary arteries is typically the result of atherosclerosis. Atheromatous plaques may lie in two possible positions:

1. Eccentric—fibrolipid plaques affecting only one side of the wall of a coronary artery. Improvement of flow at the site of such plaques may be achieved by the use of vasodilator drugs. These drugs, such as glyceryl trinitrate, produce relaxation of the unaffected part of the vessel wall.
2. Concentric—collagenous plaques affecting the whole of the arterial wall circumference. As the whole wall is abnormal, drug therapy cannot improve flow over a narrowed segment.

## Cardiac referred pain

Pain of angina (and myocardial infarction) commonly radiates from the substernal and left pectoral regions to the left shoulder and the medial aspect of the left arm; this is known as cardiac referred pain.

Afferent fibres of the heart, and sensory fibres of affected cutaneous zones, enter the same spinal cord segments (T1 to T4/T5 on the left side) and ascend in the CNS along a common pathway. The brain is unable to discern the origin of the pain, hence the phenomenon of cardiac referred pain.

Less commonly, pain radiates to the right shoulder and arm, with or without concomitant pain on the left side.

## Types of angina

### Stable angina

This is a predictable angina that occurs at a fixed level of exercise, as a result of an increased demand in myocardial work, usually in the presence of impaired perfusion by blood. It is caused by a fixed obstruction of one or more of the coronary arteries, therefore limiting any increase in coronary blood flow. Pain can usually be relieved by 1 or 2 minutes of rest. A stenosis of at least 75% of the lumen of the arteries is required to produce angina on exercise.

## Unstable angina

Unstable anginal pain is unpredictable and not related to exercise. It reflects reversible ischaemia due to variable luminal stenosis of some segments of the coronary arteries: so-called dynamic obstruction.

The condition is usually the result of active fissuring and/or rupture of plaques with intimal surface thrombus deposition, microembolization and occlusion. Unstable angina is an acute event, often preceding the development of acute myocardial infarction.

### Prinzmetal's angina (vasospastic angina)

This is angina at rest caused by an increase in the coronary vasomotor tone. The mechanism for coronary spasm is unknown. Prinzmetal's angina is particularly common in the early morning. Attacks are usually self-limiting and, although pain may be severe, they rarely lead on to myocardial infarction.

---

**HINTS AND TIPS**

- Stable angina is predictable (i.e. it occurs at a fixed level of exercise), and it is caused by a fixed arterial obstruction.
- Unstable angina is unpredictable (i.e. it is unrelated to exercise), and it is caused by a variable luminal stenosis of the coronary arteries.
- Prinzmetal's angina is also unpredictable, and this is caused by coronary artery spasm.

---

## Management of angina

Stable angina can be managed as follows:

- Modification of risk factors for atherosclerosis.
- Combination drug therapy with low-dose aspirin and—potentially—nitrates, β-blockers and $Ca^{2+}$ channel blockers.
- Invasive—percutaneous coronary intervention (PCI), using balloon angioplasty to dilate a coronary artery stenosis. If the stenosis is highly progressive or disease is very severe (e.g. involving all three key coronary arteries), coronary artery bypass grafting (CABG) may be indicated.

Patients with unstable angina should be admitted to hospital for ECG analysis and potential thrombolyis or invasive correction of their occlusion. Such active management reduces progression to infarction. Unstable anginas are included in the NSTEMI category of acute coronary syndrome.

## Myocardial infarction

Myocardial infarction (MI) is necrosis of the myocardium as a result of severe ischaemia. MI is extremely common, accounting for 10–15% of all deaths and about 60% of sudden unexpected deaths. It typically affects middle-aged individuals, between 50 and 60 years, but 10% occur in 35- to 50-year-olds. MI affects males more than premenopausal women (by 5:1), but there is an increasing incidence in women postmenopausally.

Clinical features are chest pain accompanied by breathlessness, vomiting and collapse or syncope. Pain occurs in the same sites as angina, but it is usually more severe and lasts for longer.

## Regional infarcts

Infarcts occurs in the territory supplied by one major common artery, involving only one segment of the ventricular wall. The cause of infarction is nearly always thrombus formation on a ruptured or eroded unstable atheromatous plaque. Patterns of regional MI and sites of MI are shown in Figures 6.17 and 6.18

## ST-segment elevation MI (STEMI) and non-STEMI (NSTEMI)

An acute MI should be classified as STEMI when there is:

- ST elevation (2 mm in two or more chest leads, or 1 mm in two or more limb leads)
- chronic MI with Q wave formation
- imaging evidence of a full thickness scar.

Other MIs that do not meet these criteria should be classified as NSTEMI. The main difference between the two classification are their emergency mangement protocols.

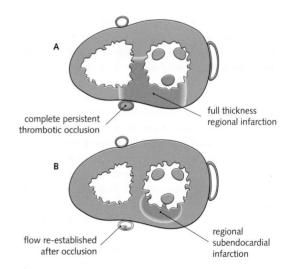

**Fig. 6.17** Patterns of regional myocardial infarction (MI). (A) Transmural or full thickness infarct. (B) Regional subendocardial infarct.

complete persistent thrombotic occlusion

full thickness regional infarction

flow re-established after occlusion

regional subendocardial infarction

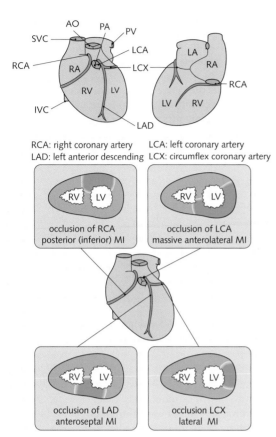

RCA: right coronary artery   LCA: left coronary artery
LAD: left anterior descending   LCX: circumflex coronary artery

occlusion of RCA
posterior (inferior) MI

occlusion of LCA
massive anterolateral MI

occlusion of LAD
anteroseptal MI

occlusion LCX
lateral  MI

**Fig. 6.18**   Sites of myocardial infarction (MI) and vessel involvement.

**Fig. 6.19  Morphological changes occurring post myocardial Infarction (MI)**

| time | macroscopic appearance | microscopic appearance |
|---|---|---|
| 0–12 hours | not visible | infarcted muscle appears uncolored on staining with nitroblue tetrazolium due to loss of oxidative enzymes; non-infarcted muscle stains blue |
| 12–24 hours | pale with blotchy discoloration | infarcted muscle is brightly eosinophilic with intercellular oedema |
| 24–72 hours | dead area appears soft and pale with a slight yellow colour | infarcted area excites an acute inflammatory response neutrophils infiltrate between dead cardiac muscle fibres |
| 3–10 days | hyperaemic border develops around the yellow dead muscle | organization of infarcted area replacement with vascular granulation tissue |
| weeks to months | white scar | progressive collagen deposition infarct is replaced by a collagenous scar |

## Histological changes following myocardial infarction

MI comprises necrosis and acute inflammation. The necrotic tissue is gradually replaced by a collagenous scar. The entire process from coagulative necrosis to scar formation takes 6–8 weeks, the macroscopic and microscopic appearances of the infarct changing with time (Fig. 6.19). The extensive necrosis of cardiac muscle is associated with the release of cardiac enzymes and proteins that can be used as clinical markers for a MI event. Examples include troponin T creatinine kinase (CK-MB cardiac isoform) and lactate dehydrogenase.

## Sequelae of myocardial infarction

The effects and sequelae of MI are variable, and they can be classified into:

- immediate effects—sudden cardiac death (described below)
- short-term complications—occurring in the first 2 weeks post MI
- long-term complications.

### Short-term complications

There are six short-term complications:

1. Arrhythmias—due to the involvement of conduction tissue, leading to ventricular fibrillation, atrial fibrillation, heart block and sinus bradycardia. Nearly all MI patients have some form of arrhythmia, usually resolving spontaneously.
2. Left ventricular failure—this is common with large areas of infarction; the necrotic wall softens in organization leading to cardiac dilatation. Ventricular remodelling is the process of thinning and stretching of the infarcted segment, with progressive dilatation and hypertrophy of the remaining ventricle.

3. Rupture, which can be:
   I. external (majority)—blood bursts through the external wall into the pericardial cavity (haemopericardium); the sudden rise in intrapericardial cavity pressure prevents cardiac filling (cardiac tamponade), leading to rapid death
   II. internal (rarely)—intracardiac rupture through the septum leads to an acquired septal defect, causing a left-to-right shunt and the development of left ventricular failure.
4. Papillary muscle dysfunction—when one or more valve leaflets are unable to close during systole there is mitral valve incompetence.
5. Mural thrombosis—on the inflamed endocardium over the area of infarction; there is a high risk of embolization producing infarction of various organs, e.g. cerebral, renal, splenic, mesenteric and lower limbs.
6. Acute pericarditis—caused by inflammation over the infarct surface.

### Long-term complications
There are four long-term complications:

1. Chronic intractable left-heart failure—the long-term effects of ventricular remodelling result in inadequate left ventricular pumping action; common when the infarct is extensive and full thickness.
2. Ventricular aneurysm (in 10% of long-term survivors)—gradual distension of the weakened fibrotic part of the left ventricular wall with thrombus formation, embolism or severe functional deficit.
3. Recurrent MI—risk of developing a further episode due to underlying coronary artery insufficiency.
4. Dressler's syndrome—a form of autoimmune-mediated pericarditis associated with a high erythrocyte sedimentation ratio (ESR) and persistent fever; develops in a very small number of cases after infarction.

#### Clinical Note
After diagnosis of STEMI management involves:
• oxygen and analgesia (morphine)
• aspirin (300 mg), nitrates and β-blockers
• early thrombolytic therapy, e.g. streptokinase
• percutaneous coronary intervention—primary angioplasty likely to become first-line treatment where resources permit
• anticoagulation to prevent reinfarction and reduce thromboembolic risk (e.g. heparin)
• bed rest for the first 24–48 hours on the coronary care unit.
   Long-term therapy—daily low-dose aspirin, β-blockers, angiotensin-converting enzyme (ACE) inhibitors and statins.

## Sudden cardiac death
Sudden cardiac death is the most important immediate consequence of myocardial ischaemia. It is usually due to ventricular fibrillation. This may be the result of:

• previous ischaemic heart disease, e.g. angina or previous infarction; cardiac arrhythmias can arise from muscle adjacent to an area of old scarring
• acute myocardial ischaemia, which, due to a new thrombotic event, may precipitate arrhythmia.

   Other causes of sudden death include ruptured or dissecting aneurysms of the aorta and pulmonary emboli.

## Heart failure
Heart failure can result from many different types of heart disease. It develops when the heart is no longer able to maintain an adequate cardiac output, or can only do so by increasing the filling pressure. The prognosis of heart failure is worse than many cancers; half of those with severe left-ventricular impairment die within 2 years.
   Heart failure may develop acutely (e.g. following myocardial infarction) or chronically (e.g. gradually progressing ischaemic heart disease).

## Classification
### Left-sided heart failure
This occurs due to either reduced output from the left ventricle or increased input pressure from the left atrium. Common causes include:

• ischaemic heart disease—including the effects of ventricular remodelling after infarction
• hypertension—pressure overload produces initial ventricular hypertrophy, but this compensatory change cannot be maintained indefinitely and the ventricle eventually dilates
• valve disease—either aortic or mitral.

   Eventually, the increased pressure in the left atrium works back through the vasculature resulting in pulmonary hypertension. Pulmonary oedema (also termed pulmonary congestion) and eventual right-sided heart failure may follow, resulting in symnptoms of dyspnoea (breathlessness), orthopnoea (breathlessness on lying flat) and paroxysmal nocturnal dyspnoea (attacks of extreme breathlessness, usually at night).

### Right-sided heart failure
The most common cause is progression of left-sided failure, so-called biventricular heart failure. In these cases, the right ventricle has to pump against increased resistance in the pulmonary circulation.

Isolated right heart failure may rarely develop due to:

- chronic lung disease (cor pulmonale)
- pulmonary emboli (usually multiple)
- pulmonary valve stenosis.

This many result in clinical symptoms of peripheral oedema, congestive hepatomegaly, and congestive splenomegaly.

## DISORDERS OF THE HEART VALVES

## Concepts of heart valve disease

### Types of valve disorder

Valve disorders can be:

- stenosis—narrowing or abnormal rigidity of a valve
- regurgitation (or incompetence)—failure of a valve to close fully.

Both types may coexist in one valve but one type is usually dominant.

Factors that may cause heart valve damage:

- congenital abnormality
- postinflammatory scarring, e.g. after rheumatic heart disease
- degeneration with ageing
- dilatation of the valve ring, e.g. in dilated cardiomyopathy
- degeneration of collagenous support tissue of the valve
- acute destruction by necrotizing inflammation.

### Commonly affected valves

The mitral and aortic valves are the most frequently affected; the tricuspid and pulmonary valves only infrequently.

Figure 6.20 outlines the major causes and basic features of acquired valve disease.

### Abnormalities of flow and their effects

Diseased valves often cause regurgitant jets of blood, with concomitant development of endocardial lesions opposite the jet's origin. These lesions (jet lesions) are typically seen on the septum opposite the aortic valve.

## Degenerative valve disease

### Calcific aortic stenosis

There are two types:

1. Degenerative calcific aortic valve stenosis—calcification of the aortic valve associated with increasing age; typically affects the elderly

2. Bicuspid calcific aortic valve stenosis—calcification of the congenital bicuspid aortic valve (present in 1% of people); quite common, usually manifesting by 40–50 years of age.

In both types, the valves become thick and fibrotic with a fusion of the commissures. Large nodular masses of calcium may be found subendothelially within the sinuses of Valsalva, so restricting the opening of the aortic cusps.

### Effects

There are two effects:

1. Aortic stenosis—thickening and fusion of valves → decreased valve lumen → reduced systolic flow
2. Aortic regurgitation—increased rigidity of valves → failure to close properly → backflow into the left ventricle during diastole.

Stenosis and regurgitation result in left ventricular hypertrophy, coronary insufficiency (often angina), and syncope or sudden death due to acute left-sided heart failure.

### Mitral annular calcification

This is 'wear and tear' of the mitral valve with calcification of the valve leaflets. Massive calcification can immobilize the valve and predispose to the development of either thrombosis or bacterial endocarditis.

### Mitral valve prolapse ('floppy valve syndrome')

The changes here are due to myxomatous degeneration. The leaflets are thickened and redundant, containing large amounts of mucopolysaccharides and abnormal collagen. It most commonly involves the posterior mitral leaflet, which is soft and bulges upwards into the atrium during systole. The net result is mild valvular incompetence and an increased risk of rupture of one of the chordae, which may lead to sudden, severe valvular incompetence.

Mitral valve prolapse can also be a feature of connective tissue disorders such as Marfan's syndrome.

## Rheumatic heart disease

Rheumatic fever is an immune disorder that follows 2–3 weeks after a streptococcal infection, usually tonsillitis or pharyngitis.

### Epidemiology

This disease occurs mainly in children aged 5–15 years. It was once prevalent in Europe, including the UK, and in the USA. Its incidence has now decreased in the

**Fig. 6.20** Major causes and basic features of acquired valve disease

| Valve lesion | Causes | Effects | Physical findings |
|---|---|---|---|
| Mitral stenosis | Rheumatic | Left-sided cardiac failure with predisposition to atrial thrombosis Left atrial hypertrophy and dilation leads to: <br>• pulmonary vascular congestion <br>• pulmonary hypertension <br>• right ventricular hypertrophy <br>• 'nutmeg liver' and congested kidneys | Loud $S_1$ Opening snap Diastolic rumble |
| Mitral regurgitation | Acute: <br>• papillary muscle dysfunction <br>• cusp damage by endocarditis <br>Chronic: <br>• postinflammatory scarring, commonly rheumatic <br>• left ventricular dilation <br>• floppy mitral valve syndrome (prolapse) | Acute: <br>• pulmonary oedema <br>Chronic: <br>• left ventricular hypertrophy and dilation <br>• giant left atrium <br>• progressive left-sided cardiac failure develops with time | Pansystolic murmur Widely split $S_2$ |
| Aortic stenosis | Calcification of congenital bicuspid aortic valve Rheumatic Senile calcific degeneration | Early: <br>• asymptomatic but with slowly <br>• progressive left ventricular hypertrophy <br>Late: <br>• left ventricular failure <br>• low cardiac output → breathlessness <br>• coronary artery insufficiency → angina <br>• cerebrovascular insufficiency → syncope sudden death | Systolic ejection murmur reaching peak intensity in mid- or late systole Narrow pulse pressure Slow-rising carotid pulse |
| Aortic regurgitation | Rheumatic Endocarditis Senile calcification Aortic root dilation | Left ventricular hypertrophy Progressive left ventricular failure | Diastolic murmur Wide pulse pressure Collapsing pulse |

developed world and it is now most frequently seen in parts of central Africa, the Middle East and India.

## Pathogenesis

Susceptible individuals develop antibodies to antigens produced by specific strains of group A streptococci; these antibodies then cross-react with host antigens. The disease is a systemic disorder affecting:

• heart—pericarditis, myocarditis and endocarditis (collectively known as pancarditis)
• joints—polyarthritis
• skin—subcutaneous nodules and erythema marginatum
• arteries—arteritis.

The most important target organ is the heart. Repeated attacks of rheumatic fever lead to progressive fibrosis of the endocardium and valves, which is the main cause of chronic scarring of the valves.

### Aschoff's nodules

These pathognomonic heart lesions consist of multinucleate giant cells surrounded by activated macrophages and lymphoid cells (predominantly T cells). Lesions stimulate fibroblast proliferation and lead to scarring.

## Acute rheumatic heart disease

In the acute phase, rheumatic fever causes a pancarditis, the components of which are:

• rheumatic pericarditis—acute inflammation of the pericardium

- rheumatic myocarditis—mild inflammation with occasional muscle fibre necrosis
- rheumatic endocarditis—mitral valves are most prone to the development of severe lesions.

## Chronic rheumatic heart disease

The main morbidity of rheumatic fever is the long-term effects of the immune damage causing chronic scarring of valves, particularly the mitral valve. Chronic valvular heart disease develops in about 50% of those affected by rheumatic fever with carditis. Lesions may develop after 10–20 years in Western countries, but much earlier in developing countries.

### Pathogenesis

Endocardial valvular damage from the acute phase heals by progressive fibrosis. Valve leaflets and chordae tendineae become thickened, fibrotic and shrunken, often with fusion to their partners; there is frequent secondary deposition of calcium.

Once damage has developed, the altered haemodynamic stresses extend the damage even in the absence of continued autoimmune processes.

## Infective endocarditis

This is an acute or subacute disease resulting from infection of a focal area of the endocardium, which usually has pre-existing damage. It can affect almost any age group, but it is increasing in incidence in the elderly population. Predisposing factors in susceptible individuals include genitourinary infection, diabetes, tooth extraction, pressure ulcers and surgical procedures. It is more common in males than females (3:1).

## Morphological features

The characteristic lesions of endocarditis are termed vegetations. These are formed from deposits of platelets, fibrin and bacteria. The mechanism of formation is outlined in Figure 6.21. Vegetations may form in areas of high-pressure gradients, for example at an incompetent valve.

Almost all vegetation occurs on valve leaflets or chordae tendinae. The size varies from a small nodule to a large mass that may occlude the valve orifice. The mitral and aortic valves are the most commonly affected.

## Causative organisms

### Bacteria

Pathogens such as *Staphylococcus aureus,* alphahaemolytic streptococci, pneumococci, meningococci and *Escherichia coli* are commonly responsible.

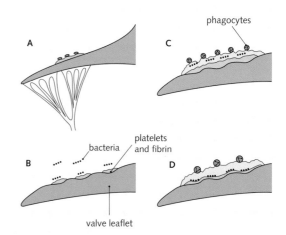

**Fig. 6.21** Pathogenesis of vegetation formation in infective endocarditis. (A) Abnormality on endocardium of valve leaflet is coated with small deposits of platelets and fibrin (thrombus). (B) Circulating bacteria or fungi colonize the platelet thrombus. (C, D) Further layers of platelets and fibrin are deposited, and the microorganisms proliferate in the superficial layer of the vegetation. They are separated from blood by a thin layer of fibrinous material, which protects against immune destruction but allows diffusion of nutrients. (Adapted from Underwood, 2009.)

### Fungi

Fungi such as *Candida* and *Aspergillus* can occasionally cause endocarditis, particularly in drug addicts, the immunosuppressed or those with valve prostheses.

The type of causative organism responsible depends on whether the affected valve is structurally normal or abnormal.

## Infection of structurally normal valves

Infective organisms are pathogenic and directly invade the valve causing rapid destruction. This is commonly seen in intravenous drug addicts (often affecting the tricuspid valve), after open heart surgery and following septicaemia from other causes. Highly virulent forms of *Staphylococcus aureus* are often responsible for such infections.

## Infection of structurally abnormal heart valves

Infective organisms are of low pathogenicity and are derived from normal commensal organisms of the skin, mouth, urinary tract and gut. Following trivial episodes of bacteraemia, organisms become enmeshed in platelet aggregates on the surface of the abnormal endocardium, growing to cause persistent infection. The main underlying abnormalities in this group are:

- congenital bicuspid aortic valves
- postinflammatory scarring

- mitral valve prolapse syndrome
- prosthetic valves.

The incidence has increased in Western countries in recent years, mainly as a result of patients surviving with structurally abnormal hearts and heart valves.

## Types of infective endocarditis

### Acute

The cause is usually a virulent organism, such as *Staphylococcus aureus*. It can affect either normal or abnormal heart valves.

The bacteria proliferate in the valve, causing necrosis and the generation of thrombotic vegetations. Consequently, there is destruction of valve leaflets with perforation and acute disturbance of valve function leading to acute heart failure.

*Prognosis*—disease is rapidly progressive and often fatal due to the incidence of embolic events, renal failure and heart failure.

### Subacute

The typical cause here is when less virulent organisms, such as *Streptococcus viridans* are involved.

The bacteria proliferate slowly in the thrombotic vegetation on damaged valve surfaces. Gradual valve destruction occurs, stimulating further thrombus formation with the potential for systemic embolization.

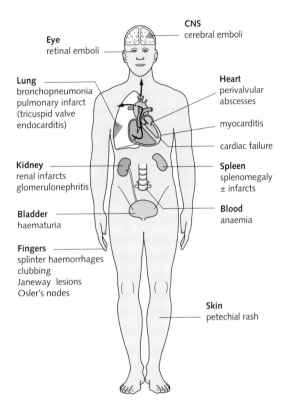

**Fig. 6.22** Complications of infective endocarditis.

> **Clinical Note**
>
> Key clinical features of endocarditis are:
> - systemic symptoms—fever, weight loss and malaise due to cytokines (low-grade infection)
> - skin petechiae and microhaemorrhages in the retina and skin, particularly around the fingernails (splinter haemorrhages), caused by the deposition of immune complexes in small vessels—they also cause glomerulonephritis
> - finger clubbing (cause unknown), occasionally with characteristic Janeway lesions and/or Osler 's nodes
> - splenomegaly and anaemia due to persistent bacteraemia.

### Sequelae

The sequelae are as follows:

- Valvular regurgitation due to gradual destruction of valves leading to cardiac failure.
- Perivalvular abscesses following extension of the infection into the valve ring and myocardium,

producing sinuses, fistulae, septal defects and abnormalities of conduction.
- Mycotic aneurysms—infection of the muscular wall of a medium-sized artery caused by emboli to the vasa vasorum.
- Multi-organ infarction—small emboli of infected thrombotic material enter the systemic circulation producing infarction of many organs especially the brain, spleen and kidneys. Infarcted organs may in turn become infected by organisms within the occluding thrombus.

Complications of infective endocarditis are summarized in Figure 6.22.

## Non-bacterial thrombotic (marantic) endocarditis

Non-bacterial thrombotic endocarditis is inflammation of the valves with the formation of sterile thrombotic vegetations (marantic vegetations) on the closure lines of valve cusps. It occurs in severely debilitated patients with serious systemic disease, particularly malignancy.

# Endocarditis of systemic lupus erythematosus (Libman–Sacks disease)

Thrombotic vegetations complicate SLE in 50% or more of fatal cases. The vegetations are small, meaning that valvular changes rarely give rise to any appreciable functional deficiency, but thrombotic material can fragment and cause embolic infarction.

# Carcinoid heart disease

Carcinoid syndrome is caused by excess 5-hydroxy-tryptamine secretion by a carcinoid tumour (usually of the small intestine, which has metastasized to the liver) and can result in endocardial fibrosis of the tricuspid and pulmonary valves, in turn resulting in stenosis or incompetence.

# Complications of artificial heart valves

## Prosthetic valve diseases

The prosthetic valve diseases are:

- thrombosis leading to valve obstruction or embolism
- valve failure due to breakage of a mechanical prosthesis, or tissue calcification and cusp rupture of bioprosthesis
- infective endocarditis from turbulence and prosthetic material; its incidence is 1–2% per year
- obstructive gradients—the valve may be too small or there may be tissue ingrowth of the pannus onto the valve ring
- haemolysis of red blood cells passing through a mechanical valve, occasionally leading to jaundice.

## Precautions necessary to avoid complications of artificial heart valves

The precautions are lifelong anticoagulation (with warfarin) and appropriate prophylactic antibiotic therapy to protect against infective endocarditis, e.g. before dental procedures.

## DISEASES OF THE MYOCARDIUM

# Concepts of myocardial disease

## Cardiomyopathy

This is a group of disorders in which the structural or functional abnormality primarily affects the myocardium. It should only be considered if all other potential causes of myocardial impairment have been excluded.

## Effects of cardiomyopathy

Cardiomyopathies usually cause progressive development of cardiac failure. The time scale varies from weeks to years depending on the specific pathology. In some instances, sudden cardiac death is the first manifestation of disease.

## Classification

Cardiomyopathies can be grouped into two types according to aetiology:

1. Primary idiopathic cardiomyopathies—unknown aetiology
2. Secondary cardiomyopathies—diseases of the heart muscle associated with/caused by a systemic disease.

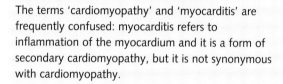

**HINTS AND TIPS**

The terms 'cardiomyopathy' and 'myocarditis' are frequently confused: myocarditis refers to inflammation of the myocardium and it is a form of secondary cardiomyopathy, but it is not synonymous with cardiomyopathy.

# Primary idiopathic cardiomyopathy

Primary cardiomyopathies follow three main patterns according to the dysfunction of the myocardium—dilated, hypertrophic obstructive or restrictive.

## Dilated (congestive) cardiomyopathy

These are abnormalities of the myocardium causing poor systolic contraction. They are characterized by:

- dilatation of the ventricles—usually left more than right
- thin, stretched chamber walls
- hypocontractile muscle.

Aetiology is often unidentifiable but the condition may represent end-stage myocardial damage for known causes, including viral myocarditis, alcohol and other forms of secondary cardiomyopathies.

## Hypertrophic cardiomyopathy

A familial condition (usually autosomal dominant) resulting in systolic function with marked reduction in systolic volume and difficulty in diastolic filling. This is characterized by:

- gross hypertrophy of the heart walls, particularly affecting the interventricular septum
- loss of the normal parallel orientation of hypertrophied muscle fibres—disorganized branching.

The genetic mutations identified tend to affect the production of proteins making up the myocardial muscle unit (sarcomere). This condition may present in young adults and juveniles with sudden unexplained death on exertion (hypertrophic obstructive cardiomyopathy, HOCM). Less dramatic presentations include angina and breathlessness on exertion in a young person or repeated fainting attacks.

## Restrictive cardiomyopathy

Abnormal stiffness of the myocardium results in impaired ventricular filling during diastole. The stiffness is caused by infiltration of the myocardium, for example:

- amyloid in amyloidosis
- fibrosis in endomyocardial fibrosis (fibrosis of thrombotic material deposited on the endocardial surfaces).

The condition causes high atrial pressures resulting in atrial hypertrophy → atrial dilatation → atrial fibrillation.

## Secondary cardiomyopathies

### Myocarditis

This rare disease is characterized by the presence of inflammatory cells in the myocardium. The clinical picture is highly variable, from an asymptomatic disorder with minor ECG changes, to rapidly progressing heart failure.

### Aetiology

The vast majority of cases of myocarditis are either infectious or immune-mediated. The infectious causes are:

- viruses—viral infection is the commonest cause of myocarditis in the UK. Coxsackie virus is the commonest. Other agents include influenza, echovirus, HIV, CMV, poliomyelitis or mumps virus
- bacteria, e.g. *Corynebacterium diphtheriae* (diphtheria), Borrelia (Lyme disease)
- *Chlamydiae* and *Rickettsiae*
- fungi, e.g. Candida
- protozoa, e.g. toxoplasmosis, *Trypanosoma cruzi* (Chagas' disease)
- helminths, e.g. trichinosis.

The immune-mediated causes are:

- post-streptococcal, e.g. acute rheumatic fever
- post-viral
- SLE
- drug hypersensitivity, e.g. sulphonamides, doxorubicin, cyclophosphamide.

Other less common causes include sarcoidosis (see Chapter 7) and giant cell myocarditis, an acute fulminating form of fatal acute myocarditis.

**Fig. 6.23** Aetiology of secondary cardiomyopathies

| Causes | Example |
|---|---|
| Infection and inflammation | Myocarditis |
| Multisystem disease | Diabetes<br>Amyloidosis<br>Thyroid dysfunction<br>Haemochromatosis |
| Toxic and metabolic disturbances | Alcohol<br>Catecholamines<br>Drugs, e.g. adriamycin |
| Primary muscle disorders | Muscular dystrophy<br>Mitochondrial cytopathy |

## Other secondary cardiomyopathies

Other causes of secondary cardiomyopathies are listed in Figure 6.23.

## Neoplasms of the heart

Tumours of the heart are extremely rare. Examples include:

- myxoma—a benign tumour of stellate cells, typically arising from the endocardium (usually of the left atrium)
- connective tissue tumours, such as lipomas, fibromas and fibroelastomas
- malignant tumours, such as rhabdomyosarcomas
- metastatic or local-spread tumours.

## DISEASES OF THE PERICARDIUM

## Accumulation of fluid in the pericardial sac

### Pericardial effusion

This is the accumulation of fluid within the pericardial cavity. Effusions may be:

- serous—transudate has a low protein content ($<2$ g/100 mL) and usually contains only very scanty mesothelial cells. Caused by heart failure, hypoalbuminaemia or myxoedema
- serosanguinous—exudate with high protein content ($>3$ g/100 mL). Occurring with infection, uraemia, neoplasia or connective tissue disorders
- chylous—accumulation of lymphatic fluid occurring in the presence of lymphatic obstruction of pericardial drainage, most commonly due to neoplasms and tuberculosis.

The aetiology is of two types: inflammatory (e.g. acute pericarditis) and non-inflammatory. If non-inflammatory, at least one of the following effects must have occurred:

- ↑ capillary permeability, e.g. severe hypothyroidism
- ↑ capillary hydrostatic pressure, e.g. congestive heart failure
- ↓ plasma oncotic pressure, e.g. cirrhosis and the nephrotic syndrome.

Clinical effects depend on the increase in pressure within the pericardium which, in turn, depends on:

- volume of effusion—the greater the volume the greater the interference with cardiac function
- rate at which the fluid accumulates—sudden increase → marked elevation of pressure → severe cardiac chamber compression. Slow effusion (over weeks to months) → pericardium stretches → no elevation of pressure
- compliance characteristics of the pericardium—even small effusions may cause marked elevation of pressure if there is stiffness of the pericardium, e.g. chronic constrictive pericarditis.

The condition is often asymptomatic, but it may present with a dull constant ache in the left side of the chest. Unlike ischaemic cardiac pain, it is accentuated by inspiration, by movement, and by lying flat.

## Haemopericardium

This is the accumulation of blood in the pericardial sac. The causes of haemopericardium are outlined in Figure 6.24. In most cases, death occurs rapidly due to the sudden rise in intrapericardial cavity pressure, which prevents cardiac filling (cardiac tamponade): as little as 200–300 mL usually being sufficient.

## Cardiac tamponade

Fluid (of any kind) accumulates under high pressure, compressing the cardiac chambers to such an extent that filling of the heart is severely limited, resulting in acute

**Fig. 6.24** Aetiology of haemopericardium

| Causes | Example |
| --- | --- |
| Rupture of heart | Traumatic, e.g. stab wound Spontaneous, e.g. myocardial infarct |
| Rupture of intrapericardial portion of aorta | Dissecting aneurysm Syphilitic aneurysm Traumatic |
| Haemorrhagic tendencies | Purpura Scurvy Hypoprothrombinaemia Anticoagulant therapy |

heart failure. The condition is often associated with malignant disease.

### Diagnosis
The physical signs are:

- sinus tachycardia
- increased jugular venous pulse (often with a further rise on inspiration—Kussmaul's sign)
- decreased systemic blood pressure (producing shock in severe cases)
- cyclical decrease in systolic blood pressure during each inspiration—pulsus paradoxus.

Investigations include echocardiography (which shows the presence of pericardial effusion with right ventricular diastolic collapse) and cardiac catheterization combined with pericardiocentesis.

The management of cardiac tamponade depends on the extent of haemodynamic compromise. Severe cases may be rapidly fatal and require relief by emergency paracentesis; less critical cases require formal surgical drainage.

## Pericarditis

Pericarditis, i.e. inflammation of the pericardium, is the main disorder of the pericardium. The condition is often complicated by the development of an effusion.

## Acute pericarditis

In acute pericarditis both pericardial surfaces (visceral and parietal layers) are coated with a fibrin-rich acute inflammatory exudate. The loss of smoothness leads to the clinical sign of a friction rub. The causes of acute pericarditis are listed in Figure 6.25.

Variants can be:

- serous, non-bacterial inflammation—the exudate is a clear, straw-coloured and protein-rich fluid
- serofibrinous or fibrinous—occurs with MI. The exudate contains plasma protein including fibrinogen. This is the most common form of acute pericarditis
- suppurative (or purulent) pericarditis—associated with pyogenic bacterial infection, serosal surfaces are erythematous and coated with thick, creamy pus
- haemorrhagic—blood is mixed with inflammatory exudate
- caseous—fibrinous exudate with granulation tissue and areas of caseation caused by tuberculosis.

### Clinical features
The clinical features of acute pericarditis are:

- pleuritic chest pain—typically retrosternal pain radiating to the shoulders and neck
- fever
- pericardial friction rub
- ECG abnormalities.

**Fig. 6.25** Aetiology of acute pericarditis

| | |
|---|---|
| Infarction | Myocardial infarction: local pericarditis over infarct is the commonest cause of pericarditis |
| Infective | Viral infections: second most common cause, usually clinically mild, rarely requiring hospital treatment<br>Pyogenic: e.g. staphylococci, streptococci, haemophilus septicaemia or pneumonia<br>Tuberculosis: spread to pericardium from tuberculous lymph nodes in mediastinum; now rare |
| Injury | Postoperative: following open heart surgery<br>Pericarditis is diffuse, involving entire pericardial surface<br>Heals by fibrosis → obliteration of pericardial cavity |
| Invasive | Malignant pericaritis: usually due to infiltration of pericardium by local spread from a primary bronchial tumour; less commonly the cause is blood-borne metastases from a distant site, e.g. malignant melanoma |
| Immuno-logical | Immune pericarditis: associated with rheumatic fever or may present in patient with systemic autoimmune disease, e.g. SLE, rheumatoid disease |

**HINTS AND TIPS**

Remember the 'Five Is' of possible causes of acute pericarditis: infarctive, infective, injury, invasive and immunological.

## Chronic pericarditis

### Adhesive pericarditis
Although fibrinous pericarditis may resolve completely, it occasionally results in fibrinous adhesions or even in complete obliteration of the pericardial sac.

### Constrictive pericarditis
Progressive fibrosis and calcification of the pericardium cause restriction of ventricular filling and interference with ventricular systole. The heart is effectively encased in a solid shell and filling is impaired. Calcification may extend into the myocardium, producing impaired myocardial contraction.

This condition often follows tuberculous pericarditis, but it can also complicate haemopericardium, viral pericarditis, rheumatoid arthritis and purulent pericarditis.

### Clinical features
In chronic pericarditis, the fibrous tissue impairs venous return resulting in symptoms and signs of systemic venous congestion, namely raised jugular venous pressure, enlarged liver and ascites. Atrial fibrillation is also common.

## Rheumatic disease of the pericardium

Rheumatic disease of the pericardium is an acute form of pericarditis occurring with generalized pancarditis following streptococcal infection.

## ANEURYSMS

## Definitions and concepts

### Aneurysm
An aneurysm is an abnormal localized, permanent, dilatation of an artery. The term can also be applied to the wall of the heart. Types of aneurysm are shown in Figure 6.26:

- True aneurysms—the wall is formed by one or more layers of the affected vessel. These can be saccular or fusiform
- False aneurysms (pseudoaneurysms)—the vascular wall is breached (usually following trauma or infection), allowing communication with an extravascular space that is limited by surrounding tissue (usually an organized haematoma).

### True aneurysm morphology

Saccular aneurysms take the form of globular sacs, whereas fusiform aneurysms are spindle-shaped due to long segments of the vessel wall being affected around the whole circumference.

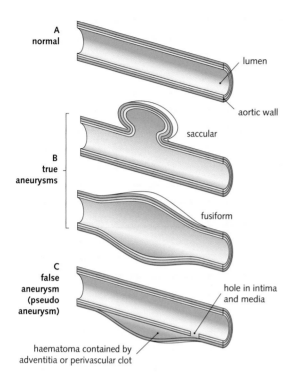

A
normal

lumen

aortic wall

saccular

B
true
aneurysms

fusiform

C
false
aneurysm
(pseudo
aneurysm)

hole in intima
and media

haematoma contained by
adventitia or perivascular clot

**Fig. 6.26** Aortic aneurysms. (A) Normal. (B) True aneurysms. (C) False aneurysm (pseudoaneurysm).

## Main causes of aneurysms

Any abnormality that weakens the media may produce an aneurysm:

- Atherosclerosis—the most common cause, typically affecting the abdominal aorta causing thinning and fibrous replacement of media.
- Cystic medial degeneration—focal degeneration of media with the formation of small cyst-like spaces filled with mucopolysaccharide. Aetiology may be idiopathic or associated with connective tissue diseases, e.g. Marfan's syndrome and Ehlers–Danlos syndrome.

The condition is generally confined to the aorta and the origins of its major branches. Extensive disease leads to dissecting aneurysm. These diseases include:

- infectious aortitis, e.g. syphilitic aortitis (rare, typically affecting the ascending and transverse portions of the aortic arch causing inflammatory destruction of the media with fibrous replacement) and mycotic aneurysms (small saccular dilatations with destruction of the wall caused by bacteria in infected thrombus)
- vasculitic syndromes (see pages 82)—inflammation of the vessels caused by immune complex deposition or cell-mediated immune reactions of the arterial wall leading to a weakening of the vessel wall then aneurysmal dilatations
- congenital aneurysms.

## Pathogenesis

The majority of aneurysms occur because of a weakening of the arterial wall with loss of elasticity and contractility. Stretching of the weakened wall is gradually progressive due to haemodynamic pressure forces producing an increased thinning of the wall until eventual rupture occurs.

The build-up of layers of thrombus within the lumen of the aneurysmal sac is protective, but not usually sufficient to repair the defect and reconstitute a normal lumen to the artery.

**HINTS AND TIPS**

The most frequent cause of an aneurysm is an atheroma. However, any abnormality that weakens the media may predispose a patient.

## Main complications

The main complications of aneurysms are rupture with critical haemorrhage and predisposition to thrombosis. The risk of rupture is usually greater with an increased size of aneurysm; high blood pressure is the most important factor in increasing the rate of growth.

## Abdominal aortic aneurysms

Abdominal aortic aneurysms (AAAs) are more common in men, especially over 60 years of age.

*Aetiology*—Atherosclerosis is the most common cause of abdominal aneurysms. However, they may also arise as a result of inflammation (vasculitis) or infection (mycotic aneurysms).

*Site*—80% of AAAs are situated below the origin of the renal arteries and are thus amenable to resection and replacement by graft.

*Morphology*—Atherosclerotic aneurysms produce a fusiform dilatation of the wall.

## Symptoms and signs

The majority of AAAs are asymptomatic, but occasionally patients are aware of a pulsatile mass. It is often first suspected because of aortic dilatation observed on radiographs, especially if the walls of the aneurysm are calcified. It may also come to attention by careful palpation during physical examination.

Symptoms may occur because of compression of neighbouring structures by the expanding aneurysm, e.g. back pain from vertebral compression, or vomiting following duodenal obstruction.

Confirmation of an AAA is achieved by ultrasonography CT, MRI or arteriography.

## Consequences

Rupture is the most devastating consequence and is often fatal. This may occur suddenly without warning or, alternatively, blood may slowly leak into the vessel wall resulting in pain and local tenderness.

Haemorrhage can occur into the retroperitoneal space, abdominal cavity or erode into the intestines resulting in massive gastrointestinal (GI) bleeding.

Thrombus formation on large atheromatous plaques is favoured, increasing the risk of embolic events, e.g. stroke.

## Prognostic factors

Fifty per cent of all abdominal aortic aneurysms that are more than 6 cm in transverse diameter rupture within 2 years if not surgically resected. Aneurysms less than 6 cm across may also rupture, albeit less frequently.

## Mortalities of emergency and elective surgery

Elective surgical repair has a much lower mortality than emergency surgery for rupture and it is, therefore, recommended for most AAAs greater than 5.5 cm in diameter, or those which are rapidly progressing or symptomatic. Mortality for surgical repair of abdominal aneurysms is also lower than that of thoracic aneurysms.

## Aortic dissection

An aortic dissection is a tear in the intima of the aorta allowing the entry of blood into media with separation of a 'flap' of intima from the rest of the aortic wall. A false lumen is created, usually between the inner two-thirds and outer third of the medial thickness giving the appearance of a doublebarrelled aorta.

## Types of dissecting aneurysms

There are two types:

1. Type A (67% of dissecting aneurysms)—arise in the ascending aorta with or without extension into the descending aorta.
2. Type B (33% of dissecting aneurysms)—are confined to the descending aorta, distal to the origin of the left subclavian artery.

*Epidemiology*—there are approximately 600 cases per year in the UK, occurring most commonly in people between 50 and 70 years old and affecting males more than females by 2:1.

Predisposing factors are:

- hypertension
- aortic atherosclerosis
- aortic aneurysm

- connective tissue disorders (e.g. Marfan's syndrome)
- pregnancy
- congenital abnormalities of the aortic valve.

## Consequences

The false lumen inevitably ruptures, either:

- externally—external rupture leads to massive fatal bleed into the thoracic cavity or, less commonly, the pericardial sac, pleural cavity or abdomen

or

- internally—rarely, blood tracks back into the lumen by rupturing through the inner media and intima forming a double-channelled aorta.

### Clinical Note

Aortic dissection:
- sudden onset severe chest pain, radiating back between the shoulder blades
- usually hypertension
- asymmetry of brachial, carotid, or femoral pulses
- mediastinal broadening and aortic 'knuckle' distortion on chest radiography
- Left-sided pleural effusion.

*Diagnosis*—echocardiography (transthoracic and/or transoesophageal), CT or MRI.

*Management*:

- Type A—emergency surgical repair
- Type B—hypertension control with bed rest; surgical intervention may be needed if there is leakage or organ ischaemia.

*Prognosis*—this condition is fatal without treatment: 25% die within 24 hours, 50% within the week, and almost all by 1 year.

## INFLAMMATORY AND NEOPLASTIC VASCULAR DISEASE

## Concepts and classification

### Vasculitides

This is a group of disorders characterized by inflammation of the blood vessel walls (vasculitis). Vasculitis can affect capillaries, venules, arterioles, arteries and, occasionally, large veins.

## Effects

The effects are:

- mild cases—transient damage to the vessel wall, which produces leakage of red blood cells
- severe cases—irreversible vessel wall destruction resulting in ischaemia and organ damage with associated systemic disturbances, commonly fevers, myalgias, arthralgias and malaise.

## Classification

Vasculitis can be classified either according to the size of the vessel affected (Fig. 6.27) or according to the pathogenesis of the inflammation (Fig. 6.28).

## Idiopathic vasculitis

The aetiology is unknown but the disorders are as follows:

- Giant cell arteritis (see below).

**Fig. 6.27** Classification of vasculitis according to size of affected vessel

| Size of vessel | Disorders |
| --- | --- |
| Large, medium and small | Syphilitic aortitis<br>Takayasu's disease<br>Giant cell arteritis<br>Kawasaki's disease<br>Rheumatoid disease |
| Medium and small | Wegener's granulomatosis<br>Polyarteritis nodosa<br>Buerger's disease<br>SLE |
| Small | Small vessel disease of arterioles, capillaries and venules<br>Henoch–Schönlein purpura |

**Fig. 6.28** Classification of vasculitis by pathogenesis

| Pathogenesis | Disorders |
| --- | --- |
| Idiopathic | Giant cell arteritis<br>Scleroderma (systemic sclerosis)<br>Takayasu's (pulseless) disease<br>Kawasaki's disease<br>Buerger's disease |
| Immune-mediated | Polyarteritis nodosa<br>Wegener's granulomatosis<br>Rheumatoid vasculitis<br>Systemic lupus erythematosus<br>Henoch–Schönlein purpura |
| Infectious | Syphilitic aortitis<br>Bacterial aortitis |

- Scleroderma (systemic sclerosis)—vascular changes are similar to those of benign or malignant hypertension, but only about 25% of patients are hypertensive. The condition is associated with progressive subcutaneous fibrosis leading to a marked tightening of the skin of the arms and hands; there are no effective treatments.
- Takayasu's (pulseless) disease—a rare chronic inflammatory and granulomatous disorder of the aorta and its proximal branches, typically affecting young or middle-aged females. The condition is characterized by severe necrotizing inflammation of all layers of affected vessel walls with fibrous replacement of muscle and a reduction of lumen. It presents clinically with hypertension or ischaemic symptoms of the arms, with loss of arm pulses.
- Kawasaki's disease—a disease of infants, primarily in Japan, affecting the main aortic branch arteries particularly the coronary arteries. It is characterized by medial fibroblastic thickening and, sometimes, aneurysm formation.
- Buerger's disease (thromboangitis obliterans)—a rare disease with a strong association with smoking, usually in young males. The condition mainly affects the small arteries of the arms and lower leg which show intimal fibrosis, thrombus formation and adventitial tissue changes affecting adjacent veins and nerves. Clinically, peripheral gangrene develops in the fingers and toes; the disease is progressive and amputations are often required.

## Immune-mediated vasculitis

Pathogenesis is due to immune complex formation between antigens and antibodies, which become trapped in venule walls and stimulate an acute inflammatory response with neutrophil chemotaxis. Neutrophils release enzymes that destroy the vessel wall. There are two main types:

1. Hypersensitivity (neutrophilic) vasculitis—most common pattern affecting capillaries and venules; usually manifests as a skin rash, often as a result of an allergy to a drug or occasionally arising as an allergic rash in viraemia or bacteraemia. It also occurs in Henoch–Schönlein purpura, serum sickness and cryoglobulinaemia.
2. Multi-organ autoimmune diseases, e.g. SLE and rheumatoid disease (mainly affects the aorta).

Autoantibodies that react against neutrophils (antineutrophil cytoplasmic antibodies; ANCA) can be detected in 90% of patients with Wegener's granulomatosis and in other types of immune-mediated vasculitis. Identification of these antibodies in serum is used in diagnostic evaluation of patients with possible vasculitis.

### Infectious vasculitis

These disorders include:

- syphilitic aortitis—tertiary manifestation of syphilis typically affecting the ascending and transverse portions of the aortic arch causing inflammatory destruction of media with fibrous replacement
- other infections—bacteria in infected thrombi can cause destruction of vessel walls with the development of small saccular dilatations and mycotic aneurysms.

## Giant cell (temporal) arteritis

Giant cell arteritis is a systemic disease that mainly involves arteries in the head and neck region, particularly the temporal arteries (hence the alternative name of temporal arteritis).

*Epidemiology*—the disease is relatively common, affecting 10 per 100 000 per year in the general population in Europe. Incidence increases with age, and it is rare in people under 50 years; it affects females more than males by 2:1.

*Aetiology*—an idiopathic disease with associations with certain types of human leucocyte antigen (HLA) DR (HLA-DR).

The microscopic appearance of vessels is as follows:

- thickened nodular vessel wall → decreased lumen
- necrosis of inner media and gradual replacement with fibrosis
- fragmentation of internal elastic lamina
- inflammatory cell infiltration—mainly T lymphocytes but also histiocytes and giant cells (hence the name)
- often complicated by thrombosis.

*Clinical features*—patients have ill-defined symptoms of:

- malaise
- tiredness
- severe headaches
- visual disturbance from involvement of the ophthalmic arteries. This is a medical emergency requiring prompt treatment to prevent blindness
- an association with polymyalgia rheumatica, a musculoskeletal condition causing muscle pain and stiffness classically in the upper body.

Investigations characteristically reveal high ESR and/or C-reactive protein (CRP). Diagnosis is made by biopsy of the temporal artery with histological investigation. Management is with high-dose corticosteroid therapy to control the disease.

## Polyarteritis nodosa

This systemic disease is characterized by inflammatory necrosis of the walls of small and medium-sized arteries. Although the disease is systemic, it causes patchy and focal inflammation with only parts of some arteries being involved.

*Epidemiology*—a rare disease (about 5–10 per million per year in most populations), but it can occur in all age groups; males more than females by 2 : 1.

*Aetiology*—the cause is unknown but the presence of antineutrophil cytoplasmic antibodies (i.e. ANCA positive) suggests an autoimmune pathogenesis. There is also an association with chronic hepatitis B infection.

*Pathogenesis*—inflammatory destruction of the vessel wall with necrosis of muscle cells and destruction of the elastic lamina. Healing occurs with fibrous replacement of the muscular media. Extensive damage to the intima predisposes to thrombosis, which is often followed by vessel occlusion and downstream infarction.

Microscopically, the artery wall shows:

- inflammatory cell infiltration—neutrophils and eosinophils are most numerous
- fibrinoid necrosis of segments of artery wall
- thrombosis, which is common.

Clinical features include systemic features of inflammation (fever, weight loss, myalgia and muscle wasting) and the effects of vessel occlusion producing small areas of infarction. Tissues most seriously affected are the kidneys, GI tract and liver.

Diagnosis is by:

- blood—neutrophilia and raised ESR
- ANCA, which are present in most cases
- tissue biopsy, usually of a kidney or asymptomatic muscle.

Management is by cyclophosphamide with corticosteroids, which has significantly improved the outcome. Antihypertensive drugs reduce morbidity from hypertensive complications.

Prognosis is variable; many patients relapse after treatment.

## Neoplastic vascular disease

### Benign

#### Haemangiomas

Haemangiomas are common developmental malformations composed of dilated vascular spaces derived from blood vessels.

There are three types of haemangioma:

1. Capillary haemangiomas (strawberry naevi), which are composed of small, capillary-like vessels.
2. Cavernous haemangiomas, which are composed of cavernous, endothelial-lined spaces (vein-like vessels).
3. Sclerosing haemangiomas, which are fibrous nodules containing iron pigment produced as a result of fibrosis or sclerosis of a capillary haemangioma.

Haemangiomas are not 'true' tumours, but they are often grouped with neoplasms because they appear as localized tissue masses. They are more accurately described as hamartomas, i.e. non-neoplastic overgrowths of tissue.

### Telangiectasias

Dilatations of capillaries are often seen in the elderly and those with irradiated skin or liver failure (spider naevi). Vessels are dilated but histologically normal.

## Malignant

### Angiosarcoma

A malignant tumour of blood vessel endothelium. This most commonly occurs as a raised bluish-red patch on the face or scalp of elderly people, which is often confused with a benign haemangioma.

Progressive enlargement of the tumour is accompanied by ulceration and, later, metastasis to regional lymph nodes.

## DISEASES OF THE VEINS AND LYMPHATICS

### Varicose veins

Varicose veins are persistently distended superficial veins in the lower limbs (long and short saphenous veins). They result from incompetent valves that allow the veins to become engorged with blood under the influence of gravity.

*Epidemiology*—the condition affects 10–20% of the general population at some age. There is an increasing incidence with age, and it is most common above 50. It affects females more than males by 4:1.

Figure 6.29 lists the predisposing factors of varicose veins.

*Anatomy of varicose veins*—the superficial and deep venous plexuses of the lower limb are connected by perforating veins (Fig. 6.30).

*Pathogenesis*—the return of blood from the deep veins is aided by normal contraction of the calf and thigh muscles. If the valves in the perforating veins become incompetent, blood is forced from deep venous plexuses to superficial venous plexuses resulting in increased pressure in the superficial veins. Combined

| Fig. 6.29 Predisposing factors of varicose veins |
| --- |
| **Defective support of vessel wall** |
| Familial tendency: in approx. 40% of all cases<br>Sex: significantly increased incidence in females<br>Obesity: adipose tissue = poor venous support;<br>muscle = good venous support<br>Age: degenerative changes in surrounding tissues and<br>decreased activity of muscles → loss of venous support |
| **Increased venous pressure** |
| Standing occupations: increased incidence in occupations<br>involving prolonged standing<br>(venous pressure is greater on standing)<br>Pregnancy<br>Intravascular thrombosis<br>Tumour masses pressing on veins<br>(e.g. uterine fibroids and ovarian tumours)<br>Garters and other constrictions |

with prolonged blood stasis, there is a tendency towards the development of varicosities.

Varicose leg ulcers are a common clinical condition, and they are associated with chronic venous insufficiency.

## Morphological changes

The morphological changes are:

- increased pressure produces a dilatation of the lumen and an increased tension on vessel walls with compensatory hypertrophy of the muscle and elastic tissues
- prolonged increased pressure produces irregular atrophy of muscle and elastic lamina with fibrous replacement leading to stretched, tortuous veins with localized bulging.

## Sequelae of varicose veins

The sequelae are:

- oedema (of lower limbs) due to increased hydrostatic pressure
- stasis dermatitis—varicose dermatitis with pigmentation due to haemosiderin deposition
- varicose ulcers—dermatitis may proceed to ulceration, which is very slow to heal. Usually on the medial aspect of the ankle or lower leg

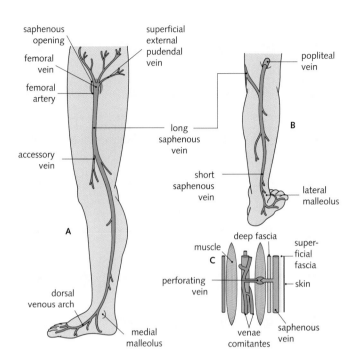

• thrombosis and embolism are very rare sequelae; these tend to affect deep veins.

## Lymphangitis and lymphoedema

### Lymphangitis

Lymphangitis is inflammation of lymphatic channels draining any focus of infection. The channels are dilated and contain inflammatory cells. The condition may result in the spread of the infection in some cases, e.g. in tuberculosis.

### Lymphoedema

Lymphoedema is oedema of the tissues caused by obstruction of the lymphatics.

#### Causes
The causes of obstructive lymphoedema are:

• metastatic spread of tumours causing mechanical blockage
• surgical removal of nodes
• post-irradiation fibrosis
• filariasis (elephantiasis)—nematode infection of lymph nodes (most common organism is *Wuchereria bancrofti);* transmitted by the bite of an infected mosquito
• post-inflammatory thrombosis and scarring, e.g. lymphogranuloma venereum
• primary lymphatic disorders (rare).

#### Effects
The effects of obstructive lymphoedema are:

• gross swelling
• increased predisposition to attacks of lymphangitis and ulceration
• severe cases result in thickening of skin and overgrowth of dermal connective tissues leading to elephantiasis.

# Pathology of the respiratory system  ⑦

## Objectives

In this chapter, you will learn to:
- Describe common disorders of the upper respiratory tract affecting the nose, nasopharynx and larynx.
- Define the differences between obstructive and restrictive lung diseases.
- Describe the pathological processes in chronic obstructive pulmonary disease, including emphysema and chronic bronchitis.
- Recognize asthma as a common cause of obstructive lung disease and describe the differences between intrinsic and extrinsic forms.
- Describe cystic fibrosis and bronchiectasis.
- Understand the effect of interstitial lung diseases on producing a restrictive pattern of lung function.
- Describe infections of the lung, most notably the pneumonias and tuberculosis.
- Recall the neoplastic diseases of the lung, particularly the four most common pathological patterns.
- Describe lung disorders of vascular and iatrogenic origin.
- Understand disorders of the pleura, notably effusions, pneumothorax and neoplasms.

## DISORDERS OF THE UPPER RESPIRATORY TRACT

### The nose and nasopharynx

### Rhinitis

Rhinitis, inflammation of the nasal mucosa, is the most common nasal disorder seen in family practice. The condition may be either acute or chronic.

#### Acute rhinitis

Aetiology of acute rhinitis is either:
- Infective
- Allergic.

Infectious rhinitis is usually of viral origin, e.g. the common cold (rhinoviruses, adenoviruses). Virally induced inflammation of surface epithelial cells is followed by exudation of fluid and mucus from the damaged surface ('runny nose'). Later, submucosal oedema produces swelling, which may lead to a partial blockage of the nasal airways.

Allergic rhinitis ('hay fever') is a type I (IgE-mediated) hypersensitivity reaction to inhaled materials such as grass and pollens, producing a mixed serous-mucous exudate and submucosal oedema leading to nasal blockage. Eosinophils are prominent in the inflammatory infiltrate.

### Chronic rhinitis

Chronic rhinitis can be caused by repeated attacks of acute rhinitis, which often develop a secondary bacterial infection. It may result in the development of nasal polyps.

Macroscopically, nasal polyps are typically smooth-surfaced, creamy, semi-translucent, ovoid masses.

Microscopically, they have oedematous tissue with scattered infiltrate of chronic inflammatory cells including plasma cells. Eosinophils are often very numerous in allergic polyps.

### Sinusitis

Sinusitis, is inflammation of the paranasal sinuses (maxillary, ethmoidal, frontal, etc.), usually secondary to acute or chronic rhinitis. Rhinitis usually results in the inflammation of the sinus linings; swelling of the mucosa around the drainage foramen of the maxillary sinus in the nasal cavity and may cause stasis of maxillary sinus secretions. Stasis predisposes to secondary bacterial infection with alteration of the static maxillary fluid from seromucous to purulent.

In severe cases, the infection may spread into the ethmoid and frontal sinuses with a risk of spread of infection to the meninges. Orbital cellulitis may also complicate acute sinusitis.

Chronic sinusitis is characterized by chronically thickened and inflamed mucosa of the sinuses and by persistent fluid accumulation.

### Kartagener's syndrome

This is a syndrome of bronchiectasis, sinusitis and situs inversus (transposition of viscera). Sinusitis is caused by abnormal ciliary function resulting in a failure to clear mucus and bacteria.

## Necrotizing lesions

### Wegener's granulomatosis

This autoimmune granulomatous vasculitis frequently presents with nasal lesions.

### Lethal midline granuloma (lymphoma)

This is a condition presenting with progressive granulomatous inflammation, ulceration and destruction of the structures in the upper respiratory tract, i.e. the nose, nasopharynx, palate and sinuses. It is thought to be a form of lymphoma affecting natural killer cells, and may occur alongside lymphomatous disease elsewhere in the body.

Untreated, death occurs from systemic disease caused by erosion of blood vessels, local infection or the development of pneumonia.

## Neoplasms

### Nasopharyngeal carcinoma

This is a squamous or anaplastic carcinoma of the nasopharynx (part of the pharynx that lies immediately behind the nasal cavities) with characteristic abundant lymphoid tissue in the stroma.

It is strongly associated with Epstein–Barr virus infection, the virus being demonstrable in tumour cells in most cases. The carcinoma is most commonly found in East Africa and South East Asia, but is rare elsewhere in the world.

The tumours often remain small and undetected until metastasis to the lymph nodes in the neck has occurred.

The prognosis is good with radiation therapy: the 5-year survival rate is 80% for localized disease and 50% for advanced disease.

### Plasmacytomas

This malignant tumour is composed of monoclonal plasma cells. It presents as a soft, haemorrhagic nasal/nasopharyngeal mass.

### Olfactory neuroblastoma

This is a rare tumour presenting in the upper part of the nasal cavity, often as a haemorrhagic mass with evidence of bone destruction. The tumours usually develop from neuroendocrine cells found in the olfactory mucosa. They are highly malignant and may metastasize widely.

## Nasopharyngeal angiofibroma

This rare benign tumour (also known as juvenile angiofibroma) occurs almost exclusively in males between 10 and 25 years old. The lesions are typically located in the nasopharynx rather than the nose, and may mimic a malignant tumour due to their rapid growth and tendency to erode bone. Ulceration and bleeding are common.

# The larynx

## Acute laryngitis

This acute inflammation of the larynx may be as a result of viruses, bacteria, irritants (cigarette smoke), mechanical factors (endotracheal intubation), or overuse of the voice.

### Sequelae of acute laryngitis

- Resolution—infective causes typically resolve without complications.
- Spread of infection may occur throughout the respiratory tract with the development of tracheobronchitis, bronchopneumonia or lung abscesses; this is more common in the elderly or debilitated due to a poor cough reflex
- Airway, obstruction—laryngeal oedema can result in a life-threatening narrowing of the airway especially in children (whose airways are narrower) suffering from *Haemophilus influenzae* epiglottitis or in cases of corrosive chemical ingestion.

### Chronic laryngitis

Chronic inflammation of the larynx is most commonly seen in heavy cigarette smokers. It may lead to a permanent thickening of the laryngeal mucosa and submucosa, particularly where there is associated excess production of keratin ('smoker's keratosis').

Overlying epidermis may also undergo keratotic thickening with dysplastic change in the basal layer; this is a predisposing factor in the development of squamous carcinoma of the larynx.

### Acute laryngotracheobronchitis (croup)

Croup is life-threatening acute inflammation and obstruction of the respiratory tract involving the larynx, trachea and epiglottis. It usually affects young children aged 6 months to 3 years and is typically caused by viral infection.

Characteristics include symptoms of laryngitis accompanied by signs of obstruction: inspiratory stridor, a rising pulse rate, restlessness and cyanosis.

Treatment is by reassurance and humidification of inspired air, which usually reverses the symptoms. In severe cases, the obstruction may require emergency intubation or tracheostomy.

### Reactive nodules/polyps

This common benign lesion is associated with upper respiratory tract infection or occurs after vocal abuse, e.g. shouting. Presentation is with hoarseness that will not resolve until the polyp is removed.

### Singer's nodules

These are small, benign bilateral laryngeal nodules located at the nodal point (junction between the anterior third and posterior two-thirds of the vocal cords). Nodules are especially common in singers and professional voice users, and they can alter the character of the voice even when only a few millimeters in diameter. They consist of oedematous connective tissue with submucosal fibrosis covered by squamous epithelium.

### Papilloma and papillomatosis

*Papilloma*

Warty papillomas on the larynx are usually due to infection by the human papillomavirus (HPV 11 and 16). The lesions are usually solitary and confined to the true vocal cords.

*Juvenile laryngeal papillomatosis*

These multiple, soft, pink papillomas on the vocal cords are largely confined to children. Lesions often extend into other parts of the larynx, sometimes even down the trachea, and they have the histological features of florid viral warts. Spontaneous regression often occurs at puberty, although the lesions are typically difficult to eradicate if this does not happen.

### Squamous cell carcinoma of the larynx

This is the most common malignant tumour of the larynx and accounts for 1–2% of cancers with an incidence of 1–2 per 100 000 per year worldwide. It typically presents after 40 years of age, affecting males more than females (but the incidence is rising in females). The risk factors are smoking, radiation to the head and neck, carcinoma in situ and keratosis (see above). The affected sites are:

- glottic region (60%)—arises from true vocal cords. The best prognosis follows early detection because this area is alymphatic, which restricts the routes for metastasis. The earliest symptom is hoarseness, which should always be investigated if persisting for more than 4 weeks.

- supraglottic region (30%), i.e. the lower epiglottis, false cords, ventricles and arytenoids. Less common laryngeal carcinoma and has a worse prognosis.
- subglottic region (10%)—arising below the true vocal cords and above the first tracheal ring; poor prognosis as late presentation is common (rich lymphatic supply to this area).

Macroscopically, they are ulcerated, diffuse, grey solid or papillary lesions.

Microscopically, the majority are well-differentiated, keratinizing squamous carcinomas; a minority are poorly differentiated with spindle cells.

Spread can be:

- local—to adjacent laryngeal structures but often confined by laryngeal cartilages for a considerable time. The presence of a palpable neck lump usually indicates metastatic disease.
- lymphatic—to regional lymph nodes.
- haematogenous—occurs late if at all; lungs are the most common site.

The prognosis depends on location, extent of spread and the presence of lymph node metastasis. The overall 5-year survival is as follows:

- glottic tumours—80%
- supraglottic tumours—65%
- subglottic tumours—40%.

## DISORDERS OF THE LUNGS

## Atelectasis

This is a defective expansion and collapse of the lung. It may occur as a result of:

- obstruction
- compression
- scarring
- surfactant loss.

## Obstructive causes

Obstruction of the larger bronchial tubes leads to resorption of air from the lung distal to the obstruction. Causes of obstruction can be within the lung (e.g. mucus plugs in bronchiectasis, inhaled foreign bodies) or outside the lung (enlarged lymph nodes as in tuberculosis or lung cancer).

Patchy atelectasis describes the pattern of atelectasis associated with chronic obstructive airway diseases.

## Compressive causes

Compressive atelectasis is the compression of the lung caused by the accumulation of fluid or air in the pleural cavity, e.g. following a pneumothorax.

## Scarring

Scarring of the lung may cause contraction of the parenchyma and lung collapse.

## Surfactant loss

Surfactant is a surface active agent produced by type 2 pneumocytes (alveolar cells). It reduces surface tension and gives the lung sufficient compliance to expand without collapse. Surfactant loss can be either developmental or acquired and leads to a generalized failure of lung expansion, termed microatelectasis.

Lack of surfactant causes respiratory distress in premature infants; steroids may be administered to the mother to aid fetal lung development (and surfactant production) if premature labour is inevitable.

## Consequences of atelectasis

The collapse of a lung has important clinical consequences as respiratory function will be disturbed and there is a predisposition to infection. Expansion can be aided by physiotherapy and bronchoscopy-mediated removal of the obstructive/compressive cause. However, prolonged atelectasis becomes irreversible.

# Classification of diffuse lung disease

## Obstructive lung diseases

Obstructive lung diseases are those in which there is obstruction to the flow of air within the lungs, although the lungs themselves may be hyperinflated. Disorders include emphysema, chronic bronchitis, bronchiectasis and asthma.

Chronic obstructive pulmonary disease (COPD) is used clinically where emphysema and chronic bronchitis occur together, almost always as the result of long-term cigarette smoking.

## Restrictive lung diseases

Restrictive lung diseases are those in which there is obstruction to the expansion of the lungs (e.g. due to fibrosis or oedema) such that they can only take in a limited amount of air. In these diseases, although the lungs are often underinflated, the rate of air flow is unaffected. Causes of this restrictive pattern are covered in more detail later under 'Diffuse interstitial diseases' (see page 96).

Both obstructive and restrictive lung diseases can cause significant respiratory impairment with a characteristic pattern of pulmonary function tests (Fig. 7.1 and Fig. 7.2).

# Chronic obstructive pulmonary disease

Chronic obstructive pulmonary disease (COPD) is a chronic, slowly progressive disease of airflow limitation caused by an abnormal inflammatory response of the lungs to noxious substances (usually from cigarette smoking).

## Pathological changes

COPD classically involves three overlapping pathological processes:

1. Chronic bronchitis—this causes hyperpalsia of the bronchial submucosal glands, leading to an increased Reid index.
2. Emphysema—abnormal diltation of air spaces with destruction of alveolar walls.
3. Bronchiolitis—this describes inflammation of the small airways (bronchioles).

Chronic bronchitis and emphysema are considered in more detail in separate sections below.

## Diagnosis

Common symptoms of COPD are persistent cough, sputum production and breathlessness. If combined with a strong history of tobacco or pollutant exposure, lung function tests are performed (see Figs 7.1 and 7.2). These are suggestive of COPD if:

**Fig. 7.1** Characteristic patterns of lung function tests in obstructive and restrictive lung diseases

|  | Obstructive lung diseases | Restrictive lung diseases |
| --- | --- | --- |
| Vital capacity (VC) | ↓ or normal | ↓↓ |
| $FEV_1$ | ↓↓ | ↓ |
| $FEV_1$/VC ratio | ↓ | Normal or ↑ |
| Peak respiratory flow rate (PEFR) | ↓ | Normal |

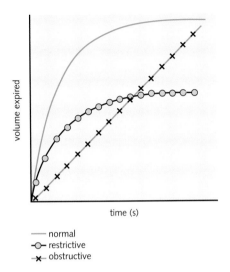

normal
—○— restrictive
—✕— obstructive

**Fig. 7.2**   Illustration of a normal, obstructive deficit and restrictive deficit vitalography.

- forced expired volume in one second ($FEV_1$) is less than 80% predicted
- FEV1/forced vital capacity (FVC) ratio is less than 70% predicted
- the limitation is incompletely reversible with bronchodilators (e.g. inhaled salbutamol). This distinguishes the result from asthma, which is fully reversible.

A chest X-ray may show hyperinflation, flat hemidiaphragms, reduced peripheral vascular markings and bullae.

**Clinical Note**

Treating stable COPD involves:
- bronchodilators—often combinations of inhaled $\beta_2$-agonists (e.g. salbutamol), anticholinergics (e.g. tiotropium) and oral theophyllines
- help smoking cessation (e.g. nicotine replacement)
- inhaled corticosteroids if very symptomatic
- long-term oxygen if in chronic respiratory failure
- nutritional support to maintain weight
- influenza and pneumococcal vaccinations.

Remember **SHONA** for the principles of treating an infective exacerbation of COPD:
- Steroids (oral)
- Heparin (prevent deep vein thrombosis in immobile patients)
- Oxygen
- Nebulized bronchodilators
- Antibiotics.

## Complications

The frequency of complications increases with progression of the disease:

- infection—this produces acute exacerbations of symptoms requiring hospital admission (see clinical sketch)
- pneumothorax—bullae are thin-walled airspaces created by alveolar collapse. Rupture of subpleural bullae may produce a pneumothorax
- respiratory failure—with hypoxia and hypercapnia (type 2 failure)
- cor pulmonale—right-sided heart failure (see Chapter 6).

Note that in COPD, the respiratory centre may become relatively insensitive to $CO_2$, relying on hypoxic drive to maintain respiratory effort. It is, therefore, potentially dangerous to give these patients high-concentration oxygen without careful observation, as hypoventilation or apnoea may result.

## Emphysema

Emphysema is a permanent dilatation of any part of the air spaces distal to the terminal bronchiole, occurring with tissue destruction but without fibrosis. It is a common condition, which usually forms part of COPD, but may occasionally present alone.

The aetiology is unclear, but risk factors are the same as for COPD, including cigarette smoking, occupational dusts or chemicals and atmospheric pollution. The inherited disorder $\alpha_1$-antitrypsin deficiency predisposes to early emphysema.

### Pathogenesis

In normal individuals, extracellular elastases secreted into the lung by inflammatory cells are inhibited by protease inhibitors (particularly $\alpha_1$-antitrypsin). In emphysema, these inhibitors are either inactivated (e.g. by cigarette smoke) or absent (inherited disorder), resulting in continued activity of the elastases with destruction of lung parenchyma. Destruction of respiratory tissue leads to a loss of elastic recoil in the lungs and a decreased area available for gaseous exchange. About one-third of lung capacity must be destroyed before clinical symptoms of emphysema appear.

### Types of emphysema

There are several forms of emphysema, defined by the location of damage in the respiratory acinus (Fig. 7.3):

- Centrilobular—dilatation of the respiratory bronchioles at the centre of acinus. It is most common in men and is closely associated with cigarette

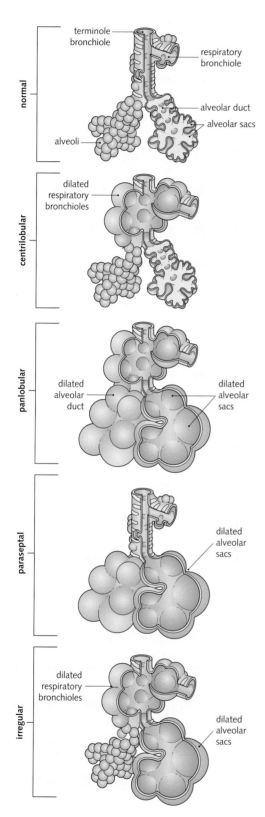

**Fig. 7.3** Diagrams of the main types of emphysema.

smoking. Lesions are most commonly found in the upper lobes.

- Panacinar—dilatation of the terminal acinus, which later affects the respiratory bronchioles, thereby affecting the whole acinus. Typically affects the lower lobes. This pattern is typically seen in inherited $\alpha_1$-antitrypsin deficiency (caused by variants of the *pi* gene with the homozygous **piZZ** state resulting in hepatic cirrhosis as well).
- Paraseptal—involves air spaces at the periphery of lobules, typically adjacent to the pleura. Usually affects the upper lobes adjacent to areas of scarring or atelectasis.
- Irregular—irregular involvement of the respiratory acinus and almost always associated with scarring. It is thought to be caused by the trapping of air following lung fibrosis and it is, therefore, commonly present around old healed tuberculous scars at the lung apices.

## Clinical features

In the early stages of emphysema, a rapid respiratory rate enables individuals to maintain blood oxygenation, such that levels of $PaCO_2$ and $PaO_2$ are near normal. Patients are breathless but not cyanosed (so-called 'pink puffers'). However, on the slightest exertion patients become increasingly breathless and ultimately hypoxic (type 1 respiratory failure). Complications are the same as described for COPD.

The lungs are hyperinflated, the trachea is often descended (i.e. there is decreased cricosternal distance between the cricoid cartilage and the sternal notch) and the accessory muscles may be hypertrophied. Associated chronic bronchitis may produce cough and sputum. Breath sounds are quiet, especially over bullae, often with crepitations or wheezes.

## Chronic bronchitis

Chronic bronchitis is defined as a cough productive of sputum on most days for 3 months of the year for at least 2 successive years. It typically affects middle-aged men and normally forms part of COPD; most cases are due to cigarette smoking.

### Pathogenesis

Constant irritation by cigarette smoke causes chronic inflammation of the respiratory bronchioles (bronchiolitis) and increased mucous secretion.

Hypersecretion of mucus is associated with hyperplasia of the submucosal mucus-secreting glands. Proteases stimulate this hypersecretion following their release by neutrophils recruited as part of the inflammatory response. The Reid index gives the ratio of gland to wall thickness in the bronchus, and it is significantly increased in cases of chronic bronchitis.

## Clinical features

Bronchiolar obstruction must be extensive and widespread to give clinical symptoms. Eventually, extensive mucus plugging leads to the clinical obstructive features of the disease with typical cough and sputum production.

In later stages of the disease, progressive obstruction may result in patients with hypercapnia, hypoxaemia and cyanosis (so-called 'blue bloaters'). Other complications include:

- recurrent low-grade bronchial infections caused by bacteria such as *Haemophilus influenzae* and *Streptococcus pneumoniae*, or viruses such as respiratory syncytial virus and adenovirus
- squamous metaplasia—loss of ciliated cells as a result of squamous metaplasia can further exacerbate the problem
- malignancy—persistent injury by smoking may invoke dysplastic changes in metaplastic squamous epithelium, which may ultimately become malignant (squamous cell carcinoma of the bronchus).

The late complications of COPD discussed previously may also occur.

## Asthma

Asthma is an increased irritability of the bronchial tree with paroxysmal narrowing of the airways, which may reverse either spontaneously or after treatment with bronchodilators.

This is a common disorder, affecting around 15% of children and 7% of adults. Its incidence is thought to be rising, possibly due to environmental atmospheric pollution.

## Classification

Asthma can be classified into two categories, depending on whether there is an allergic basis to the disease:

1. Extrinsic asthma (atopic)—early-onset asthma triggered by environmental allergens. Individuals often have a family history of allergic disorders. IgE levels are raised and an immediate type 1 hypersensitivity to the allergen is produced on skin challenge. This is the most common type of asthma.
2. Intrinsic asthma (non-atopic)—adult-onset asthma often associated with chronic bronchitis, as well as other asthma triggers such as cold or exercise. IgE levels are normal, there is no family history of allergic disorders and skin testing is negative.

However, there is often much overlap between the two types and many patients do not fit neatly into any one type.

## Pathogenesis

There are three key features in both types of asthma:

1. Airflow limitation—obstruction is caused by a combination of bronchospasm, oedema and mucous plugging. This may be spontaneously reversible, or reversible with bronchodilator treatment.
2. Airway hyper-responsiveness to bronchoconstrictor trigger factors.
3. Airway inflammation—it appears that the allergic inflammation process of extrinsic asthma is driven by type 2 helper T cells (Th2). With time, airway remodelling occurs so that the smooth muscles of the bronchial wall become hypertrophied, increasing airflow limitation.

### HINTS AND TIPS

Remember that both asthma and COPD are obstructive lung diseases, but there are key differences between them:
- Asthma is due to a sensitizing agent; COPD is due to a noxious agent.
- Asthmatic airway inflammation is predominated by CD4+ T cells and eosinophils; COPD occurs with predominantly CD8+ T cells, macrophages and neutrophils.
- Asthma airflow limitation is completely reversible with bronchodilator medication; COPD is only partially reversible.

### The three phases of extrinsic asthma
- Early (15–20 minutes)—a rapid onset of bronchoconstriction caused by histamine release from mast cells. The allergen binds to IgE antibodies on the surface of mast cells causing cross-linking and degranulation (Fig. 7.4).
- Late (4–6 hours)—following recovery from the early phase, inflammatory mediators released by mast cells cause activation of macrophages and chemotaxis of polymorphs and eosinophils into the bronchial mucosa. These cells release inflammatory mediators causing a secondary wave of bronchoconstriction unrelated to exposure to the original antigen (Fig. 7.4).
- Prolonged hyper-reactivity (over days)—an exaggerated response of the airway on further re-exposure to the allergen or other bronchoconstrictor trigger factors over ensuing days. Persistence of inflammatory cells within the bronchial wall leads to damage and loss of epithelial cells.

**Fig. 7.4**   Pathogenesis of the early and late stages of asthma. (CI, cellular infiltration; M, mucus; SM, smooth muscle.)

## Structural changes

The main structural changes that take place in asthmatic airways are listed below and illustrated in Figure 7.5:

- Immune cell infiltration—the bronchial mucosa is infiltrated by eosinophils, mast cells, lymphoid cells and macrophages

- Mucosal oedema—extravasation of plasma into submucosal tissues produces a narrowing of the airways
- Mucus hypersecretion leads to plugging of airways
- Hypertrophy of bronchial smooth muscle due to recurrent bronchoconstriction
- Focal necrosis of the airway epithelium, caused by prolonged inflammation

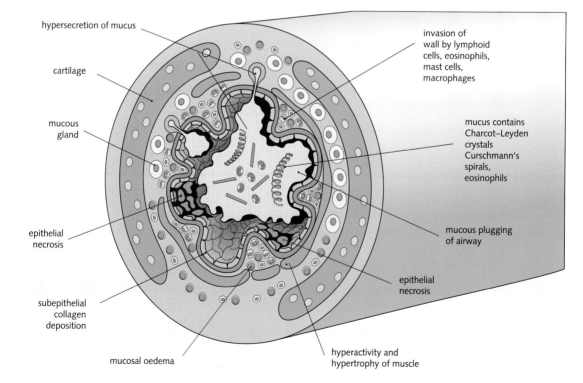

**Fig. 7.5**   Morphological changes in the airways in asthma.

- Deposition of collagen beneath the bronchial epithelium in long-standing cases
- Sputum contains Charcot–Leyden crystals (derived from eosinophil granules) and Curschmann's spirals (composed of mucus plugs from small airways).

## Clinical features

Clinical features are as follows:

- Mild disease (majority of cases)—acute, intermittent episodes of bronchospasm (wheezing, dyspnoea or coughing) are triggered by well-recognized causes.
- Moderate to severe disease (small percentage)—increasingly severe and irreversible asthma in middle or old age (chronic asthma); patients may present with signs of respiratory distress.
- Acute severe asthma (formerly status asthmaticus)—severe, acute disease usually presenting with tachypnoeic distress, tachycardia and pulsus paradoxus. Air entry may be inadequate to generate any wheeze (the silent chest is an ominous sign) and death may result from acute respiratory insufficiency.

The main complication is cor pulmonale. Pulmonary vasoconstriction caused by chronic alveolar hypoventilation results in pulmonary hypertension leading to right ventricular hypertrophy.

### Clinical Note

The clinical signs of asthma include widespread, polyphonic, high-pitched wheezes. In severe chronic asthma, a barrel chest may develop.

The disease can usually be controlled by treatment including $\beta_2$-agonists, corticosteroids, theophyllines and leukotriene receptor antagonists.

Acute severe asthma can be life-threatening. It requires immediate oxygen, nebulized $\beta_2$-agonists and anticholinergics and systemic corticosteroids. Arterial blood gases should be taken to determine severity; if life-threatening, intravenous aminophylline or magnesium sulphate may be of use.

## Prognosis

- Remission—approximately 50% of cases of childhood asthma resolve spontaneously but may recur later in life; remission in adult-onset asthma is less likely.
- Mortality—death occurs in approximately 0.2% of asthmatics accounting for about 2000 deaths per year in the UK. Mortality is usually (but not always) preceded by an acute attack and about 50% are more than 65 years old.

## Bronchiectasis

This is an irreversible dilatation of the bronchi or their branches. Its causes are:

- congenital—cystic fibrosis, primary ciliary dyskinesia and Kartagener's syndrome (bronchiectasis, situs inversus and sinusitis)
- acquired—infection (especially whooping cough, necrotising pneumonia or measles in childhood) and obstruction (either by an inhaled foreign body or by tumour).

Widened bronchi are more prone to infections, *Haemophilus influenzae* and *Pseudomonas aeruginosa* being the most common pathogens. Patients often cough up purulent sputum, which may contain blood.

Treatment consists of antibiotics (often long-term) for infections and postural drainage physiotherapy to drain sputum.

## Cystic fibrosis

Cystic fibrosis (CF) is a hereditary multisystem disease characterized by the production of abnormally thick mucus, and primarily affects the lung and the pancreas. It is the most common autosomal recessive disorder affecting 1 in 2000 newborns. Approximately 1 in 25 Caucasians are heterozygous carriers of the CF gene.

## Pathogenesis

The mutated gene is found on chromosome 7 and encodes for a protein termed the cystic fibrosis transmembrane regulator (CFTR). The most common mutation is deletion of the phenylalanine residue at position 508, which is found in 70% of cases. This protein normally enables the transport of chloride ions across cell membranes. In cystic fibrosis, defective CFTR results in impaired chloride transport, which prevents the release of sodium and water to liquefy mucus. The net result is the production of extremely thick and viscous mucus by the exocrine glands.

The epithelial dysfunction of cystic fibrosis affects the following systems:

- Bronchi—abnormally viscid mucus cannot be cleared from the lungs
- Intestine—causing meconium ileus in newborn babies and distal intestinal obstruction syndrome later in life
- Pancreas—causing deficiency of the pancreatic enzymes, resulting in malabsorption and failure to thrive
- Liver—causing biliary cirrhosis
- Vas deferens—failure to develop leads to male infertility.

In the respiratory tract, the bronchi and bronchioles become obstructed by abnormally viscid mucus, which leads to four main problems:

1. Infections—obstruction and stagnation of secretions leads to repeated bouts of infection, particularly with *Staphylococcus aureus* and *Pseudomonas aeruginosa*. *Burkholderia cepacia* infection is often intrinsically resistant to multiple antibiotics and some forms are transmissible between patients. This has resulted in the segregation of CF patients in hospitals and the community.
2. Bronchiectasis—a frequent complication (see above).
3. Hyperinflation of the lungs due to air trapping behind mucin plugs; increased risk of developing spontaneous pneumothorax.
4. Hypoxia, scarring and destruction of the pulmonary vascular bed, leading to pulmonary hypertension and cor pulmonale.

## Prognosis

The median age of survival is just over 30 years, but newly born CF sufferers are now expected to live beyond 40 years. Newer drugs, such as DNAase mucolytics and nebulized tobramycin (an antibiotic), appear to reduce the rate of decline. Future treatment goals include the replacement of the defective gene using gene therapy strategies.

# Diffuse interstitial diseases

Interstitial lung diseases are a group of non-infectious, non-malignant disorders in which there is inflammation of the alveolar walls with a thickening of the interstitium between the alveoli, usually with fibrosis. This large group of diseases occurs with a mainly restrictive pattern (see Fig. 7.1).

Disorders can be classified into broad groups, as shown in Figure 7.6. There are thought to be over 200 distinct diffuse interstitial conditions. The most important of these are discussed below.

## Idiopathic pulmonary fibrosis

This disease, of unknown aetiology, is rare but increasing in incidence. It mainly affects the elderly, and males more than females. Fibrosis occurs at the lung bases, resulting in peripheral 'honeycombing'. This describes the appearance of the cut surface of the lung (and can be seen using high-resolution CT scanning).

As with all diseases causing interstitial fibrosis, there is some inflammation involving neutrophil and lymphocyte infiltration. Even the earliest lesions show focal accumulation of fibroblasts; such foci become more collagenous as the disease progresses. Fibrosis results in alveolar wall collapse and the production of cystic spaces.

Macroscopically, the lung is converted into a mass of cystic airspaces separated by areas of dense collagenous scarring.

**Fig. 7.6** A classification scheme for interstitial (parenchymal) lung diseases

| | |
|---|---|
| Known cause or association | Connective tissue disease, e.g. rheumatoid disease, scleroderma<br>Drug- or toxin-induced disease, e.g. nitrofurantoin, amiodarone, methotrexate<br>Pneumoconiosis, e.g. coal-worker's pneumoconiosis, silicosis or asbestosis<br>Extrinsic allergic alveolitis, e.g. farmer's lung, bird fancier's lung |
| Idiopathic interstitial pneumonias | Idiopathic pulmonary fibrosis (IPF)<br>Idiopathic bronchiolitis obliterans organizing pneumonia (BOOP) |
| Granulomatous disease | Sarcoidosis |
| Eosinophilic disease | Idiopathic eosinophilic pneumonia<br>Allergic bronchopulmonary aspergillosis |
| Infections | Miliary tuberculosis<br>Cytomegalovirus<br>*Pneumocystis carinii* |
| Others | Part of a systemic inflammatory disease, e.g. acute respiratory distress syndrome (ARDS)<br>Acute or chronic radiation pneumonitis<br>Diffuse intrapulmonary haemorrhage, e.g. Goodpasture's syndrome<br>Rare disorders, e.g. alveolar proteinosis, histiocytosis |

The clinical feature of the early-stage disease is a slowly increasing respiratory insufficiency due to reduced lung capacity and residual volume, reduced compliance and reduced diffusion capacity.

The characteristic signs are dyspnoea, cough and finger clubbing. There is a restrictive pattern of lung function tests. Median survival is 4 years, although the response to traditional end-stage drug regimens is very variable (usually corticosteroids and azathioprine).

## The pneumoconioses

This is a group of interstitial lung diseases resulting from chronic exposure to inorganic dust. The three most common types of pneumoconioses are coal-worker's pneumoconiosis (CWP), silicosis and asbestosis.

In the normal lung, inhaled dust is coughed out, or ingested by macrophages. However, if the dust is toxic to macrophages there is local inflammation, secretion of cytokines and stimulation of fibrosis. The end result is a restrictive pattern of respiratory dysfunction.

### Coal-worker's pneumoconiosis

CWP is an interstitial lung disease caused by inhaling coal dust. It has three types of pathology:

1. Simple coal-worker's pneumoconiosis—not usually associated with any clinically significant impairment of respiratory function, despite focal aggregates of dust-laden macrophages. The condition does not progress if the affected individual leaves the mining industry.
2. Progressively massive fibrosis—large nodules and scarring results in severe respiratory impairment. The upper lobes are predominantly affected and there may be cavitation of the nodules. This condition may progress even after leaving the mining industry.
3. Caplan's syndrome—associated with rheumatoid disease, where the nodules appear large, carbon pigmented and rheumatoid.

### Silicosis

This is caused by the inhalation of quartz-containing dust (quartz being silicon dioxide), which is abundant in stone and sand.

It is associated with occupations such as slate mining, quarrying and stone masonry.

*Pathogenesis*—silicates are toxic to macrophages, which stimulate cytokine generation precipitating inflammation with fibrosis and nodule formation.

Tuberculosis is a common complication of silicosis (silicotuberculosis). This is thought to be due to impaired local defences as a consequence of accumulated silica in macrophages.

### Asbestosis

This interstitial lung disease is caused by the inhalation of asbestos, a fibrous silicate mineral that was widely used between 1890 and 1970. It is associated with occupations involving asbestos mining/processing, the building industry, insulating and fire-resistant material and shipyard and ship's engine-room work. There are two main forms of asbestos:

1. Serpentine asbestos (white asbestos)—this is the most common form; fibres persist in the lung for a limited time.
2. Amphibole asbestos (blue and brown asbestos)—fibres persist in the lung for many years and are the main cause of malignant mesothelioma.

Risk of disease depends on the duration and intensity of exposure, and the type of asbestos (short fibres are less pathogenic).

The characteristics of asbestosis are:

• there is usually a latent period of 25 years before clinical symptoms become evident
• interstitial fibrosis is maximal at lung bases and asbestos bodies may be seen histologically. Asbestos bodies are fibres coated in acid mucopolysaccharides and haemosiderin
• the disease progresses with an increasing restrictive defect associated with interstitial fibrosis
• pulmonary hypertension and cor pulmonale develop in the late stages.

## Sarcoidosis

Sarcoidosis is a multisystem disease of unknown aetiology characterized by the presence of non-caseating granulomas primarily affecting the lymph nodes and lungs.

Maximum incidence is in people between 30 and 40 years of age, affecting slightly more females than males.

Other affected sites are the skin, eyes, liver, spleen, nervous system, phalanges, parotid glands and (rarely) the heart.

The aetiopathogenesis is unknown but thought to involve the type IV hypersensitivity reaction. The disease seems to be less common in smokers and more common with increasing geographical distance from the equator.

Histology shows non-caseating histiocytic granulomas in the lung interstitium. Patients with lung involvement present with slowly progressive dyspnoea and cough and are found to have lung shadowing on chest radiograph with enlargement of the hilar lymph nodes.

*Diagnosis*—there are no diagnostic blood tests for sarcoidosis, but there is often hypercalcaemia, raised serum angiotensin converting enzyme and a reduced tuberculin skin test. The definitive diagnosis is histological, requiring a tissue sample, e.g. skin lesion biopsy, transbronchial biopsy.

Treatment involves steroid therapy in progressive disease.

**Fig. 7.7** Causes of extrinsic allergic alveolitis (Redrawn with permission from medicshandbook.com)

| Disease | Inhaled antigen |
|---|---|
| Bird-fancier's and pigeon-fancier's lung | Proteins in bird droppings |
| Farmer's lung (exposure to mould hay) | *Micropolyspora faeni, Thermoactinomyces vulgaris* |
| Malt worker's lung | *Aspergillus clavatus* |
| Bagassosis (exposure to molasses) | *Thermoactinomyces sacchari* |

## Other interstitial lung diseases

Other interstitial lung diseases of note are:

- Goodpasture's syndrome—a diffuse pulmonary haemorrhagic syndrome caused by complement activation following autoantibody binding to the basement membrane.
- Idiopathic pulmonary haemosiderosis—a rare condition with type II pneumocyte hyperplasia.
- Rheumatoid disease—the lung and pleura are affected in 10–15% of patients.
- Extrinsic allergic alveolitis—immune mediated interstitial granulomatous inflammation caused by inhalation of organic agents (type III and type IV hypersensitivity). Examples include farmer's lung and pigeon-fancier's lung. See figures 7.6, 7.7.

## INFECTIONS OF THE LUNGS

### Pneumonia

Pneumonia is defined as the infection of alveolar tissue resulting in the consolidation of lung tissue with an intra-alveolar inflammatory exudate.

Pneumonia is the fifth most common cause of death in the USA. It is most common in the very young and the elderly.

## Predisposing factors

Although pneumonia frequently occurs in previously healthy individuals, it is also predisposed by the presence of debility and immobility:

- Suppressed cough reflex, e.g. in coma, anaesthesia and neuromuscular junction disorders
- Impaired mucociliary clearance, e.g. through cigarette smoke, irritant gases, viral diseases (e.g. influenza) and genetic conditions (e.g. immotile cilia syndrome)
- Pulmonary oedema, e.g. due to right-sided cardiac failure

- Impaired alveolar macrophages—alcohol, cigarette smoke, oxygen toxicity
- Retention of secretions due to COPD
- Immunosuppression, e.g. drugs (cytotoxics and immunosuppressives), AIDS, congenital immunodeficiencies and leukaemias
- Drugs—previous course of broad-spectrum antibiotics or cytotoxics
- instrumentation—endotracheal intubation or mechanical ventilation
- prior viral respiratory tract infection
- other—prolonged hospitalization, general debility, immobility.

> **HINTS AND TIPS**
>
> Remember **INSPIRATION** for the predisposing factors of pneumonia:
> - **I**mmunosuppression
> - **N**eurological impairment of the cough reflex
> - **S**ecretion retention
> - **P**ulmonary oedema
> - **I**mpaired mucociliary clearance
> - **R**espiratory tract infection (viral)
> - **A**ntibiotics and cytotoxics
> - **T**racheal instrumentation
> - **I**mpaired alveolar macrophages
> - **O**ther
> - **N**eoplasia.

## Classification

Pneumonia can be classified according to:

- microbiology—causative organism may be bacterial, viral, fungal or protozoal
- pattern of spread of infection—either lobar or bronchopneumonia
- clinical classification—according to circumstances surrounding the development of disease, e.g. community acquired, hospital acquired, disease of immunosuppression or aspiration pneumonia.

## Causative organisms

Bacterial infection is the most common type of pneumonia, accounting for 80–90% of cases. Knowledge of the circumstances in which a person develops pneumonia is a strong clue as to the likely organism causing the infection (Fig. 7.8).

The clinical features are fever, shortness of breath, cough, pleuritic pain and sputum (occasionally with haemoptysis). There are signs of consolidation with bronchial breathing and/or coarse crackles. Confusion, uraemia, tachypnoea (raised respiratory rate) and hypotension are signs suggestive of severe infection requiring hospital admission.

As a general rule of thumb, community-acquired pneumonia is usually caused by Gram-positive bacteria whereas hospital-acquired pneumonias are mainly due to Gram-negative bacteria.

## Bronchopneumonia

Infection is centred on the bronchi but with the extension of the inflammatory exudate into the alveoli, causing a patchy consolidation of the lung (lobular distribution). Bronchopneumonia is illustrated in Figure 7.9.

The condition primarily affects the very young, very old or debilitated patients.

The infecting organism depends on whether the infection is hospital or community acquired, but it is quite often of the hospital-acquired variety due to underlying disease.

### Pathogenesis

Patients develop retention of secretions, which gravitate to dependent parts of the lungs and become infected, hence bronchopneumonia most commonly involves the lower lobes.

Macroscopically, multiple areas of consolidation usually occur distributed bilaterally around bronchi/bronchioles in dependent parts of the lung. Affected areas are firm and airless and have a dark red or grey

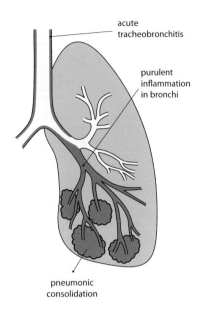

**Fig. 7.9** Bronchopneumonia.

appearance. Bronchial mucosa is inflamed and pus may be present in the more peripheral bronchi. Patchy collapse is associated with bronchial obstruction. Involvement of the pleura is common with purulent pleuritis.

Microscopically, there is acute inflammation of the bronchi and bronchioles with an acute inflammatory neutrophil-rich exudate present in the lumina and extending into the peribronchial alveoli.

Complications and sequelae are as follows:

- resolution—complete resolution occurs only if treatment is instituted early, before the onset of structural damage
- bronchial damage—imperfect repair of the bronchial mucosa results in scarring of the bronchial wall, with increased predisposition to further infection and to bronchiectasis

**Fig. 7.8** Common pathogenic bacteria in hospital- and community-acquired pneumonia

| Community-acquired infection | Hospital-acquired infection |
|---|---|
| Streptococcus pneumoniae (> 60%) | Klebsiella |
| Haemophilus influenzae | Pseudomonas |
| Legionella pneumophilus | Acinetobacter |
| Staphylococcus aureus | Methicillin resistant Staphylococcus aureus (MRSA) |
| Mycoplasma pneumoniae | Escherichia coli |
| Chlamydia pneumoniae | Proteus |
| Chlamydia psittaci | Serratia<br>As well as organisms responsible for community-acquired pneumonia (but much less frequently) |

- lung fibrosis—inflammatory exudate is often not completely absorbed but is organized with residual fibrous scarring
- lung abscesses—single or multiple areas of suppurationa
- empyema—pus in the pleural cavity as a result of extension of infection into the pleural cavity
- pericarditis—direct extension of infection to the pericardium
- death—very common cause of death, particularly as a terminal manifestation of debilitating diseases.

## Lobar pneumonia

This is a uniform or homogenous consolidation of part of a lobe or of the whole lobe caused by infection (Fig. 7.10). The condition often affects otherwise healthy adults, primarily between the ages of 20 and 50 years old. Individuals living in poor social conditions, and alcoholics who have reduced access to good medical care, are particularly prone to this pattern of pneumonia, which is often caused by *Streptococcus pneumoniae*.

### Pathogenesis

Organisms gain entry to distal air spaces without colonization of bronchi. Infection spreads rapidly through the alveolar spaces and bronchioles, causing acute inflammatory exudation into air spaces.

Macroscopically, the whole lobe becomes consolidated and airless.

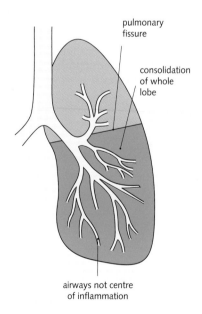

pulmonary fissure

consolidation of whole lobe

airways not centre of inflammation

**Fig. 7.10** Lobar pneumonia.

Microscopically, the alveoli are filled with an acute inflammatory exudate, which is limited by the pulmonary fissures.

There are four pathological stages of lobar pneumonia:

1. Congestion—outpouring of protein-rich exudate into the alveolae
2. Red hepatization—massive accumulation of red cells and polymorphs in the alveolar spaces, giving a liver-like consistency (hence 'hepatization')
3. Grey hepatization—accumulation of fibrin in the lung spaces with red-cell disintegration
4. Resolution—most patients recover with their lungs returning to normal structure and function.

Complications and sequelae are as follows:

- Lung fibrosis—inflammatory exudate is often not completely absorbed but is organized with residual fibrous scarring and permanent lung dysfunction.
- Bacteraemia—bacterial dissemination of organisms can lead to septicaemia with meningitis, arthritis, endocarditis or pyemic abscesses.
- Lung abscesses—single or multiple areas of suppuration.
- Empyema—pus in the pleural cavity as a result of extension of infection into the pleural cavity.
- Pleural effusion—non-infected effusion is common.
- Death.

## Primary atypical pneumonia

This is an inflammation of the alveolar septa by inflammatory cells (acute interstitial pneumonitis) in the absence of any consolidation. Patients develop fever, dry cough and dyspnoea, but there is little sputum and few signs of consolidation, hence the term 'atypical' pneumonia. It may be caused by several factors including infection by viruses, *Mycoplasma*, *Chlamydia* and *Rickettsia* species.

### Viral pneumonia

This is a common cause of pneumonia in early childhood but is much less frequent in healthy adults. The majority of viral lung infections cause an atypical pneumonia, which is typically self-limiting (e.g. cytomegalovirus, measles or varicella). However, these infections can prove fatal in an immunocompromised host.

A minority of viruses cause a much more severe pattern of infection. The influenza viruses can cause an acute fulminating pneumonia with pulmonary haemorrhage; the clinical course may be rapidly fatal.

A common complication is secondary infection with pyogenic bacteria, due to the stripping of the respiratory epithelium by the initial viral infection. This can transform a mild viral lung infection into a severe suppurative bronchopneumonia, particularly after influenza infection.

### Mycoplasma

*Mycoplasma* species account for 15–20% of community-acquired pneumonia. It is more common in children between 5 and 15 years old, but more serious in adults. The organisms cause a low-grade, chronic, atypical pneumonia that can result in pulmonary fibrosis. It may occur in epidemics.

### Chlamydia and Rickettsia

A number of chlamydial and rickettsial infections are complicated by the development of pneumonia. Such infections include typhus, psittacosis and Q fever. Fatal cases are rare, except in psittacosis.

## Pneumonia in the immunocompromised

The lungs of immunocompromised patients are extremely prone to disease by opportunistic infections, i.e. infections caused by microorganisms that are non-pathogenic to healthy, immunocompetent individuals.

Common opportunistic agents include:

- viruses—cytomegalovirus, respiratory syncytial virus, varicella-zoster virus, measles (see primary atypical pneumonia, above). Cytomegalovirus pneumonitis is particularly common after bone marrow transplantation
- fungi—both *Candida* and *Aspergillus* can cause widespread areas of necrosis with the formation of microabscesses containing characteristic hyphae, e.g. invasive pulmonary aspergillosis. Mortality is high
- protozoa—*Pneumocystis carinii* pneumonia (PCP) is common in AIDS patients, affecting 30–50% of cases. Alveoli are filled with a fine, honeycomb-like material in which the small fungal yeasts of the infection can be seen. This disease has a very high mortality rate in patients with AIDS if not treated.

## Pulmonary tuberculosis

Pulmonary tuberculosis (TB) is a chronic granulomatous infection of the lung caused by *Mycobacterium tuberculosis*. It is overall uncommon in the UK and other developed countries (at about 10 per 100 000, although over 40 per 100 000 in London), but extremely common worldwide (up to 500 per 100 000 in parts of Africa) where it is a leading cause of death.

Rates in the UK are increasing as a result of HIV infection, the increasingly elderly population, overcrowding and social deprivation, immigrant populations and a reduced priority for control. The development of multi-drug-resistant (MDR) tuberculosis has exacerbated this problem.

### Spread

Spread is by various means:

- Inhalation *of Mycobacterium tuberculosis* in the form of droplets (by far the most common mode)
- Ingestion of food or milk
- Inoculation of the skin
- Transplacental spread, i.e. congenital TB.

### Diagnosis

The main form of definitive diagnosis is a positive Ziehl–Neelsen stain of a patient sample (e.g. sputum). Such samples should be cultured and tested to assess drug sensitivity.

### Predisposing factors

These are:

- close contact with infected individuals—increased risk for those living/working in crowded or unhygienic conditions and for healthcare workers
- immunosuppression—the very young, very old, immunosuppressive therapy and other diseases of immunodeficiency, particularly AIDS
- malnourishment
- other diseases—pre-existing chronic lung disease (especially silicosis), diabetes mellitus and alcoholism.

### Pathogenesis

The destructive effects of infection are entirely due to the hypersensitivity reaction of the host directed against bacterial cell-wall constituents. The following sequence of events occurs:

1. 0–10 days—mycobacteria excite a transient but marked acute inflammatory response. Neutrophils phagocytose the organisms but are unable to destroy them, as the cell walls are resistant to degradation. Instead, engulfed bacteria are drained into local lymph nodes.
2. After 10 days—development of a T-cell-mediated immune response (type IV hypersensitivity reaction) to the bacillary cell-wall constituents results in cytokine release and macrophage activation. Gradually a chronic inflammatory pattern develops, which is dominated by aggregates of macrophages called epithelioid cells, which form variable numbers of granulomas (see Chapter 2) with a central core of necrotic caseous tissue containing viable mycobacteria. Tuberculous granulomas are termed tubercles.

Macroscopically, the granulomas appear as pinhead-sized white or greyish foci (tubercles) in the tissues.

Microscopically, granulomas are the histological hallmark of TB infection. A granuloma consists of a central area of amorphous caseous necrosis, surrounded by three cellular layers:

1. An inner layer of activated macrophages (epithelioid cells) with Langhans' giant cells
2. A middle layer of lymphocytes
3. An outer layer of fibroblastic tissue, which merges with surrounding structures and increases with the age of the lesion.

The healing of a granuloma occurs slowly, with progressive fibrosis and later calcification. The central necrotic area remains caseous for some time and mycobacteria may remain viable indefinitely within a healed lesion. This is partly due to the ability of the *Mycobacterium tuberculosis* to remain latent within macrophages (inside phagosomes), inhibiting the fusion of lysosomes. Reactivation results in secondary (or post primary) tuberculosis.

TB can be classified into two types, according to the pattern of infection:

1. Primary infection—the first encounter with the organism, resulting in the development of a small parenchymal peripheral focus with a large response in the draining lymph nodes.
2. Secondary infection—reactivation or reinfection of a previously infected individual, resulting in the development of a large, localized, parenchymal reaction but with minimal lymph-node involvement.

## Primary tuberculosis

The lung is by far the most common site of primary infection, usually occurring in a child or young adult with no specific immunity. Other sites include the pharynx, larynx, skin and intestine.

Inhaled organisms proliferate in the alveoli at the periphery of the lung, often just beneath the pleura. This primary parenchymal tubercle is termed the Ghon focus. It is often associated with enlarged caseous hilar lymph nodes. The combination of lung and lymph node lesions together constitutes the primary complex or Ghon complex.

Primary tuberculosis will either resolve or progress as shown below.

### Resolution

This occurs in the majority of cases (85–90%) and the episode is often entirely asymptomatic. The Ghon focus and caseating granulomas in the lymph nodes heal with fibrosis. The disease does not progress due to the confinement of organisms within a fibrotic shell. However, walled-off bacteria may remain viable within the healed primary complex (latent tuberculosis). A tuberculin skin test becomes positive 1–2 months after the onset of infection.

### Progression

In patients with poor immunity, the disease is progressive. There is a further spread of mycobacteria with continuing enlargement of the caseating granulomas in the lymph nodes (progressive primary TB). Enlarging nodes spread the infection by eroding into adjacent structures in two ways:

1. Bronchus—erosion of an infected lymph node into a bronchus results in tuberculous bronchopneumonia (Fig. 7.11A). The bacilli pass down into the bronchi of one lung where infection can then spread into the opposite lung. There is further spread of infection into the bronchioles and alveoli with the development of extensive, confluent, caseating, granulomatous lesions. This condition is known as 'galloping consumption' and it is usually rapidly fatal.
2. Blood vessel—erosion of an infected lymph node into a blood vessel results in haematogenous spread of mycobacteria to many parts of the body, including the remainder of the lung, causing miliary tuberculosis (Fig. 7.11B).

Direct lymphatic spread (i.e. without erosion) may allow spread to the pleura and pericardium.

## Secondary tuberculosis

This occurs as a result of the reactivation of quiescent but viable mycobacteria in hosts with weakened immune responses, or as a result of reinfection by additional organisms. Reactivation occurs in 5–10% of those with latent infection, usually in the lungs.

Caseous granulomas typically develop in the apical segments of the lungs, spreading directly and locally but without lymph node lesions. The initiating apical lesion is often called an Assmann focus, and it is histologically similar to the Ghon focus.

Secondary tuberculosis will either resolve or spread as shown below.

### Resolution

Spontaneous healing with fibrosis and calcification occurs, though viable organisms may remain without producing any clinical symptoms.

### Spread

In adults with poor immune responses, secondary tuberculosis progresses locally with direct extension and continuing caseation. Further spread of mycobacteria produces various types of progressive tuberculosis:

- Apical cavitation fibrocaseous tuberculosis—a direct extension of the infection. Continuing caseation results in the formation of a large caseous mass

**Fig. 7.11**  Patterns of progressive pulmonary tuberculosis. (A) Tuberculous bronchopneumonia. (B) Miliary tuberculosis of the lung.

A

B

surrounded by a thin cellular wall. If caseous material is expectorated, a cavity results. The lesion can heal at this stage but it may spread further into the bronchi, bloodstream or directly into the pleura.

- Tuberculous pneumonia (see above).

- Miliary tuberculosis—the disease becomes widely disseminated with numerous small granulomas in many organs. Common target tissues are the kidneys, liver, bone marrow and meninges; disease can, therefore, occur in any of these tissues.

Complications are usually the result of extensive fibrosis involved in the healing process:

- Pulmonary fibrosis—lung lesions typically heal with fibrosis, which may be extensive, producing localized honeycombing. This is common in relapsing and progressive untreated disease.
- Pleural fibrosis with obliteration of the pleural space.
- Bronchiectasis—scarring of the bronchial walls can cause distal pulmonary collapse, secondary infection and bronchiectasis.

Immunization with the BCG vaccine is common practice in the UK, with a protective efficacy of 80%. Treatment of infected individuals involves initial therapy with three drugs (rifampicin, isoniazid and pyrazinamide), followed by continued therapy with rifampicin and isoniazid only. Total treatment lasts 6 months. Ethambutol is added to the regimen where drug resistance is likely (e.g. in HIV-positive patients) and the total treatment time may be extended.

### HINTS AND TIPS

Tuberculosis is a good example of a chronic inflammatory disease. Remember that primary pulmonary tuberculosis has a small granulomatous focus but large lymph node response. By contrast, secondary disease presents with large granulomatous disease (potentially in a number of different tissues) and minimal lymph node involvement.

## NEOPLASTIC DISEASES OF THE LUNGS

## Bronchogenic carcinoma

Bronchogenic carcinoma is the most common cause of death from neoplasia in the UK, affecting 30 000 people per year. Males are affected more than females, but there is an increasing incidence in women. The peak incidence is between the ages of 40 and 70 years, reflecting the cumulative exposure to several potential causative carcinogens. The risk factors include:

- cigarette smoking—the earlier the age at which smoking starts and the more cigarettes smoked result in an increased risk. Cigarette smoke contains a large number of carcinogens, e.g. polycyclic hydrocarbons. There is a steady decline in risk if smoking stops
- occupational factors, such as exposure to radioactive material, asbestos, nickel, chromium, iron oxides and coal gas plants
- environmental factors, such as radon (a natural radioactive gas in certain geographic areas)

- pulmonary fibrosis—somewhat controversial, but it appears that there is an increased risk of carcinoma development in areas of lung affected by fibrosis.

There are four main histological types of lung carcinoma (Fig. 7.12):

1. Squamous cell carcinoma—35%
2. Small cell carcinoma ('oat cell carcinoma')—20%
3. Adenocarcinoma (including bronchioalveolar carcinoma)—30%
4. Large cell anaplastic carcinoma—15%.

A small proportion of tumours are mixed adenosquamous carcinoma.

Tumours may be central (all types) or peripheral (mainly adenocarcinomas).

Central or hilar tumours (70%) arise in relation to the main bronchi extending into the bronchial lumen and invading the adjacent lung.

Peripheral tumours (30%) arise in peripheral airways or alveoli, often occurring in relation to scars and frequently extending to the pleural surface.

The routes of spread are as follows:

- Local—central tumours invade locally either through the bronchial wall into the surrounding lung or along the outside of the bronchi (peribronchial spread) to distant parts of the lung. Direct extension into pleura and adjacent mediastinal structures is a feature of advanced disease. Apical lung tumours (Pancoast tumours) may invade local sympathetic ganglia and produce Horner's syndrome (ptosis, miosis and anhidrosis).
- Lymphatic spread—carcinomas spread to the ipsilateral and contralateral peribronchial and hilar lymph nodes. Compression of adjacent tissues by infiltrated nodes may then cause symptoms.
- Transcoelomic spread—tumour cells may seed within the pleural cavity, causing a malignant pleural effusion.
- Haematogenous spread—most commonly to the brain, bone, liver, adrenal glands and skin.

## Histological types

### Squamous cell carcinoma

This is the most common type of lung cancer. It is thought to be derived from metaplastic squamous epithelium, which develops to line the main bronchi as a result of exposure to agents such as cigarette smoke.

Tumours are typically central and close to the carina, frequently presenting with features related to bronchial obstruction. Compared with other types, they are relatively slow growing and metastasize outside the thorax late; they may be resectable.

Histologically, the tumours show a range of differentiation, from well-differentiated lesions producing lots

**Fig. 7.12** Summary of histological types of lung cancers

| | Small cell | Squamous | Large cell | Adenocarcinoma |
|---|---|---|---|---|
| Relative incidence | 20% | 35% | 15% | 30% |
| Sex differences | Males > females | Males > females | Males > females | Males = females |
| Associated with cigarette smoking | Yes | Yes | Yes | No? (passive smoking) |
| Most common site | Centrally located | Centrally located | Centrally located | Peripherally located; often originating in areas of pre-existing lung scarring |
| Non-metastatic symptoms | ADH secretion Ectopic ACTH secretion Lambert–Eaton myasthenic syndrome | Hypercalcaemia HPOA | — | HPOA |
| Rate of growth | Fast; metastases usually present at diagnosis | Slow growing; metastasizes late | Fast | Slow growing; metastasizes early |

*Note: ACTH, adrenocorticotrophic hormone; ADH, antidiuretic hormone; HPOA, hypertrophic pulmonary osteoarthropathy*

of keratin through to poorly differentiated lesions with only a few keratin-producing cells.

## Small cell (oat cell) carcinoma
These highly malignant tumours arise from the bronchial endocrine or APUD cells. They contain a few dense secretory granules that are also seen in greater numbers in bronchial carcinoid tumours. Therefore, small cell carcinoma is thought to represent a type of neuroendocrine tumour.

Due to their endocrine nature, this form of cancer can be associated with paraneoplastic syndrome, the most frequent of which is adrenocorticotropic hormone (ACTH); also of note is the syndrome of inappriopriate ADH secretion (SIADH). Squamous cell carcinoma is associated with parathyroid hormone-like activity.

Macroscopically, these tumours are usually centrally located and they are associated with a rapid rate of growth. Metastases are usually present at the time of diagnosis.

Microscopically, the cells are round to oval and have little cytoplasm. All small cell carcinomas are considered high grade.

## Large cell anaplastic carcinoma
This poorly differentiated tumour is thought to be of either squamous or adenocarcinoma origin. Lesions may be central or peripheral and they are composed of large cells with nuclear pleomorphism and frequent giant cell forms. They have a poor prognosis and are frequently widely disseminated at the time of diagnosis.

## Adenocarcinoma
This tumour is derived from glandular cells, such as mucous goblet cells, Clara cells, or type II pneumocytes. A proportion of adenocarcinomas are thought to originate in areas of pre-existing lung scarring or fibrosis (scar cancers). Adenocarcinoma has the slowest rate of growth and is the most common form of lung cancer in women. It can be linked to passive cigarette smoking and characteristically develops peripherally. There are four main histological patterns:

1. Acinar—prominent gland-like spaces lined by columnar epithelium
2. Papillary—fronds of tumour on thin septa
3. Solid carcinoma with mucin production—poorly differentiated lesions
4. Bronchioalveolar carcinoma (see below).

### HINTS AND TIPS

Cigarette smoking is the major risk factor for the development of neoplastic diseases of the lung. It is thought to be responsible for over 90% of all lung carcinomas. Passive smoking has been linked to approximately 5% of all lung cancers.

## Clinical features of lung cancer

There are no early symptoms of lung cancer; it is usual for a lesion to have been growing for many years before clinical presentation. The presentations of lung cancer are outlined in Figure 7.13 and they can be classified into:

- pulmonary symptoms—most common types of presenting symptom including cough, dyspnoea, chest pain and haemoptysis
- metastatic symptoms—metastatic spread is present in 70% of patients at presentation; 30% present with symptoms caused by metastatic disease
- local symptoms—local spread within the thorax can cause superior vena cava syndrome (compression of SVC results in facial swelling), Horner's syndrome and hoarseness
- non-metastatic extrapulmonary syndromes (paraneoplastic syndromes)—lung cancer frequently causes systemic syndromes that are not associated with metastatic effects and these may rarely be a presenting feature of disease
- asymptomatic: finding a lesion on chest X-ray or CT scan.

Diagnosis is through clinical features (see above), imaging (chest X-ray and CT scans) and histological confirmation techniques:

- Bronchoscopy—tumour biopsy obtained
- Cytology of pleural effusion.

**Fig. 7.13** Clinicopathological features of lung cancer

| Cause | Clinical features |
|---|---|
| **Pulmonary involvement** | |
| | Cough (80%): infection distal to airway blocked by tumour<br>Haemoptysis (70%): ulceration of tumour in bronchus<br>Dyspnoea (60%): local extension of tumour<br>Chest pain (40%): involvement of pleura and/or chest wall<br>Wheeze (15%): narrowing of airways<br>Systemic features: weight loss, anorexia and malaise |
| **Local spread** | |
| | Horner's syndrome: local invasion of cervical sympathetic ganglion<br>Hoarseness: spread to the left hilar region may cause recurrent laryngeal nerve palsy<br>Pain in T1 dermatome and wasting of intrinsic hand muscles: caused by brachial neuritis as a result of direct invasion of plexus by apical tumours<br>Pericarditis: due to direct tumour invasion |
| **Metastatic spread** | |
| | Pathological fracture<br>CNS symptoms (brain metastasis)<br>Hepatomegaly or jaundice (liver metastasis) |
| **Non-metastatic extrapulmonary syndromes** | |
| Endocrine disturbances | Inappropriate ADH secretion: by small cell carcinoma and characterized by low sodium and plasma osmolality with high urine osmolality<br>Ectopic ACTH secretion: caused by small cell carcinoma and associated with Cushing's syndrome<br>Hypercalcaemia: caused by secretion of parathyroid hormone-related peptide by a squamous cell carcinoma |
| Neurological syndromes | Peripheral sensory motor neuropathy<br>Cerebellar degeneration causing ataxia<br>Proximal myopathy<br>Dermatomyositis<br>Lambert–Eaton myasthenic syndrome: associated with small cell tumours |
| Hypertrophic pulmonary osteoarthropathy (HPOA) | Finger clubbing<br>Swelling of wrists and ankles with periosteal new bone formation (seen in 2–3% of squamous cell carcinomas and adenocarcinomas) |

Note: ACTH, adrenocorticotrophic hormone.

## Prognosis and staging

Histological types and the stage of lung cancer determine the outcome and its likely response to treatment. Survival is better for early stage disease, except for small cell carcinoma (very early metastases).

The staging system used for lung cancer is shown in Figures 7.14 and 7.15.

## Treatment

### Surgical intervention

Tumours are classified as either operable or inoperable, according to the stage of the disease. For example, distant metastases and advanced local spread are contraindications for surgical resection.

Only 10% of all lung tumours are considered operable at diagnosis. Many patients are unsuitable for surgery due to comorbidities (e.g. poor cardiac status). However, 5-year survival rates are as high as 75% in carefully selected patients with early disease (stage 1).

### Radiotherapy and chemotherapy

Tumours are grouped into two categories according to differences in prognosis and response to radiotherapy and chemotherapy:

1. Small cell lung carcinoma—very sensitive to radiotherapy and chemotherapy. However, the disease is usually extensive at diagnosis such that survival is still poor despite local control of tumour growth. Treatment offers good palliation of pain, cough and dyspnoea. Therapy produces a median survival of 11 months (compared with 3 months if untreated) and a 1-year survival of 45%.
2. Non-small cell lung carcinoma (squamous, large-cell and adenocarcinoma); inoperable cases may be treated with radiotherapy depending on clinical circumstances. The role of chemotherapy is limited. Overall prognosis is poor with only a 50% 2-year survival without spread, 10% with spread.

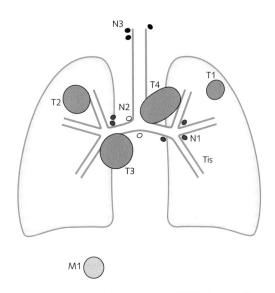

**Fig. 7.15**   Tumour, node, metastasis (TNM) staging of lung cancer.

Figure 7.12 summarizes the main histological types of lung cancer.

**Clinical Note**

Combination chemotherapy for small cell lung cancer often involves intravenous cyclophosphamide, doxorubicin and vincristine given in cycles lasting 3 weeks each. Although small cell cancer is very sensitive to this therapy, it has almost always metastasized by the time of treatment. Radiotherapy alone is rarely radical (curative) in lung cancer but is of great use in the palliation of symptoms such as superior vena cava obstruction and pain caused by invasion of the chest wall.

**Fig. 7.14** Tumour, node, metastasis (TNM) staging of lung cancer

| Stage | TNM group | Clinical |
|---|---|---|
| Stage I | TI N0 M0<br>T1 N1 M0 | Tumour < 3 cm; distal to origin of lobar bronchus (T1)<br>With (N1) or without (N0) spread to ipsilateral hilar nodes<br>No metastases (M0) |
| Stage II | T2 N0 M0<br><br>T2 N1 M0 | Tumour > 3 cm, 2 cm distal to the carina, which invades visceral pleural (T2)<br>With (N1) or without (N0) spread to ipsilateral hilar nodes<br>No metastases (M0) |
| Stage III | All T3/T4 cases<br><br>All N3 cases<br>All M1 cases | All tumours involving the carina; involving mediastinal structures (T3/T4)<br>All tumours with spread to contralateral nodes (N3)<br>All cases of metastases (M1) |

## Bronchioalveolar carcinoma

This is a special type of adenocarcinoma derived from alveolar or bronchial epithelial cells (Clara cells and type II pneumocytes). There are two types:

1. Multifocal diffuse infiltrative tumours—replace areas of lung in a manner resembling pneumonic consolidation. Cells are tall, columnar, have few mitoses and secrete mucin.
2. Single, grey masses of tumour up to 10 cm in diameter—cells are cuboidal with hyperchromatic nuclei and mitoses. Cells form papillary structures; there is often no mucin secretion. In the absence of metastases, this subtype has a better prognosis than other forms of lung cancer.

## Secondary tumours of the lung

Metastatic deposits may spread to the lungs from distant primary sites, most often from carcinomas of the breast, kidney, uterus, ovary, testes and thyroid. Spread is usually via the blood, most commonly resulting in bilateral deposits.

## Carcinoid tumours

These are neuroendocrine tumours of the lungs, representing about 5% of all pulmonary neoplasms. The majority are benign, although a minority has the potential for local recurrence or metastasis (atypical pulmonary neuroendocrine tumours).

In contrast to intestinal carcinoid tumours, most pulmonary lesions do not secrete 5-hydroxytryptamine (serotonin).

## Bronchial hamartomas

These are common but benign lesions of the lung, usually 1–3 cm in diameter and consisting largely of cartilage. They are firm and glistening white in appearance (often termed chondromas). Other elements are bronchial epithelium, fat and muscle. Bronchial hamartomas are asymptomatic and are mainly discovered at post-mortem examination.

## Miscellaneous mesenchymal tumours

These tumours can be either benign (e.g. neurofibromas, lipomas) or malignant (sarcomas are extremely rare in the lung).

## DISEASES OF VASCULAR ORIGIN

## Pulmonary congestion and oedema

Pulmonary oedema is defined as an increase in extravascular fluid in the alveolar walls (pulmonary interstitium), which, if severe, subsequently affects the alveolar spaces.

## Pathogenesis

Normally, a balance exists between hydrostatic pressure and colloid osmotic (oncotic) pressure such that only a small amount of fluid passes into the interstitium. This fluid is drained from the lung via lymphatic channels.

Pulmonary oedema can result from increased hydrostatic pressure (left ventricular failure) or increased alveolar capillary permeability (inflammatory aloveolar reactions) where the lymphatic drainage capacity is exceeded, resulting in a net accumulation of fluid within the interstitium.

Macroscopically, the lungs are heavy and congested. In fatal cases, fluid flows from the cut surfaces and it can often be seen in the large airways.

Microscopically, the interstitium is widened, the capillaries are congested and the alveoli are filled with proteinaceous fluid.

## Acute respiratory distress syndrome

Acute respiratory distress syndrome (ARDS) is a clinical syndrome of diffuse alveolar capillary damage, characterized by pulmonary exudation and oedema with widespread systemic metabolic derangements.

Many conditions predispose to ARDS, most commonly systemic sepsis and severe trauma. The causes are listed in Figure 7.16.

The exact pathogenesis is unknown in many cases, but events are thought to occur in two phases: an acute exudative phase (with capillary and alveolar endothelium injury) and a late organization phase (cell proliferation and fibrosis). This forms a characteristic intra-alveolar hyaline membrane composed of fibrin and cellular debris, resulting in severe hypoxia.

In severe cases of ARDS, cytokines liberated from the lung vascular bed can enter the systemic circulation and these may cause systemic endothelial activation with massive neutrophil recruitment leading to multiorgan failure.

Figure 7.17 shows the main events and outcomes in ARDS.

**Fig. 7.16** Causes of ARDS

| Cause | Clinical features |
|---|---|
| Blood borne | Major trauma, especially associated with raised intracranial pressure<br>Septicaemia<br>Major burns<br>Disseminated intravascular coagulation<br>Massive blood transfusion<br>Amniotic fluid embolism<br>Acute pancreatitis<br>Cardiac surgery with bypass<br>Antitumour chemotherapy<br>Paraquat poisoning |
| Air borne | Pulmonary aspiration of gastric contents<br>Inhalation of toxic fumes or smoke<br>Near drowning<br>Pneumonia from many causes requiring ventilation |

## Embolism, haemorrhage and infarction

### Pulmonary embolism

Pulmonary embolism (PE) is the occlusion of a pulmonary artery, most commonly by thromboemboli originating in the systemic veins (Fig. 7.18). The condition accounts for 1% of all hospital deaths, but this rises to 30% in patients with severe burns or trauma.

The vast majority of cases are caused by emboli arising from thrombosis of the deep leg veins (calf, popliteal, femoral and iliac veins). Venous thrombosis is considered in more detail in Chapter 6.

The consequences of PE are pulmonary hypertension (which puts a strain on the right side of the heart) and infarction of the lung (which occurs in only about 10% of cases of PE, as dual circulation protects against ischaemic necrosis).

### Clinical features
The effect of PE depends on the extent of the pulmonary vasculature blockage and the time scale involved:

- Massive PE (5% of cases) is a sudden blockage of more than 60% of the pulmonary vasculature, resulting in electromechanical dissociation of the heart, i.e. the heart continues to beat but there is no output as pulmonary vascular resistance is too high. This results in cardiovascular collapse and rapid death. One example is a saddle embolus at the bifurcation of the left and right pulmonary arteries.
- Major PE (10% of cases) is a blockage of the middle-sized pulmonary arteries. These patients commonly

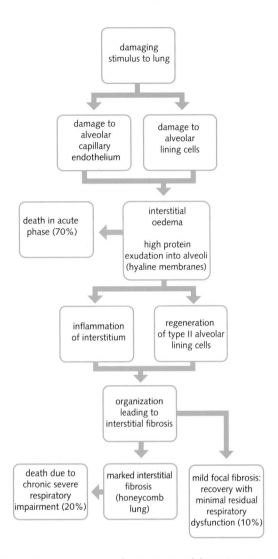

**Fig. 7.17** Main events and outcomes in adult respiratory distress syndrome.

experience breathlessness. Lung infarction develops in about 10% of such cases, which may lead to haemoptysis and pleuritic chest pain, if adjacent to the pleura. If untreated, patients may develop a subsequent massive thromboembolism.

- Minor PE (85% of cases) is a blockage of the small peripheral vessels by small emboli. Patients may be asymptomatic or may experience breathlessness and pleuritic chest pain as a result of small infarcts. As with major pulmonary embolism, patients may develop a subsequent massive thromboembolism if untreated.
- Recurrent minor PE (minority) is a blockage of the many small peripheral arteries over a period of many months by recurrent small emboli. The condition

**Fig. 7.18** Pulmonary thromboembolism. (Adapted from Underwood, 2000.)

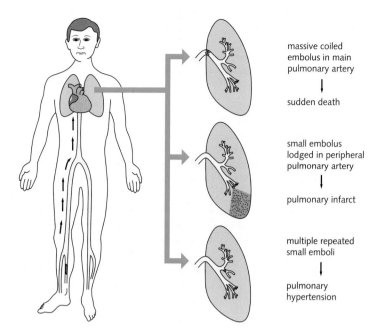

massive coiled embolus in main pulmonary artery

↓

sudden death

small embolus lodged in peripheral pulmonary artery

↓

pulmonary infarct

multiple repeated small emboli

↓

pulmonary hypertension

can lead to the obliteration of the vascular bed with the development of pulmonary hypertension and right heart strain.

### Prevention and treatment

Pulmonary thromboembolism is the most common preventable cause of death in hospital patients. Prevention involves:

- mobilizing early following surgery
- anti-embolic (TED) stockings
- heparin prophylaxis.

Treatment is with oxygen, analgesia and anticoagulation therapy (heparin, warfarin).

### Non-thrombotic emboli

These are rare, but include:

- fat, following a bone fracture
- amniotic fluid during labour
- air (after trauma or surgery)
- decompression sickness, e.g. in deep sea divers ('the bends' or Caisson disease). Rapid decompression releases nitrogen bubbles, which cause problems in the CNS and bones and can produce functional obstruction of the pulmonary vessels
- foreign bodies
- tumour embolism—renal or bronchial cell carcinoma.

## Pulmonary infarction

Infarction of lung tissue is usually associated with embolism.

The lower lobes are involved in 75% of cases. Macroscopically, pulmonary infarcts are typically haemorrhagic (because of blood entering from the bronchial circulation) and wedge shaped, and there is often an associated pleural reaction, which causes chest pain. With time, the infarct becomes organized to form a fibrous scar.

Microscopically, there is extravasation of blood into the necrotic lung.

Common sequelae include:

- pulmonary dysfunction due to the loss of lung tissue
- pulmonary vascular obstruction leading to right heart failure (cor pulmonale)
- pleurisy and pleural effusion
- healing, with fibrous scarring
- septic infarction due to either a primary septic embolism or secondary infection leading to abscess formation.

## Pulmonary hypertension and vascular sclerosis

This is increased pressure of the lung vasculature, the most important being:

- chronic obstructive airways disease
- interstitial fibrosis of the lungs
- chronic pulmonary venous congestion.

Pulmonary hypertension causes irreversible structural changes to:

- pulmonary vasculature—medial hypertrophy of the muscular arteries (increased smooth muscle) and pulmonary veins (arterialization); occlusion of the pulmonary arteries caused by intimal proliferation
- lungs; interstitial fibrosis
- right side of the heart—increased workload of the right side of the heart causes ultimate development of right heart failure (cor pulmonale).

The clinical effects are breathlessness and the symptoms and signs of right-sided cardiac failure.

## Diffuse pulmonary haemorrhagic syndromes

A few interstitial lung disorders may produce diffuse haemorrhage, often with rapid patient deterioration. Important examples include:

- Goodpasture's syndrome—an autoimmune disease resulting in the breakdown of collagen in both lung alveoli and kidney glomeruli
- Wegener's granulomatosis—an autoimmune granulomatous vasculitis affecting blood vessels of the upper respiratory tract and lung
- idiopathic pulmonary haemosiderosis—a rare disorder, probably of immunological origin, that can produce repeated diffuse alveolar haemorrhage, particularly in children.

## DISEASES OF IATROGENIC ORIGIN

## Drug-induced lung disease

Many drugs have pulmonary side effects, such as some anticancer agents that produce chronic pulmonary fibrosis. The calcium channel blocker and antiarrhythmic drug amiodarone can have similar effects.

Asthma can by induced by aspirin (the mechanism for this is unknown) and certain β-blockers (by bronchoconstriction caused by an antagonistic effect on $\beta_2$-receptors of bronchial smooth muscle).

## Complications of radiotherapy

### Acute radiation pneumonitis

Excessive exposure to radiation causes diffuse alveolar damage and is an established cause of ARDS.

### Chronic radiation pneumonitis

Less severe exposure occurring over a longer period of time results in progressive pulmonary fibrosis with the typical restrictive defect of pulmonary function.

## DISORDERS OF THE PLEURA

## Inflammatory pleural effusions

### Serofibrinous pleuritis

This acute inflammation of the pleura is accompanied by an accumulation of high-protein fluid ($>30$ g protein/L; exudate) containing fibrinogen/fibrin between the pleural surfaces.

The condition is commonly due to infection, infarction or tumour.

#### Pathogenesis

Effusion is the result of movement of fluid through damaged vessel walls.

In serofibrinous pleuritis, the effusion is typically unilateral, with the pleural surface covered by a fibrinous exudate. The fluid consists of a straw-coloured fibrinous fluid containing mesothelial cells, lymphocytes and polymorphs. In neoplastic diseases, malignant cells can also be identified within the pleural fluid.

#### Sequelae

Common sequelae include:

- atelectasis—compression of the lungs causes pulmonary collapse and respiratory impairment
- adhesions—formation of fibrous adhesions between the visceral and parietal pleura
- fibrosis—obliteration of the pleural space by fibrosis, which is common in long-standing effusions
- empyema (see below).

### Suppurative pleuritis (empyema)

This is an acute inflammation of the pleura with accumulation of pus in the pleural cavity. Typically caused by pulmonary infection (e.g. pneumonia, tuberculosis, lung abscess), it can also complicate thoracic surgery or penetrating chest wall injury.

Common sequelae include septicaemia (haematogenous spread of infection to other organs) and atelectasis (lung collapse as a result of compression).

### Haemorrhagic pleuritis

This acute inflammation of the pleura occurs with the accumulation of a blood-stained exudate and is often caused by tumour or pulmonary infarcts.

## Non-inflammatory pleural effusions

### Hydrothorax

This collection of low-protein fluid ($<30$ g protein/L; transudate) is due to the movement of excess fluid through normal vessel walls. Common causes are:

- cardiac failure (most common)—increased hydrostatic pressure in pulmonary hypertension
- hypoalbuminaemia—decreased oncotic pressure.

Effusions are usually bilateral and the pleural surface appears normal. Fluid is straw coloured and contains occasional lymphocytes and mesothelial cells.

The condition can cause pulmonary collapse (compression of the lungs causing respiratory impairment) or it may resolve completely (resorption of fluid on correction of the cause with no structural alterations).

## Haemothorax

Bleeding into the chest is called haemothorax. It is most commonly the result of:

- trauma, especially with rib fractures
- surgery
- pulmonary infarction
- spontaneous rupture of diseased arteries, e.g. atheromatous and dissecting aortic aneurysm.

If blood remains within the pleural cavity, the result is organization and pleural fibrosis.

## Chylothorax

The accumulation of chyle (milky white emulsified fat) within the pleural cavity, caused by a leakage from the thoracic duct, is typically the result of malignant infiltration, surgery or trauma.

## Pneumothorax

This is the presence of air in the pleural cavity, the causes of which are described in Figure 7.19.

Spontaneous pneumothorax can be either primary (of unknown cause occurring in otherwise healthy individuals) or secondary (i.e. secondary to lung disease).

Traumatic pneumothorax is a result of chest injury or is iatrogenic.

Complications of pneumothorax include:

- Atelectasis—lung collapse due to compression of the underlying lung.
- Tension pneumothorax—progressive increase in air pressure within the pleural cavity, causing massive collapse of the affected lung, mediastinal shift and compression of the contralateral lung producing life-threatening respiratory insufficiency. The condition occurs as a result of a one-way valve-like mechanism at the point at

**Fig. 7.19** Causes of pneumothorax

| Cause | Type | Clinical features |
|---|---|---|
| Spontaneous | Primary | Idiopathic rupture of pulmonary 'bleb'; most common in thin young males |
| | Secondary | COPD: emphysema, chronic bronchitis and asthma<br>Pneumonia<br>Cystic fibrosis<br>Whooping cough<br>Pleural malignancy |
| Traumatic | Chest injury | Penetrating chest wounds<br>Rib fractures<br>Oesophageal rupture |
| | Iatrogenic | Subclavian cannulation<br>Positive pressure artificial ventilation<br>Pleural aspiration<br>Oesophageal perforation during endoscopy<br>Lung biopsy |
| Note: COPD, chronic obstructive pulmonary disease. | | |

which air enters the pleural cavity. Air that enters the cavity in inspiration is unable to escape during expiration.

## Pleural neoplasia

### Pleural fibroma

This is a benign tumour of submesothelial connective tissue. The causes are unknown but there is no association with asbestos. The tumour is well circumscribed, localized and attached to the pleural surface by a pedicle. Histologically, it is composed of fibroblast-like cells with abundant collagen fibres.

### Metastatic neoplasms

These are the most common pleural tumours, most frequently arising from the lungs, breast or ovary, but they can arise from any malignant tumour. They are usually associated with a high-protein exudate (see above).

### Malignant mesothelioma

This primary neoplasm of the pleura is rare, but is an important cause of death in people previously exposed to asbestos, such as those from the ship building industry. There is a latent interval between asbestos exposure and disease presentation of between 25 and 45 years. Fibres of crocidolite (blue asbestos) are thought to be most important in the development of mesothelioma. These asbestos fibres become trapped in the lung following inhalation and they are particularly resistant to macrophage and neutrophil destruction.

Macroscopically, the tumours are highly malignant and they spread locally around the pleural cavity and pericardium. However, haematogenous/lymphatic metastasis is rare.

Microscopically, mesotheliomas have spindle cells and glandular patterns.

Clinical features include chest pain and breathlessness and there are commonly recurrent or persistent pleural effusions, which may be bloodstained.

### Clinical Note

Asbestos exposure also increases risk of lung cancer. Indeed, an individual exposed to asbestos has a far greater risk of dying from lung cancer than mesothelioma, particularly if they also smoke. However, the number of mesothelioma cases has rapidly risen in the UK over the last 20 years and it is estimated that this trend will continue until at least 2010. No curative treatment is possible and death usually occurs within 10 months of diagnosis.

In this chapter, you will learn to:
- Describe disorders of the upper gastrointestinal tract, most notably those of the oesophagus.
- Understand congenital abnormalities, inflammation, ulceration and neoplasia of the stomach.
- Describe patterns of liver injury, including cirrhosis, and reflect on the resulting complications.
- Recall the causes and mechanisms of liver injury, including infection, alcohol and cancer.
- Describe disorders of the biliary tree and gall bladder.
- Understand pancreatitis and carcinoma of the pancreas.
- Recognize congenital abnormalities, infection and inflammation as potential disorders of the intestine.
- Describe the causes of intestinal malabsorption, obstruction and vascular compromise.
- Discuss neoplastic disease of the intestine and how it develops.
- Understand common pathology of the peritoneum, namely inflammation and tumours.

## DISORDERS OF THE UPPER GASTROINTESTINAL TRACT

## The mouth and oropharynx

### Cleft palate and cleft (hare) lip

These are the most common major congenital malformations of the mouth. They frequently occur together as a result of the same process, namely a failure of fusion during the embryonic period.

*Aetiology*—a few cases are associated with a chromosomal abnormality (e.g. trisomy 13 or 18), but the majority have no identified cause. Retinoic acid (vitamin A) has recently been proposed as having teratogenic activity in the developing palate.

*Morphology*:

- Cleft lip—may be unilateral or bilateral, involving the lip only or extending upwards and backwards to include the floor of the nose and the alveolar ridge (Fig. 8.1).
- Cleft palate—considerable variation, from a small defect in the soft palate (bifid uvula) that causes little disability, to a complete separation of the hard palate combined with a cleft lip (Fig. 8.2).

The effects are an abnormal facial appearance, defective speech and feeding difficulty with extensive lesions (child is unable to suck).

Management is by artificial feeding, with plastic surgery recommended between 1 and 2 years of age.

## Stomatitis

This describes inflammation of the oral cavity, which can be non-infective or infective.

### Non-infective stomatitis

Aphthous ulcers are tiny, painful and shallow, occurring on a background of red mucosa typically on the lips, tongue or buccal mucosa. The ulcer crater is covered by a creamy exudate composed of fibrin and inflammatory cells, mainly neutrophils.

Aetiology and pathogenesis are unknown. These ulcers may be associated with Crohn's disease, coeliac disease and Behçet's syndrome; they also occur in 20% of the normal population.

Most aphthous ulcers spontaneously heal within a week, although they often recur. Occasionally, large ulcers may persist for several weeks before healing by fibrosis.

### Infective stomatitis

The majority of infections of the lips and buccal cavity are due to either viruses or fungi:

- Herpes simplex virus (herpetic stomatitis)—viral infections of the lips and mouth. Usually manifest as large blisters or crops of small painful vesicles, which eventually erode to form shallow tender ulcers. Severe herpetic stomatitis is important in the immunosuppressed (e.g. HIV-positive patients).
- Oral candidiasis—*Candida albicans* infection of the mouth (also known as 'oral thrush'). Common in

**Fig. 8.1** Different types of cleft lip. (A) Median cleft upper lip. (B) Median cleft lower lip. (C) Unilateral cleft lip. (D) Bilateral cleft lip. (E) Oblique facial cleft.

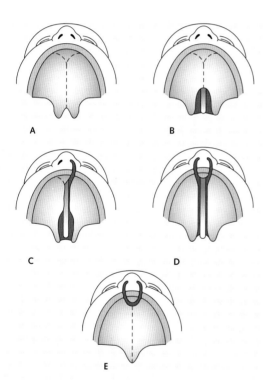

**Fig. 8.2** Different types of cleft palate. (A) Cleft uvula. (B) Cleft soft and hard palate. (C) Total unilateral cleft palate and cleft lip. (D) Total bilateral cleft palate and cleft lip. (E) Bilateral cleft lip and jaw.

infants but less so in adults without diabetes mellitus or immunosuppression. The condition develops as white patches on palatal, buccal and tongue surfaces. Lesions are composed of tangled fungal hyphae mixed with acute inflammatory cells and some desquamated epithelium. Underlying epithelium is acutely inflamed and red.

### Glossitis

This inflammation of the tongue arises either as a result of infective stomatitis (see above) or is due to a deficiency of nutritional factors, especially niacin, riboflavin, folic acid and vitamin $B_{12}$:

- Acute deficiency—tongue is 'beefy-red,' raw and painful because of atrophy of papillae.
- Chronic deficiency—tongue appears moist and unduly clean.

## Precancerous and benign neoplastic disease

### Leucoplakia (keratosis)

This premalignant epithelial dysplasia may precede the development of carcinoma. The condition is characterized by a white patch or plaque (hyperkeratosis) of the oral cavity that cannot be scraped away. The condition usually affects the tongue. All lesions are considered precancerous unless proven otherwise by histological evaluation.

### Erythroplakia (erythroplasia)

Less common than leucoplakia, this is characterized by the presence of red velvety patches of epithelial atrophy and pronounced dysplasia. It is seen mainly in elderly males on the buccal mucosa or the palate.

Malignant transformation is far more common than with leucoplakia. The development of erythroplakia is associated with heavy tobacco use.

## Malignant neoplastic disease

### Squamous cell carcinoma

This is the most common tumour of the mouth, and it is derived from lining epithelium. It may arise from pre-existing dysplasia such as described above. Carcinoma affects 2 per 100 000 in the UK, occurring in men more than women by about 2:1. The risk factors are:

- smoking—direct relationship between number of cigarettes smoked per day and the risk of developing oral cancer
- alcohol—moderate intake = decreased risk; excessive intake = increased risk
- nutritional deficiencies
- viral infections, particularly some forms of human papilloma virus (HPV).

Macroscopically, there are raised nodular lesions and central ulceration with hard raised edges.

Microscopically, the tumour is typically well-differentiated and keratinizing.

The sites are:

- lips (most common)—usually recognized early and amenable to surgery
- tongue—typically occurring on the lateral border of the anterior two-thirds

- cheek or floor of the mouth (less common in the UK)—generally asymptomatic, resulting in extensive local invasion making surgical removal difficult.

*Prognosis*—may infiltrate locally and metastasize to regional lymph nodes in the neck. Five-year survival is about 50%.

## The oesophagus

## Congenital abnormalities

### Oesophageal atresia

In oesophageal atresia, the upper end of the oesophagus is intact, but it ends in a blind pouch. Oesophageal atresia affects 1 per 4000 live births, and more than 85% of cases are associated with the tracheo-oesophageal fistula—an abnormal communication between the lower oesophagus and trachea (Fig. 8.3).

The effects are:

- Fetus—inability to swallow amniotic fluid results in polyhydramnios, the accumulation of an excessive amount of amniotic fluid.
- Neonate—appears healthy initially but swallowed fluid returns through the nose and mouth and respiratory distress occurs. The condition must be surgically corrected in early life, but is also associated with other congenital abnormalities such as those of the heart.

### Webs and rings

These localized constrictions of the oesophagus are caused by mucosal folds or muscular contractions.

In Plummer–Vinson or Paterson–Brown–Kelly syndrome, upper oesophageal webs are associated with dysphagia in patients with iron-deficiency anaemia, cheilosis and glossitis. This is a rare but important condition because of an association with the development of postcricoid oesophageal carcinoma.

## Inflammation of the oesophagus (oesophagitis)

### Reflux oesophagitis

Inflammation of the oesophagus caused by gastro-oesophageal reflux disease (GORD) is the most common oesophageal abnormality and is caused by reflux

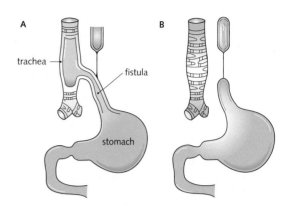

**Fig. 8.3** Oesophageal atresia. (A) Blind ending of oesophagus with fistula formed between lower part and trachea. (B) Oesophageal atresia with no fistulous communication: very rare.

of gastric acid through the lower oesophageal sphincter. The condition affects about 5% of adults; it can occur at any age (but with increased incidence over the age of 55 years), and it affects males more than females.

Figure 8.4 lists the predisposing factors of reflux oesophagitis.

Symptoms are a burning pain in the centre of the lower chest commonly known as 'heartburn'.

The complications are:

- peptic ulceration of lower oesophagus—development of small ulcers which become chronic with fibrosis
- lower oesophageal stricture—progressive fibrous thickening of the lower oesophagus wall producing difficulty in swallowing
- Barrett's oesophagus—metaplasia of lower oesophageal mucosa, with normal squamous epithelium replaced by glandular columnar epithelium composed of tall columnar cells. This increases the risk of oesophageal adenocarcinoma (see below).

Relevant investigations include endoscopy and 24-hour intraluminal pH monitoring.

Management is by:

- lifestyle alterations—weight loss, stopping smoking, avoiding late meals and decreasing alcohol intake

| **Fig. 8.4** Predisposing factors of reflux oesophagitis | |
|---|---|
| Factors that increase intra-abdominal pressure | Overeating/obesity<br>Pregnancy<br>Poor posture |
| Factors that render the lower oesophageal sphincter lax or incompetent | Hiatus hernia<br>Smoking<br>Alcohol ingestion |

- drug therapy—antacids, alginates, $H_2$-receptor antagonists and proton pump inhibitors (severe symptoms)
- surgery—for those not responding to medical therapy, repair of hiatal defects or fundoplication may be appropriate.

### Other causes

Other less common causes of oesophagitis are:

- infective agents—*Candida albicans*, herpes simplex and cytomegalovirus may cause acute oesophagitis in the immunosuppressed
- physical agents—irradiation or ingestion of caustic agents (e.g. suicide attempts)
- desquamative skin diseases, e.g. pemphigoid and epidermolysis bullosa may cause oesophageal ulceration, blistering and eventual erosion.

## Lesions associated with motor dysfunction

### Achalasia

Achalasia is a condition in which peristalsis is abnormal and lack of relaxation of the lower oesophageal sphincter. This may occur at any age but it is mainly seen in middle-aged individuals. The cause is unknown but reduced numbers of ganglion cells in the muscle plexus have been noted in long-standing cases.

The consequences are:

- difficulty in swallowing (dysphagia)—increasing slowly over years
- regurgitation of undigested food
- occasional severe chest pain caused by oesophageal spasm
- mega-oesophagus—oesophageal distension occurs over a period of time
- increased predisposition to development of squamous cell carcinoma of the oesophagus.

### Chagas' disease

Infection by *Trypanosoma cruzi* is a cause of secondary achalasia due to destruction of the myenteric plexus. It is common in South America.

### Hiatus hernia

This is a common condition in which the upper part of the stomach herniates through the diaphragmatic oesophageal opening (hiatus) into the thoracic cavity.

The incidence is 5 per 1000 in the UK but it is 50–100 times less common in Asia and Africa. It may rarely be caused by a congenitally short oesophagus but is mainly thought to arise from increased abdominal pressure and loss of diaphragmatic muscular tone.

There are two types (Fig. 8.5):

1. Sliding hiatus hernia (90%)—stomach herniates through oesophageal diaphragmatic hiatus,

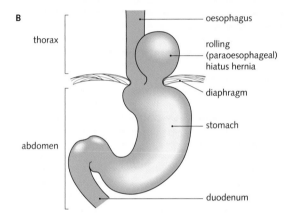

**Fig. 8.5** Types of hiatus hernia. (A) Sliding hiatus hernia. (B) Rolling hiatus hernia.

resulting in the gastro-oesophageal junction moving into the thorax (associated with reflux oesophagitis and peptic ulceration).

2. Rolling (para-oesophageal) hiatus hernia (10%)—the fundus of the stomach protrudes through the hiatus, but the gastro-oesophageal junction remains below the diaphragm (less associated with reflux).

### Lacerations

Oesophageal perforation is rare, but it may be caused by:

- traumatic rupture—usually associated with vomiting
- impaction of a sharp foreign body
- intubation of strictures.

'Mallory–Weiss tear' is a longitudinal oesophageal laceration as a result of severe retching or vomiting. This is most commonly seen in alcoholics, and classically occurs with vomiting of clear fluid (pretearing), followed by vomiting of blood (post-tearing).

# Oesophageal varices

Oesophageal varices are varicosed, dilated submucosal veins in the oesophagus.

The condition is caused by portal hypertension (most commonly associated with cirrhosis of the liver).

## Pathogenesis

Oesophageal veins normally drain into both systemic and portal venous systems.

Increased pressure in the portal venous system (e.g. as a result of severe diffuse long-standing liver disease) causes dilatation of the oesophageal veins, which often protrude into the lumen.

Rupture of these varices, or ulceration of overlying mucosa, can produce a massive haemorrhage into the oesophagus and stomach, often precipitating vomiting of blood (haematemesis).

## Management

There are three stages:

1. Local measures to control bleeding—sclerotherapy, balloon tamponade and transjugular intrahepatic portosystemic stent shunting (TIPSS). TIPSS creates a shunt directly connecting the portal and hepatic veins of the liver, so reducing portal hypertension
2. Reduction of portal venous pressure—drug therapy with terlipressin and somatostatin
3. Prevention of recurrent bleeding—sclerotherapy banding and TIPSS.

# Neoplastic disease

## Barrett's oesophagus

*Definition*—metaplastic replacement of normal squamous oesophageal epithelium with glandular columnar epithelium. Caused by persistent oesophageal reflux; approximately 10% of these patients will develop Barrett's oesophagus.

Barrett's oesophagus predisposes to the development of adenocarcinoma. Metaplastic glandular epithelium can progress to epithelial dysplasia and then to frank adenocarcinoma.

### HINTS AND TIPS

Barrett's oesophagus is a classic example of metaplasia, and is a good example to quote in an examination.

## Benign neoplastic disease

Benign tumours of the oesophagus are rare. The majority are leiomyomas derived from the smooth muscle of muscularis propria; the minority are derived from nerves, i.e. schwannomas and neurofibromas.

## Malignant neoplastic disease

The most common malignant tumours of the oesophagus are squamous carcinomas and adenocarcinomas. Incidence is 5–10 per 100 000 per year in the UK. Risk factors are:

- smoking/alcohol
- dietary (tannic acid, food colourings, nitrates and nitrosamines)
- Barrett's oesophagus—10% of these cases will develop adenocarcinoma in their lifetime
- corrosives
- achalasia
- iron-deficiency anaemia
- HPV infection—this may have a role in the development of some squamous cell carcinomas.

Squamous cell carcinomas are more common than adenocarcinomas. They mostly develop in men who are heavy alcohol drinkers or heavy smokers, and may be preceded by an epithelial dysplastic change. They usually present late, located in the middle and lower oesophagus, and often causing dysphagia.

Adenocarcinomas mainly occur in the lower oesophagus in areas of metaplasia (Barrett's oesophagus). However, some adenocarcinomas are primary carcinomas of the stomach that have infiltrated the lower oesophagus.

## Clinical features of oesophageal tumours

- Common—progressively worsening painless dysphagia, anorexia, weight loss, anaemia (acute or chronic)
- Rare—hoarse voice (involvement of larynx or left recurrent laryngeal nerve palsy), supraclavicular lymphadenopathy tracheo-oesophageal fistula.

Investigations of choice are:

- upper GI endoscopy—with cytology and biopsy
- CT of chest and abdomen—stage the tumour and so determine operability
- endoscopic ultrasound—especially good for staging disease.

Management is often palliative to relieve pain and dysphagia (intubation, dilatation, bypass). Combinations of surgery, radiotherapy and chemotherapy (often neoadjuvant) may be attempted in early disease. Squamous carcinoma has a slightly better prognosis due to its radiosensitivity, but overall 5-year survival from oesophageal cancer is just 6–9%.

# DISORDERS OF THE STOMACH

## Inflammation

Gastritis is the term used to describe inflammation of the gastric mucosa.

## Acute gastritis

This superficial acute inflammation is typically caused by ingested chemicals, the most common being alcohol, aspirin and other non-steroidal anti-inflammatory drugs (NSAIDs).

### Acute erosive gastritis

Focal loss of the superficial gastric epithelium causes dyspepsia with vomiting and possibly haematemesis, if the erosions are numerous.

Causes are:

- NSAIDs
- heavy, acute alcohol ingestion
- severe stress or shock (e.g. after major trauma or burns)
- hypotension—acute hypoxia of surface epithelium.

## Chronic gastritis

Chronic inflammation of the gastric mucosa is a common condition. It increases with age and is more common in developed countries. Mucosal atrophy occurs with intestinal metaplasia, increasing the likelihood of gastric carcinoma.

The condition is present in over 90% of patients with duodenal ulceration, in about 70% of those with gastric ulceration, and it is also common in those with gastric cancer.

There are three main aetiological types:

- Infectious—gastritis associated with *Helicobacter pylori*
- Immune—pernicious anaemia and atrophic gastritis without pernicious anaemia
- Reactive—after gastrectomy or adjacent to erosions/ulcers.

### Helicobacter-associated gastritis

This is the most common form of chronic gastritis, accounting for more than 90% of cases, and it may arise at any age. The pyloric antrum is the most severely affected area, but damage is also seen in the fundus.

Pathogenesis is as follows:

- Colonization—*Helicobacter pylori* colonizes epithelial surface beneath thin layer of mucus. This causes an initial acute neutrophilic gastritis, which gives way to chronic gastritis.
- Urease production—the bacterium produces the enzyme urease, which breaks down urea to give $CO_2$ and ammonia.
- Immune response—the presence of the organism results in an immune response $\rightarrow$ epithelial damage.
- Persistence of infection—once established, infection may persist for years.

The morphological features are:

- mucin depletion leading to damage to the underlying epithelium
- atrophy of gastric glands
- mixed acute and chronic inflammatory cell reaction in lamina propria and superficial epithelium
- intestinal metaplasia—normal gastric epithelium is replaced by a type similar to that of the small intestine.

The tests available for diagnosis of *Helicobacter pylori* infection are listed in Figure 8.6.

### Autoimmune chronic gastritis

This organ-specific autoimmune disease associated with pernicious anaemia is generally seen in elderly patients with the development of severe atrophy of the mucosa (atrophic gastritis). It particularly affects the body of the stomach.

**Fig. 8.6** Test for diagnosis of *Helicobacter pylori* infection

| Type | Test | Diagnosis |
|---|---|---|
| Non-invasive | Urea breath test | Radiolabelled urea is administered; urease produced by *Helicobacter pylori* $\rightarrow$ radioactive $CO_2$, which can be detected on the breath |
| | Serology | Antibodies to *Helicobacter pylori* can be detected in serum |
| | Stool analysis | Bacteria detected in faecal material |
| Invasive | Histology | Organisms can be seen in biopsy material |
| | Culture | Can be cultured from biopsy material |
| | CLO test | Biopsy added to test kit containing urea. If urease present $NH_3$ produced causes change in colour of indicator |

CLO, *Campylobacter*-like organism.

Antibodies are of two types:

1. Antibodies against gastric parietal cells (90%)—associated with decreased hydrochloric acid production (hypochlorhydria)
2. Antibodies against intrinsic factor (60%) → failure of absorption of dietary vitamin $B_{12}$ → interference with normal erythropoiesis in bone marrow → megaloblastic, macrocytic anaemia (pernicious anaemia).

The most common form occurs without pernicious anaemia, even though antibodies of both types are often present. This is due to a residual ability to absorb vitamin $B_{12}$, which may be lost with time producing pernicious anaemia.

The morphological features are:

- loss of specialized cells
- fibrosis
- infiltrate of plasma cells and lymphocytes
- intestinal metaplasia.

### Reactive gastritis (reflux gastritis)
In this pattern of mucosal injury the dominant feature is epithelial change with minimal inflammatory cell infiltrates. The causes are threefold:

1. Idiopathic—majority of cases
2. Reflux of alkaline bile-containing duodenal fluid into the lower part of the stomach. This may be caused by motility disturbances (e.g. due to gallstones or cholecystectomy) or pyloric incompetence (as a result of previous surgery to the pyloric area)
3. Drugs—NSAIDs may cause direct damage to the mucus layer.

Morphological features are:

- epithelial desquamation
- foveolar hyperplasia
- vasodilatation
- mucosal oedema.

### Complications of chronic gastritis
Regardless of cause, all forms of chronic gastritis can cause:

- Intestinal metaplasia—more likely to result in dysplasia and eventual carcinoma
- Peptic ulcerations—caused by damage to the gastric lining by acidic gastric secretions.

## Gastric ulceration

### Peptic ulcers
Peptic ulcers are ulcers of the oesophagus, stomach or duodenum caused by damage to the epithelial lining by gastric secretions, particularly acid.

It is estimated that about 10% of the Western population experience peptic ulceration at some time. Ulcers usually develop in adulthood and have a natural history of repeated healing and relapse over many years.

Sites of peptic ulceration, in order of decreasing frequency, are:

- duodenum—classically the first portion due to hypersecretion of acid by the stomach
- stomach—usually at the antrum due to regurgitated bile in pyloric incompetence, or surface epithelial damage by *Helicobacter pylori* infection or NSAIDs
- gastro-oesophageal junction—due to gastric reflux onto unprotected mucosa
- gastro-enterostomy sites.

Aetiology is probably multifactorial but damaging influences include *Helicobacter pylori* infection, NSAIDs and stress. Less commonly, peptic ulcers may be associated with acid hypersecretion (e.g. gastrinoma), infection, duodenal obstruction/disruption, vascular insufficiency or radiation.

Other factors, such as chronic gastritis, smoking and genetic predisposition, are also believed to play a role in the pathogenesis.

### Pathogenesis
Upper GI mucosa is normally protected by either squamous epithelium (oesophagus) or an acid-resisting mucous barrier containing neutralizing bicarbonate ions. Peptic ulceration occurs when the aggressive action of acid and pepsin is not opposed by adequate mucosal protective mechanisms.

Macroscopically, peptic ulcers are typically 1–2 cm in diameter (but they can be much larger) with sharply defined borders surrounding the ulcer crater.

Microscopically, the ulcer crater usually penetrates into the muscularis propria of the stomach and it has four histological zones, namely:

- superficial necrotic debris
- non-specific acute inflammation
- granulation tissue
- fibrosis.

Complete healing of the ulcer leads to fibrous replacement of muscle with regrowth of epithelium over the scar. Clinical features include episodic epigastric pain (alleviated by antacids) which is worsened by eating and may occur with nausea and heartburn (oesophageal ulcers).

### Sequelae
Complications and sequelae are as follows:

- Healing—slow process hastened by acid-inhibiting agents or mucosal protectants.

- Haemorrhage—may be small and undetected (causing chronic anaemia) or occur as an acute episode of haematemesis.
- Adherence and erosion—ulcer penetrates full thickness of the stomach or duodenal wall, adhering to and eroding into underlying tissue, particularly the pancreas or liver.
- Perforation—may lead to peritonitis.
- Fibrous strictures—caused by the healing of peptic ulcers, which may obstruct the oesophagus or stomach (acquired pyloric stenosis).
- Malignant change (very rare).

---

**Clinical Note**

Peptic ulcer management:
- General—stopping smoking, avoiding NSAIDs, alcohol in moderation.
- Medical—eradication of *Helicobacter pylori* [triple therapy with a proton pump inhibitor (e.g. omeprazole), plus two antibiotics, e.g. clarithromycin and metronidazole]. If no infection is present, acid suppression medications include antacids, PPI and $H_2$-receptor antagonists.
- Surgical—rarely in acute ulcer haemorrhage or where medical control is impossible. A partial gastrectomy is used for gastric ulcers but complications are common.

---

## Acute gastric ulcer

Acute peptic ulcers usually develop in areas of erosive gastritis, and they are predisposed by the same factors that promoted erosion (e.g. NSAIDs). In contrast to chronic ulcers, they are generally multiple and shallow with minimal surrounding inflammation or fibrosis.

Acute ulcers may heal without scarring or they may progress to chronicity.

## Hypertrophic gastropathy

### Ménétrier's disease

This rare disease of unknown cause is characterized by gross hyperplasia of gastric pits, atrophy of glands and a marked overall increase in mucosal thickness. It is associated with hypoalbuminaemia as a result of gastric protein loss via superficial ulcerations (a form of 'protein-losing gastroenteropathy').

### Hypertrophic hypersecretory gastropathy

An extremely rare condition, this is characterized by acid hypersecretion and gastric protein loss.

## Zollinger–Ellison syndrome

A gastrin-secreting tumour (gastrinoma) of the pancreatic G cells results in gastric gland hyperplasia and gastric hypersecretion (see Chapter 10). Multiple peptic ulcers and diarrhoea also occur.

## Neoplastic disease

### Benign polyps

Benign gastric polyps are rare compared with the incidence of malignant tumours of the stomach. The types are:

- hyperplastic polyps—most common polyp of the stomach, formed by regeneration of mucosa, often at the edge of an ulcer in the stomach antrum
- adenomatous polyps—true benign tumours of the surface epithelium ranging up to 5 cm in size. Very rare, but dysplasia indicates that malignant change is possible
- fundal polyps—cystic glandular lesions seen mainly in women
- hamartomatous polyps—occur in Peutz–Jeghers syndrome (hereditary condition of multiple polyps in the small intestine associated with pigmented areas around the lips, inside mouth, and on palms and soles).

Other benign tumours of the stomach are derived from mesenchymal tissues, the most common being leiomyomas. These appear as mucosal or intramural nodules and are usually asymptomatic.

### Gastric adenocarcinoma

The vast majority of malignant tumours of the stomach are adenocarcinomas derived from mucus-secreting epithelial cells. Incidence has been falling worldwide, with 17 per 100 000 males and 7 per 100 000 females affected per year in the UK. Males are affected more than females by 3:2.

Gastric adenocarcinoma is common in the Far East and certain parts of South America, but less so in Western Europe and North America.

The sites are:

- pylorus (60%)—often produce symptoms of obstruction to the gastric outlet
- fundus (20–30%)—typically a fungating, ulcerating mass
- cardia (5–20%)—may produce dysphagia.

Unlike chronic peptic ulcers of the stomach, they are not confined to the lesser curvature.

Aetiology is unknown but dietary factors are suggested to account for geographical variation, e.g. ingestion of smoked and salted-preserved foods. Other risk factors include:

- *Helicobacter pylori* infection—chronic *Helicobacter pylori* infection increases gastric carcinoma risk 5- to 6-fold. This is thought to be the result of chronic gastritis producing intestinal metaplasia, with eventual dysplasia and carcinoma. Chronic inflammation creates reactive oxygen species capable of damaging DNA, along with gland atrophy and hypochlorhydria, which favour further bacterial growth. However, the vast majority of those with *Helicobacter pylori* infection do not develop cancer
- Chronic gastritis and intestinal metaplasia of other cause, e.g. autoimmune gastritis
- Gastric adenomatous polyps
- Postgastrectomy patients with persisting gastric inflammation
- Gastric cancer families (rare).

The sequence of events in the development of gastric carcinomas is as follows:

Normal mucosa → chronic gastritis → intestinal metaplasia → dysplasia → intramucosal carcinoma (early gastric cancer) → invasive carcinoma.

Several genetic changes have been reported in gastric cancer, including alterations of *p53* and *E-cadherin* expression, along with overexpression of oncogenes such as *c-myc*. *E-cadherin* changes appear unique to diffuse gastric cancer.

Gastric cancers are classified as either early or advanced according to the extent of their spread through the stomach wall.

### Early gastric cancer

This is confined to the mucosa and/or submucosa regardless of whether spread has occurred to regional lymph nodes. It is associated with a good prognosis. The cancer is further divided into three types according to macroscopic appearance (Fig. 8.7).

### Advanced gastric tumours

These extend beyond the submucosa, and are associated with a poor prognosis. They are further divided into three types macroscopically (Fig. 8.8):

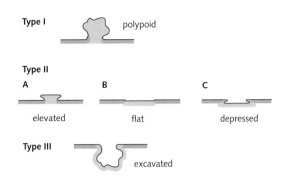

**Fig. 8.7** Macroscopic classification of early gastric cancers: type I polypoid; type II is further divided into: (A) elevated, (B) flat and (C) depressed; type III excavated.

1. Polypoid—protrudes into stomach lumen and presents early due to gastric discomfort and bleeding when traumatized. Usually amenable to surgical excision and has the best prognosis.
2. Ulcerating (most common type)—similar to benign peptic ulcers but with a raised edge, necrotic shaggy base and an absence of the radiation folds seen in benign peptic ulcers.
3. Diffuse infiltrative pattern (linitis plastica)—presents late and has the worst prognosis. Tumour spreads extensively within mucosa and submucosa producing a shrunken, inexpansible, rigid stomach. Symptoms are usually non-specific (e.g. vomiting due to small stomach capacity) and metastatic spread is common at the time of diagnosis. Surface ulceration is not a prominent feature and so haematemesis is not common until the later stages.

## Other gastric tumours

These are rare but include:

- lymphomas (see Chapter 13)—a common site for extranodal non-Hodgkin's lymphoma. *Helicobacter pylori* infection is associated with a low-grade lymphoma (so-called 'MALToma')

**Fig. 8.8** Comparison of the types of advanced gastric carcinomas

|  | Polypoid | Ulcerative | Diffuse infiltrative |
|---|---|---|---|
| Incidence | Common | Very common | Rare |
| Haemorrhage | Yes | Yes | Not until late stage |
| Prognosis | Good | Intermediate | Poor |
| Involvement | Focal | Focal | Diffuse |

- carcinoid tumours (page 154)
- gastrointestinal stromal tumours (GISTs)—relatively rare tumours that are thought to arise from interstitial cells that control gastrointestinal peristalsis. GISTs may be benign or malignant; it appears that 85% of cases display *c-KIT* mutations.

## GENERAL ASPECTS OF HEPATIC DAMAGE

### Patterns of hepatic injury

Following hepatic injury, the liver has a limited set of responses:

- Necrosis
- Inflammation
- Regeneration
- Fibrosis.

All pathological processes of the liver result in one or more of the above reactions.

### Necrosis

Acute hepatocellular injury can result in variable forms of necrosis. The underlying type of necrosis depends on aetiology.

#### Coagulative necrosis
This is typically a result of ischaemia (see Chapter 2).

#### Hydropic degeneration
This is the ballooning of individual hepatocytes, generally as a result of viral hepatitis. Mild swelling is reversible, but more advanced changes may progress to necrosis.

#### Focal necrosis
Necrosis of small groups of hepatocytes occurs in acute viral- or drug-induced hepatitis.

#### Zonal necrosis
Necrosis confined to certain zones is seen with particular conditions, e.g. centrilobular area (zone 3) is affected in acetaminophen (paracetamol) toxicity (Fig. 8.9).

#### Massive necrosis
Necrosis of the majority of hepatocytes occurs with fulminant hepatic damage and is seen in some cases of viral- and toxin-induced damage.

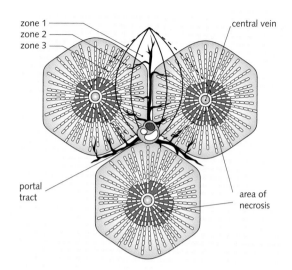

**Fig. 8.9** Centrilobular (zone 3) zonal necrosis. Zone 1 is perivenous (near portal vein) with a good oxygen supply, whereas zone 3 is pericentral (near central vein) with a poorer oxygen supply.

#### Interface (piecemeal) necrosis
Liver cells at the interface between the periportal parenchyma and inflamed portal tracts are destroyed.

### Inflammation

Inflammation of the liver is known as hepatitis, and it is a common response to a wide array of damage, e.g. viral infection, autoimmune disorders, drugs and toxins.

### Regeneration

Under normal circumstances there is very little liver cell proliferation. However, following hepatic injury, liver cell regeneration occurs to restore liver function, even if the architectural structure of the liver cannot be restored. This is a crucial phenomenon for recovery for patients with fulminant or subfulminant liver failure.

### Fibrosis

Repeated chronic damage to the liver can result in fibrosis, which is usually considered an irreversible change. Growth factors produced as part of an inflammatory response are thought to stimulate proliferation and differentiation of mesenchymal cells (the normally inconspicuous fat-storing cells of Ito located in the space of Disse) into collagen-secreting fibroblasts.

Development of fibrosis is an important complication of several liver diseases, and it is one of the characteristic features of cirrhosis.

Cleft lip & Cleft palate are diff. (Both have inability to breastfeed/suckle)

Cleft lip (Trisomy 13&18)
↳ uni/bilateral
upper/lower
nose floor & alveolar ridge

Cleft palate
↳ soft palate/uvula/hard palate

Stomatitis
↳ non-infective → Aphthous ulcers
↳ infective → Herpetic Stomatitis
→ Oral Candidiasis (Thrush)

Glossitis → Niacin/Riboflavin/Folic acid/B12 deficiency
Infective Stomatitis

Webs/Ring → Localised constrictions caused by mucosal folds/muscular contraction in the oesophagus

The liver can either; Regenerate, Necrose*, Fibrose* or inflame

# Cirrhosis

Cirrhosis is an irreversible condition in which the liver's normal architecture is diffusely replaced by nodules of proliferating hepatocytes separated by bands of scar tissue. Cirrhosis represents the end-stage of many processes—it is not a specific disease in itself. It involves:

- long-standing destruction of liver cells
- chronic inflammation that stimulates fibrosis
- regeneration of hepatocytes to cause nodules.

Macroscopically, the liver is tawny and characteristically knobbly (due to nodules). On a cut surface, parenchyma is replaced by nodules of regenerated hepatocytes separated by fine fibrosis.

Microscopically, the nodules of hepatocytes are separated by bands of collagenous tissue. Bile ducts and portal vessels run in the fibrous septa.

Cirrhosis can be classified either according to the size of regenerative nodules (Fig. 8.10) or according to its aetiology (Fig. 8.11). The aetiological classification is most useful in determining prognosis and treatment. The clinical features of cirrhosis are illustrated in Figure 8.12.

| Fig. 8.10 Classification of cirrhosis according to nodular size | |
|---|---|
| **Type** | **Nodule size** |
| Micronodular | ≤3 mm |
| Macronodular | 3 mm–2 cm |
| Mixed micro- and macronodular | Mixture of small and large |

| Fig. 8.11 Classification of cirrhosis according to incidence in the Western world | |
|---|---|
| Common | Alcoholic liver disease Cryptogenic (no cause found) Chronic hepatitis caused by hepatitis B and C viruses |
| Uncommon | Autoimmune chronic hepatitis Primary biliary cirrhosis Chronic biliary obstruction (biliary cirrhosis) Cystic fibrosis |
| Treatable but rare | Haemochromatosis Wilson's disease |
| Rare | $\alpha_1$-antitrypsin deficiency Galactosaemia Glycogenosis type IV Tyrosinaemia |

Consequences are:

- liver failure—reduced hepatocyte function (decreased synthesis of proteins, failure of detoxification)
- portal hypertension and its complications (see below)—a result of impeded blood flow through liver
- reduced immune competence → increased susceptibility to infection
- increased risk of hepatocellular carcinoma
- increased risk of portal vein thrombosis.

# Portal hypertension, ascites and splenomegaly

## Portal hypertension

This is a continued elevation in portal venous pressure, normal portal venous pressure being less than 2–5 mmHg. Causes of portal hypertension can be classified according to whether the site of obstruction to flow is:

- prehepatic—blockage of vessels before the hepatic sinusoids
- hepatic—blockage in the hepatic sinusoids
- posthepatic—blockage in the central veins, hepatic veins or vena cava.

Figure 8.13 lists the causes of portal hypertension.

*Complications*—portal hypertension causes back-pressure in the portal vascular bed leading to splenomegaly, ascites and varicose venous channels.

The causes and effects of portal hypertension are shown in Figure 8.14.

Portal hypertension can be controlled with β-blocker drugs (usually propranolol) to reduce the risk of oesophageal variceal haemorrhage.

## Portosystemic shunts

Venous communications that link portal and systemic venous systems become enlarged in portal hypertension. The four sites of portal-systemic anastomosis are:

1. Lower third of the oesophagus—left gastric vein (portal tributary) anastomoses with oesophageal veins (systemic tributary)
2. Halfway down the anal canal—superior rectal veins (portal tributary) draining upper half of anal canal anastomose with middle and inferior rectal veins (systemic tributaries)
3. Paraumbilical veins—connect left branch of the portal vein with superficial veins of anterior abdominal wall (systemic tributaries)
4. Veins of ascending colon, descending colon, duodenum, pancreas and liver (portal tributaries) anastomose with renal, lumbar and phrenic veins (systemic tributaries).

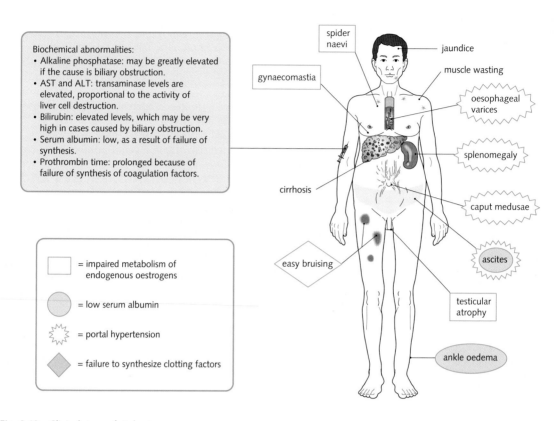

Biochemical abnormalities:
• Alkaline phosphatase: may be greatly elevated if the cause is biliary obstruction.
• AST and ALT: transaminase levels are elevated, proportional to the activity of liver cell destruction.
• Bilirubin: elevated levels, which may be very high in cases caused by biliary obstruction.
• Serum albumin: low, as a result of failure of synthesis.
• Prothrombin time: prolonged because of failure of synthesis of coagulation factors.

spider naevi
gynaecomastia
jaundice
muscle wasting
oesophageal varices
splenomegaly
cirrhosis
caput medusae
easy bruising
ascites
testicular atrophy
ankle oedema

□ = impaired metabolism of endogenous oestrogens

○ = low serum albumin

✷ = portal hypertension

◇ = failure to synthesize clotting factors

**Fig. 8.12** Clinical signs of cirrhosis.

| Fig. 8.13 Classification of portal hypertension | |
|---|---|
| Prehepatic | Portal vein thrombosis |
| Hepatic | Cirrhosis (most common cause of portal hypertension) Idiopathic portal hypertension Hepatic fibrosis: caused by schistosomiasis (important cause in endemic areas) Polycystic disease of the liver |
| Posthepatic | Disease of hepatic veins and branches, e.g. Budd–Chiari syndrome Severe right-sided heart failure Constrictive pericarditis |

*Pathogenesis*—under normal conditions, portal venous blood traverses the liver and drains into the inferior vena cava of the systemic venous circulation by way of the hepatic veins. In portal hypertension, flow through this direct route is reduced and the portal venous blood is forced through smaller communications that exist between the portal and systemic systems.

Anastomotic channels become dilated resulting in the development of varicose venous channels, namely:

• oesophageal varices—may cause severe bleeding
• caput medusae—distension of paraumbilical veins
• haemorrhoids—rectal varices develop.

## Ascites

Ascites is the accumulation of free fluid in the peritoneal cavity. Common causes are:

• peritonitis
• malignancy in the peritoneal cavity
• hypoproteinaemia—e.g. nephrotic syndrome
• portal hypertension—most commonly caused by cirrhosis
• heart failure.

*Pathogenesis of ascites in cirrhosis*—increased transudation of fluid in ascites occurs as a result of:

• ↑ hydrostatic pressure in portal veins
• ↑ plasma oncotic pressure (due to lowered albumin synthesis by damaged liver cells).

Figure 8.15 describes the types of ascites.

Clinical features are abdominal distension with fullness in the flanks, shifting dullness on percussion and fluid thrill.

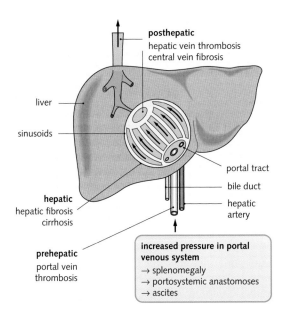

posthepatic
hepatic vein thrombosis
central vein fibrosis

liver

sinusoids

portal tract

bile duct

hepatic
hepatic fibrosis
cirrhosis

hepatic
artery

prehepatic
portal vein
thrombosis

**increased pressure in portal venous system**
→ splenomegaly
→ portosystemic anastomoses
→ ascites

**Fig. 8.14**   Causes and effects of portal hypertension.

## Splenomegaly

Increased pressure in the portal vein is transmitted to the splenic vein resulting in splenomegaly. A variety of haematological abnormalities are associated with hypersplenism (see Chapter 13).

### Clinical Note

Ascites management:
• Restrict sodium intake.
• Diuretics, e.g. spironolactone.
• Paracentesis—drain 3–5 L over 1–2 hours for immediate relief. Drainage to dryness may be supported by colloid (e.g. albumin).

• LeVeen shunt—a subcutaneous draining tube connecting peritoneum to internal jugular vein via a one-way valve. Complications of infection, thrombosis and pulmonary oedema limit use.
• TIPSS—relieves portal hypertension.
  *Prognosis*—only 10–20% survive 5 years from onset.

## Jaundice and cholestasis

### Jaundice

This presents as a yellowing of the skin, sclerae or mucous membranes, indicating excess bilirubin in the blood. It is clinically detectable when plasma bilirubin exceeds 50 µmol/L (3 mg/dL), although the biochemical definition refers to any reading above normal levels (approximately 18–24 µmol/L).

The metabolism of bilirubin is illustrated in Figure 8.16.

### Causes of jaundice
The easiest way to classify jaundice is by aetiology (Fig. 8.17):
• Prehepatic—the most common cause is haemolysis-associated jaundice, a mild form of which occurs in many neonates due to immature liver function in the first weeks of life.
• Intrahepatic—any cause of hepatocellular damage or intrahepatic cholestasis may be responsible. Hereditary enzyme defects may reduce the ability to conjugate bilirubin, so producing jaundice. Gilbert's syndrome is the most common of these conditions; it is not serious and requires no treatment.
• Posthepatic—any obstruction beyond the liver, e.g. gallstones.

| **Fig. 8.15** Types of ascites | |
| --- | --- |
| **Transudate low protein fluid (< 30 g/L)** | **Exudate high protein fluid (> 30 g/L)** |
| Cirrhosis | Malignancy |
| Constrictive pericarditis | Peritonitis |
| Cardiac failure | Pancreatitis |
| Hypoalbuminaemia, e.g. nephrotic syndrome | Budd–Chiari syndrome |
| | Hypothyroidism |
| | Lymphatic obstruction (chylous ascites) |

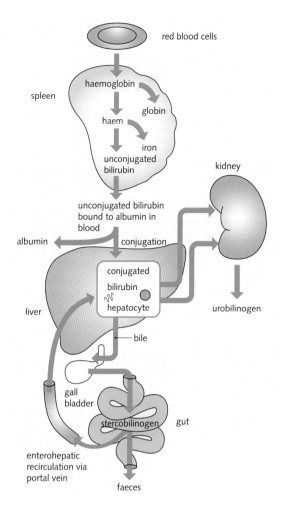

**Fig. 8.16**  Bilirubin metabolism.

## Unconjugated versus conjugated hyperbilirubinaemia

An alternative classification system is based on chemical analysis of bilirubin in the blood (Fig. 8.18).

Failure of bile flow caused by the obstruction of either small (intrahepatic) or large (extrahepatic) bile ducts is termed cholestasis. It results in jaundice due to conjugated hyperbilirubinaemia. The high levels of conjugated bilirubin pushed back into the blood result in dark urine (high urobilinogen content), while the lack of bilirubin passing through the liver produces pale faeces. Conjugated bilirubin may be deposited in the skin causing itching (pruritus).

Unconjugated hyperbilirubinaemia is caused by states such as haemolysis, where the excessive release of bilirubin overwhelms the ability of the liver to conjugate it into a water-soluble form (bilirubin-glucuronate). Insoluble bilirubin does not enter the urine and so this remains a normal colour, but faeces are darkened by the increased amount of bilirubin excreted through the liver. Pruritus does not usually occur.

**HINTS AND TIPS**

Two important points to note about jaundice:
1. Liver disease is not the only cause of jaundice; there are other causes, e.g. haemolysis.
2. Many patients with significant liver disease are not jaundiced.

## Hepatic failure

This is usually the end point of long-standing chronic liver disease, when up to 90% of hepatic function has been lost.

**Fig. 8.17** Causes of jaundice

| Cause | Clinical consequence |
| --- | --- |
| Prehepatic causes | Haemolysis (commonest cause) |
| Intrahepatic causes | Hereditary enzyme defects, e.g. Dubin–Johnson, Rotor's, Gilbert's and Crigler–Najjar syndromes<br>Drugs causing intrahepatic cholestasis<br>Pregnancy-associated cholestatis<br>Hepatocellular damage, e.g. alcohol, virus hepatitis |
| Posthepatic (obstructive) causes | Large duct obstruction as a result of:<br>• Gallstones<br>• Strictures caused by inflammation or fibrosis<br>• Extrahepatic biliary atresia<br>• Compression by extrinsic masses, e.g. carcinoma of the pancreas, enlarged lymph nodes |

| Fig. 8.18 Classification of jaundice according to chemical composition of bilirubin | | | |
|---|---|---|---|
| **Cause** | **Type** | **Example** | **Features** |
| Unconjugated hyperbilirubinaemia | Prehepatic | Haemolysis | Urine: normal<br>Faeces: dark |
| | Intrahepatic | Impaired bilirubin uptake (Gilbert's syndrome)<br>Impaired bilirubin conjugation<br>Crigler–Najjar syndrome<br>Drugs, e.g. rifampicin | Increased risk of pigment gallstones<br>No itching<br>(excess urobilinogen with haemolysis) |
| Conjugated hyperbilirubinaemia | Intrahepatic non-cholestatic | Impaired bilirubin excretion into bile:<br>• Dubin–Johnson syndrome<br>• Rotor's syndrome | Urine: dark<br>Faeces: pale<br>Itching |
| | Intrahepatic cholestatic | Small bile duct obstruction:<br>• Acute/chronic hepatitis<br>• Cirrhosis<br>• Intrahepatic tumours<br>• Pregnancy-associated cholestasis<br>• Sclerosing cholestatis<br>• Intrahepatic biliary atresia | Urine: dark<br>Faeces: pale<br>Itching |
| | Posthepatic | Large bile duct obstruction | Urine: dark<br>Faeces: pale<br>Itching |

## Hepatic encephalopathy

This is a neuropsychiatric syndrome caused by severe liver disease, occurring most often with cirrhosis but occasionally in a more acute form in fulminant hepatic failure.

Pathogenesis is:

- Liver failure—the liver is unable to remove exogenous/endogenous compounds from the circulation. Neurotoxins (e.g. ammonia) accumulate and impair neuronal transmission.
- Shunting—in portal hypertension, there is shunting of portal blood past the liver directly into the systemic circulation.

The overall effect is a biochemical disturbance of brain function. The condition is reversible and rarely shows marked pathological changes in the brain.

## Hepatorenal syndrome

Renal failure secondary to liver failure occurs in advanced cirrhosis, and almost always in conjunction with ascites.

The kidneys themselves are normal. Renal failure is thought to result from altered systemic blood flow including diminished renal flow.

*Prognosis*—recovery depends on improvement of liver function, but in chronic liver disease this seldom occurs.

## DISORDERS OF THE LIVER AND BILIARY TRACT

### Congenital errors of metabolism

### Haemochromatosis

This condition is caused by excessive deposition of iron in the tissues, including the liver. There are two types:

1. Primary (hereditary)—an autosomal recessive trait that leads to the production of abnormal HFE protein, which is linked to excessive absorption of iron from the gut. Ninety per cent of those affected are male.
2. Secondary—results from excessive iron accumulation caused by other primary diseases (such as sideroblastic anaemia and chronic haemolytic disorders).

#### Effects of iron accumulation

Iron accumulates as haemosiderin in many tissues including the liver, pancreas, pituitary, heart and skin. Affected tissues appear rusty brown due to haemosiderin within cells, as follows:

- In the liver—hepatocyte necrosis begins in the periportal region and spreads to affect the whole liver.

Free radical generation may play a key role in this reaction. Cirrhosis ultimately develops, often with hepatomegaly.

- In the heart—infiltration of cardiac muscle can cause cardiomyopathy with heart failure.
- In the pancreas—damage to pancreatic islets may result in diabetes mellitus.
- In the skin—leaden grey pigmentation of skin due to excess melanin, especially in exposed parts, i.e. the axillae, groin and genitalia.

*Diagnosis*—there is a high saturation of transferrin in the blood, and high serum iron and ferritin levels. Diagnosis is confirmed by a liver biopsy showing heavy iron deposition and hepatic fibrosis, which may have progressed to cirrhosis.

*Management*:

- Weekly venesection (bleedings) of 500 mL until serum iron is normal followed by venesection as required to maintain normal serum ferritin.
- Therapy for cirrhosis and diabetes mellitus.
- Investigation of first-degree relatives by blood testing and possible genetic screening.

### HINTS AND TIPS

The term 'bronzed diabetes' is often used to describe haemochromatosis due to the combination of diabetes and hyperpigmentation.

## Wilson disease

This autosomal recessive disorder of copper metabolism results in chronic destructive liver disease.

Normally, dietary copper is taken up by the liver, complexed to ceruloplasmin (a copper-binding protein) and then the whole complex is secreted into the plasma. Circulating ceruloplasmin is subsequently recycled by the liver, with any remaining excess copper being re-excreted into the bile.

In Wilson disease, a mutation in a copper transport ATPase gene results in failure of the liver to secrete the copper-ceruloplasmin complex into the plasma. The copper complex accumulates within the hepatocytes, saturating the available ceruloplasmin and leaving free copper to overspill into the blood, where it can cause haemolysis or be deposited in various tissues:

- liver—chronic hepatitis, which progresses to cirrhosis
- brain—psychiatric disorders, abnormal eye movements and movement disorders resembling Parkinson disease
- eye—development of greenish-brown discolouration around cornea (Kayser–Fleischer rings).

*Diagnosis*—low levels of serum ceruloplasmin and high free copper in the blood; liver effects confirmed by biopsy.

Management is by copper chelators, e.g. penicillamine.

## Alpha$_1$-antitrypsin deficiency

Affected individuals with this inherited condition fail to produce the normal active extracellular protease inhibitor $\alpha_1$-antitrypsin.

*Pathogenesis*—$\alpha_1$-antitrypsin is normally produced and secreted by the liver to inhibit the activity of protease enzymes. Mutations in the genes encoding the inhibitor prevent their secretion such that protease enzymes are not inhibited. The *PiZ* gene is most commonly affected.

In heterozygotes, there is an increased risk of lung damage, especially emphysema in smokers. Homozygotes develop emphysema and liver disease (cholestatic jaundice in the neonate; chronic hepatitis and cirrhosis in adults). This actually occurs due to the accumulation of abnormal $\alpha_1$-antitrypsin globules in the liver, which cannot be secreted into the bloodstream.

## Others

### Reye's syndrome

This rare syndrome is characterized by acute encephalopathy with cerebral oedema as a result of sudden severe impairment of hepatic function (associated with microvesicular fatty degeneration). It occurs with high-dose aspirin use in children and adolescents, often following an upper respiratory tract infection.

## Infectious and inflammatory disease

### Viral hepatitis

Viral infection is a common cause of acute hepatitis. The main so-called hepatitis viruses are a group of hepatotrophic viruses. Although all cause a primary hepatitis, they are unrelated and they belong to different viral types.

Clinical features are similar in all forms of acute hepatitis regardless of aetiology.

Symptoms are nausea, anorexia, low-grade pyrexia and general malaise. Signs are hepatomegaly with tenderness, and jaundice 1 week after onset of symptoms, peaking at about 10 days.

*Investigations*—raised serum levels of conjugated bilirubin and liver aminotransferases (both aspartate and alanine).

## Hepatitis A

This RNA enterovirus is prevalent in tropical countries, but uncommon in developed countries.

It is the most common travel related illness in the UK.

*Transmission*—faecal-oral route, e.g. from:

- nurseries or institutions where hygiene levels are inadequate (person-to-person via hand-to-hand contact)
- recreational activities in waters contaminated by sewage outfalls
- ingestion of sewage-contaminated shellfish
- (sexual) oral-anal contact.

*Time course*—illustrated in Figure 8.19.

*Prognosis*—the majority of patients recover fully with restoration of normal liver function tests. However, a small minority (1–3 per 1000) develop fulminant hepatic failure with a mortality rate of 85%.

The disease never causes chronic hepatitis and infection confers subsequent immunity. A vaccine is available for long-term immunity.

## Hepatitis B

This is a DNA virus of the Hepadna group. It can integrate into host DNA. Transmission can be:

- blood-borne—blood transfusions, IV drug abusers, tattooing, acupuncture
- sexual—sexual intercourse
- vertical—transmission from mother to child; either perinatally (transplacental) or postnatally (breast milk).

There are three clinical patterns of infection (Fig. 8.20):

1. Asymptomatic infection (65%)—transient subclinical infection with complete recovery

2. Acute self-limiting hepatitis (25%)—symptoms include jaundice, malaise and anorexia, but the majority recover and develop lifelong immunity. There is a 1% mortality associated with fulminant acute hepatitis (massive hepatocyte necrosis)

3. Chronic hepatitis B infection (10%)—the majority enter an asymptomatic carrier state, which carries a future risk of chronic hepatitis. A minority progress to chronic hepatitis after initial infection; chronic hepatitis is a strong risk factor for cirrhosis.

*Time course*—illustrated in Figure 8.21.

Complications are cirrhosis (as a result of chronic hepatitis) and hepatocellular carcinoma. Carriers of hepatitis B are 200 times more likely to get liver cancer than non-carriers. However, there is typically a latency period of 20–30 years between infection and cancer.

*Treatment*—large doses of interferon-α/β for carriers. The role of the antiviral nucleoside drug lamivudine is currently being evaluated. Prophylactic vaccination based on the hepatitis B surface antigen (HBsAg) is available but up to 10% of normal individuals fail to produce protective antibodies.

## Hepatitis C

This RNA flavivirus is a major cause of hepatitis worldwide.

*Transmission*—predominantly blood-borne spread, although sexual and vertical transmissions do occur. Hepatitis C is widespread among intravenous drug

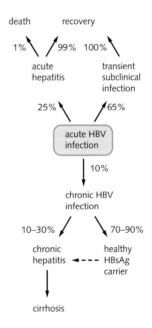

**Fig. 8.20**  Summary of the possible courses of infection. (HBV, hepatitis B virus; HBsAg, hepatitis B surface antigen.) (Adapted with permission from Clinical Medicine, 7th edn, by P Kumar and M Clarke, Baillière Tindall, 2009.)

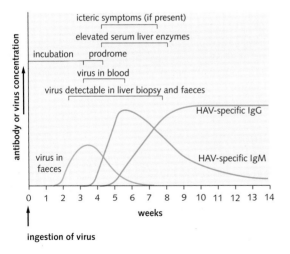

**Fig. 8.19**  Course of infection in hepatitis A. HAV-hepatitis A virus.

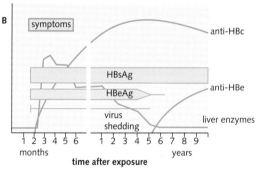

**Fig. 8.21** Course of infection in hepatitis B. (A) Acute hepatitis. (B) Chronic hepatitis. (HBsAg, hepatitis B surface antigen; HBeAg, hepatitis Be antigen; anti-HBs, antibody to HBsAg; anti-HBc, antibody to hepatitis B core antigen; anti-HBe, antibody to HBeAg.) HBsAg window is time point where neither HBsAg nor anti-HBs can be detected because of immune complex formation.

abusers and was previously spread by blood transfusions before serological screening of donated samples was introduced.

Infection is asymptomatic in 10–35% of cases, although it may progress to the carrier state. However, the majority of patients develop acute hepatitis (in 65–90% of cases).

Chronic hepatitis develops in 70–80% of those infected, increasing lifelong risk of cirrhosis and hepatocellular carcinoma.

Treatment is with interferon-cc and ribavirin, although only half of patients will respond.

### Hepatitis D

This RNA virus is incomplete and can only cause infection in the presence of hepatitis B virus; transmission is as for hepatitis B virus. Both viruses may be acquired simultaneously or hepatitis D may be acquired later as a superinfection.

The virus increases the severity of chronic hepatitis, and it may predispose to the development of fulminant hepatitis.

### Hepatitis E

This RNA virus has the same transmission pattern as hepatitis A. Infection by hepatitis E is clinically similar to hepatitis A infection.

### Other viruses

Non-hepatotrophic viruses may also cause hepatitis. Examples include group B arbovirus (yellow fever), Epstein–Barr virus and cytomegalovirus.

## Autoimmune hepatitis

It has a prevalence of about 4 per 10 000, and it typically occurs in women (70% of cases) between the ages of 20 and 40 years.

The condition is associated with hyperglobulinaemia and autoantibodies in the serum (antismooth muscle and antinuclear antibodies in type I disease; antiliver-kidney microsomal antibodies in type II). Type I disease (most common) is associated with other autoimmune disorders such as Graves disease and Sjögren's syndrome (dry eyes and mouth).

Clinically, there is insidious onset of anorexia, malaise and fatigue accompanied by abdominal distension and mild jaundice (with dark urine and itching).

Complications are cirrhosis, liver failure and hepatocellular carcinoma.

*Investigations*:

- Liver function tests—hyperbilirubinaemia, moderately raised aminotransferase levels
- Hyperglobulinaemia (mainly IgG increases), often with a raised erythrocyte sedimentation ratio (ESR)
- Serology—autoantibodies are useful if titres are high, but low levels may be found in healthy people.

The disease may run a relapsing and remitting course but it progresses inexorably to cirrhosis.

Treatment is with corticosteroids; azathioprine may help to reduce steroid dosage.

*Prognosis*—patients who do not respond to treatment will almost always progress to cirrhosis. Also, many patients develop cirrhosis despite having a response to treatment. If end-stage liver disease develops, liver transplantation is an effective procedure.

## Fulminant hepatitis

This rare syndrome of hepatic encephalopathy results from sudden severe impairment of hepatic function. It is caused by acute, severe liver damage such as:

- viral infections (most common cause), e.g. hepatitis B
- drugs and poisons, e.g. acetaminophen (paracetamol) overdose, carbon tetrachloride
- non-viral infections, e.g. *Leptospira*, *Toxoplasma gondii*, *Coxiella burnetii*
- metabolic—Wilson disease, pregnancy

- ischaemic—shock, severe cardiac failure, Budd-Chiari syndrome.

The pathogenesis of hepatic encephalopathy has already been described (see page 129).

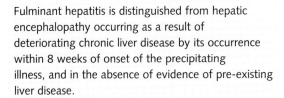

Clinical features are:

- cerebral disturbance (mental changes progressing from confusion to stupor and coma)
- weakness, vomiting and nausea
- rapidly developing jaundice with fetor hepaticus (distinctive breath odour)
- asterixis—flapping tremor
- ascites and oedema.

The liver may enlarge initially, but later it becomes impalpable; disappearance of hepatic dullness on percussion indicates shrinkage and is a bad prognostic sign.

*Complications*:

- Oedema—this may be cerebral (causing raised intracranial pressure) or pulmonary (contributing to respiratory failure)
- General vasodilatation—hypotension and hypothermia
- Infection
- Coagulation disorders
- Necrotic cirrhosis
- Pancreatitis
- Renal failure—deterioration parallels that of liver failure
- Metabolic—hypoglycaemia, hypokalaemia, hypocalcaemia, hypomagnesaemia, acid–base disturbance.

There is no specific treatment. Management is by close observation, treating complications as necessary.

*Prognosis*:

- 66% of patients with minor signs survive
- only 10% of patients with coma survive
- those who recover from fulminant hepatic failure usually regain normal hepatic structure and function.

## Postnecrotic cirrhosis

This rapidly developing cirrhosis follows extensive necrosis, e.g. postfulminant hepatitis.

## Liver abscess

This localized collection of pus within the liver is walled off and surrounded by damaged and inflamed liver tissue. Liver abscesses are rare but important, as they are inevitably fatal if untreated.

### Pyogenic abscesses

The most common causative organisms are *Escherichia coli*, various streptococci and other enterobacteria.

*Mode of infection*:

- Blood borne—via portal vein (mesenteric infections) or hepatic artery (bacteraemia). Usually solitary abscesses
- Ascending spread from colonization of biliary tract (most common)—almost always predisposed by biliary obstruction and usually resulting in multiple small abscesses
- Penetrating trauma.

Symptoms of infection and right upper quadrant pain (may radiate to the right shoulder) are common, along with hepatomegaly and a mild jaundice.

Investigations include ultrasound imaging. Needle aspiration at this time can confirm the diagnosis in addition to providing pus for culture.

Management is by prolonged antibiotics and drainage of the abscess.

*Prognosis*—the mortality of liver abscesses is 20–40%, usually through failure to make the diagnosis.

### Amoebic abscess

The most common causative organism is *Entamoeba histolytica*, which is transmitted from the bowel to the liver via the blood. The disease is rare in the UK but common worldwide, and it must be considered in patients travelling from endemic areas such as Africa, Asia and South America.

## Alcohol, drugs and toxins

### Alcoholic liver disease

Alcohol abuse is the most common cause of liver disease in Western countries. Women are more prone to alcohol-induced liver damage than men.

Alcohol is metabolized almost exclusively in the liver and liver damage is related to daily alcohol intake. Toxicity of ethanol is probably caused by the generation of its metabolic breakdown product, acetaldehyde, which binds to liver proteins and damages hepatocytes. Alcohol also stimulates collagen synthesis in the liver leading to fibrosis.

Its effects are fatty liver, acute hepatitis and cirrhosis.

### Fatty liver (hepatic steatosis)

This is the most common lesion of alcoholic liver disease. The condition is characterized by the accumulation of fat globules within the cytoplasm of hepatocytes. It is reversible on cessation of alcohol ingestion.

It is thought that alcohol stimulates hepatocyte triacylglycerol production, while impairing its excretion from the liver. The condition reflects severe metabolic derangement and it may affect a few or almost all hepatocytes.

### Alcoholic hepatitis

This is acute hepatitis with focal necrosis of liver cells. At high concentrations, alcohol causes toxic injury to hepatocytes, evoking a neutrophil-dominant inflammatory reaction, which is reversible on abstinence. Eosinophilic accumulations called Mallory bodies may be seen on liver biopsy. Continued alcohol consumption causes the development of fibrosis around central veins. The result is hepatic fibrosis that may progress to cirrhosis.

The illness resembles acute viral hepatitis and liver function tests show raised levels of aminotransferases and $\gamma$-glutamyltransferase (GGT).

### Alcoholic cirrhosis

Irreversible architectural disturbance occurs as a result of sustained alcoholic liver injury.

Normal liver architecture is diffusely replaced by nodules of regenerated liver cells separated by bands of collagenous fibrosis. This may develop after episodes of acute alcoholic hepatitis or may be insidious in its onset presenting only as end-stage liver disease.

It affects fewer than 10% of patients suffering from chronic alcoholism.

---

#### Clinical Note

Fatty change can occur without excessive alcohol intake; it is commonly seen amongst the obese and type 2 diabetic populations. There is predominantly macrovesicular change (large fat globules), although conditions such as pregnancy may be microvesicular (small fat globules). In a minority of individuals, there may be an accompanying inflammatory infiltrate, producing a non-alcoholic steatohepatitis (NASH). This is associated with the same risks of progression to cirrhosis as alcoholic hepatitis.

---

## Drugs and toxins

The liver is the main organ of drug metabolism and, consequently, drugs are a common cause of liver disease. Hepatotoxic drugs may be divided into two main

groups: intrinsic hepatotoxins and idiosyncratic hepatotoxins.

### Intrinsic hepatotoxins

These have dose-dependent, predictable toxic effects. They are responsible for a high incidence of toxic damage to the liver via either direct toxicity of an unmetabolized drug or normal hepatic conversion to a toxic metabolite.

### Idiosyncratic hepatotoxins

These have non-dose-dependent, unpredictable toxic effects. They cause liver disease in a small percentage of exposed individuals as a result of hypersensitivity (drug-mediated autoimmunity) or abnormal drug metabolism.

## Circulatory disorders of the liver

### Overview

Vascular disorders of the liver (Fig. 8.22) can be classified into one of three categories depending on their pathogenic mechanisms:

1. Obstruction to outflow—hepatic vein obstruction
2. Lobular compromise
3. Obstruction to inflow—obstruction of portal vein or hepatic artery occlusion.

### Diseases causing obstruction to outflow (hepatic vein obstruction)

- Budd–Chiari syndrome—obstruction occurs in the larger hepatic veins
- Cardiac disease—right-sided cardiac failure causes congestion of the inferior vena cava.

Clinical manifestations depend on the cause and speed with which obstruction develops, but congestive hepatomegaly and ascites are features in all patients.

### Budd–Chiari syndrome

This rare condition is caused by occlusion of the main hepatic vein or (more rarely) the intrahepatic vena cava (Fig. 8.23).

Obstruction of the hepatic vein causes severe hepatic congestion with atrophy and/or necrosis of liver cells in the affected areas. Fibrous scarring eventually occurs in areas of hepatocyte necrosis. True cirrhosis supervenes in a minority of cases.

*Clinical manifestations*—patients develop severe acute disease with:

- painful hepatomegaly
- acute portal hypertension
- rapid development of ascites
- jaundice.

Death results unless a surgical portosystemic vascular shunt is created.

**Fig. 8.22** Vascular disorders of the liver

| Cause | Example |
|---|---|
| Outflow (hepatic vein) obstruction | Veno-occlusive disease<br>Budd–Chiari syndrome<br>Right-sided cardiac failure |
| Lobular compromise | Cirrhosis<br>Non-cirrhotic fibrosis:<br>• Infective, e.g. schistosomiasis<br>• Drugs, e.g. alcohol, hypervitaminosis A, vinyl chloride, arsenic<br>• Congenital, e.g. congenital hepatic fibrosis, infantile polycystic disease<br>• Nodular regenerative hyperplasia<br>Systemic circulatory disturbances, e.g. shock |
| Inflow obstruction | Extrahepatic:<br>• Portal vein obstruction:<br>  portal vein thrombosis<br>  extrinsic compression of portal vein<br>  congenital stenosis<br>• Hepatic artery occlusion:<br>  hepatic artery thrombosis<br>  embolism, e.g. infective endocarditis<br>Intrahepatic:<br>• Occlusion of intrahepatic portal vein branches |

**Fig. 8.23** Aetiology of Budd–Chiari syndrome

| | |
|---|---|
| Idiopathic | Underlying cause cannot be found in more than half of cases |
| Thrombotic causes | Haematological diseases, for example:<br>• Primary proliferative polycythaemia<br>• Paroxysmal nocturnal haemoglobinuria<br>• Deficiencies of antithrombin III, proteins C and S<br>Pregnancy/oral contraceptives |
| Local compression of hepatic vein (rare) | Obstruction due to tumours, e.g. liver, kidneys or adrenals<br>Congenital venous webs<br>Inferior vena cava stenosis |

## Passive congestion

Congestive cardiac failure causes venous outflow obstruction in the liver due to back pressure transmitted as described below:

Inferior vena cava → hepatic vein → central veins
→ centrilobular congestion

Centrilobular sinusoids are dilated by blood and the centrilobular hepatocytes undergo atrophy and necrosis (centrilobular necrosis), giving rise to the appearance of what is described as a 'nutmeg liver' (chronic passive venous congestion).

The condition is common in tricuspid valve incompetence when the liver is pulsatile.

Arterial hypotension may increase the congestive effect of right-sided cardiac failure.

## Diseases resulting in lobular compromise

• Cirrhosis—distortion and destruction of the hepatic vascular architecture causes sinusoid occlusion
• Non-cirrhosis fibrosis—where fibrotic damage to the liver does not amount to true cirrhosis, e.g. schistosomiasis infection

- Systemic circulatory disturbances—shock from any source causes severe hypoperfusion, resulting in zonal necrosis.

## Diseases resulting in obstruction to inflow

- Extrahepatic—portal vein obstruction (thrombosis, extrinsic compression) or hepatic artery occlusion (thrombosis, embolism)
- Intrahepatic—occlusion of intrahepatic portal vein branches causes areas of venous infarction.

### Portal vein obstruction

Obstruction of the portal vein results in portal hypertension and its associated complications. The causes may be thrombotic or non-thrombotic.

Thrombotic conditions (those that predispose to portal vein thrombosis) are:

- inflammatory—thrombophlebitis and intra-abdominal sepsis (e.g. appendicitis, cholecystitis, pancreatitis)
- neoplastic—hepatocellular carcinoma, metastatic liver tumours and haematological malignancies (e.g. polycythaemia rubra vera, essential thrombocytosis, myelofibrosis)
- cirrhosis—leads to portal hypertension and stasis
- splenic vein thrombosis (often secondary to pancreatitis) may propagate into the portal vein.

Non-thrombotic conditions are external compression (e.g. by tumour masses) and cirrhosis.

### Liver infarction

True infarction of the liver is rare because of its dual blood supply and rich anastomosis of blood flow through the sinusoids. However, hepatic blood flow may be compromised in the following conditions:

- surgical trauma or accidental ligation of hepatic artery
- therapeutic arterial embolization of the liver or therapeutic hepatic arterial ligation (performed to treat isolated neoplastic masses)
- bacterial endocarditis—embolism
- eclampsia
- polyarteritis nodosa—a necrotizing vasculitis.

## Neoplasia of the liver

### Benign tumours

#### Hepatic adenomas

These typically affect premenopausal women, and they are predisposed by oestrogen-containing oral contraceptives.

The macroscopic appearance is of well-circumscribed nodules up to 20 cm in size.

The microscopic appearance closely resembles that of a normal liver, except that no portal structures are seen.

*Complications*—the majority of lesions are asymptomatic, but subcapsular adenomas are prone to rupture, leading to intra-abdominal bleeding.

#### Bile-duct adenomas

These are very common lesions composed of abnormal bile ducts in a collagenous stroma that appear as small white nodules, often beneath the liver capsule. They may be mistaken for metastatic tumour deposits at laparotomy.

#### Haemangioma

These are common hamartomas composed of abnormal vascular channels in a collagenous stroma. They are found at autopsy in 2–5% of the population and are typically seen just beneath the capsule as a dark lesion (usually 2–3 cm in size).

### Malignant

#### Hepatocellular carcinoma (liver cell carcinoma)

Carcinoma of hepatocytes is the commonest primary tumour of the liver. Uncommon in the UK (affects about 1 per 100 000) it is up to 100 times more common in parts of Africa and the Far East, probably because of the higher incidence of hepatitis B and contaminating mycotoxins. Males are affected more than females.

Predisposing factors are:

- cirrhosis—independent of cause
- hepatitis B or C infection—with chronic carrier state
- mycotoxins—these contaminate certain foods, e.g. aflatoxins produced by the fungus *Aspergillus flavus*.

Tumours may consist of a single mass or multiple nodules. Hepatocellular carcinomas often produce $\alpha$-feto-protein, which is secreted into the blood and is useful as a diagnostic marker. Prognosis is very poor with median survival of less than 6 months from diagnosis.

#### Cholangiocarcinoma

This is an adenocarcinoma anywhere in the biliary tree. Within the liver, it may arise from the intrahepatic bile duct epithelium, accounting for 5–10% of all cases of primary liver tumours.

Many cases are of unknown origin, but predisposing factors include:

- chronic inflammatory disease of the intrahepatic biliary tree, particularly sclerosing cholangitis
- disease caused by Chinese liver flukes (*Clonorchis sinensis*).

Lesions tend to be detected late and are associated with a very poor prognosis; most patients do not survive more than 6 months from diagnosis.

### Angiosarcomas

These highly malignant tumours are derived from vascular endothelium, and characterized by multifocal haemorrhagic nodules within the liver. The tumours are rare but can be associated with exposure to substances such as vinyl chloride monomer (used to make PVC) and anabolic steroids.

### Secondary tumours

The majority of malignant liver tumours are metastatic. The most common primary carcinomas, which metastasize to the liver, are of the lung, breast, colon and stomach. However, any cancer may spread to the liver, including leukaemias and lymphomas.

Mode of spread is via the bloodstream, through the portal vein (tumours of the GI tract) and the systemic circulation (other tumours). There are usually multiple nodular deposits with a central area of necrosis.

Clinically, the liver is enlarged, hard and craggy on palpation.

Extensive metastases can cause compression of the intrahepatic bile ducts leading to obstructive jaundice.

## Disorders of the biliary tree

### Disorders associated with biliary cirrhosis

Biliary cirrhosis is the result of the long-standing obstruction of bile ducts leading to the development of obstructive jaundice, liver cell necrosis and fibrosis with regenerative nodules. The main causes:

- primary biliary cirrhosis—intrahepatic bile duct destruction of unknown aetiology
- secondary biliary cirrhosis—unrelieved obstruction of the main extrahepatic bile ducts
- primary sclerosing cholangitis—inflammation and fibrosis of bile ducts (both intrahepatic and extrahepatic).

Biliary obstruction causes oedema and expansion of intrahepatic portal tracts with portal tract fibrosis. Bile droplets develop in biliary canaliculi, which may rupture and cause death of adjacent hepatocytes (so-called 'bile infarct'). Over a long period of time, liver cell death, regeneration and fibrosis result in cirrhosis.

### Primary biliary cirrhosis

This cirrhosis occurs as a result of a chronic destruction of intrahepatic bile ducts. It affects 5 per 100 000 in the UK, typically among the middle-aged population. Females are affected more than males by 10:1.

Aetiology is unknown, but it is thought to involve immune phenomena (antimitochondrial antibodies in more than 90% of cases).

It is often associated with other autoimmune diseases, e.g. rheumatoid arthritis (RA), thyroiditis, systemic lupus erythematosus (SLE), scleroderma and Sjögren's syndrome.

Pathogenesis is progressive, chronic, granulomatous and inflammatory. Inflammatory damage with fibrosis may spread from portal tracts to the liver parenchyma. The condition eventually leads to cirrhosis and its complications over a period of about 10 years.

There are four stages:

1. Florid bile—duct lesion with non-caseating granulomatous deposits
2. Ductular proliferation (periportal) upstream from damaged bile ducts
3. Scarring (bridging fibrosis)
4. Cirrhosis.

### Secondary biliary cirrhosis

This occurs as a result of prolonged mechanical obstruction to bile flow in large ducts outside the liver or within the porta hepatis. Causes are:

- gallstones—impacted in common bile duct (most common cause)
- tumours, e.g. carcinoma of bile duct, carcinoma of the pancreas
- strictures—usually following surgery
- congenital diseases—choledochal cyst, extrahepatic biliary atresia.

*Histological features*—Bile pigment accumulates in hepatocytes, in dilated biliary canaliculi and in Kupffer cells. Prolonged obstruction causes:

- 'bile infarcts'—extravasation of bile from dilated canaliculi
- 'bile lakes'—portal tract lesions from bile extravasation
- cirrhosis.

---

**Clinical Note**

Initially, primary biliary cirrhosis causes fatigue, arthralgia, pruritus and mild jaundice. This progresses following cirrhosis to:
- jaundice
- severe pruritus
- hepatosplenomegaly
- malabsorption
- xanthelasma and possible xanthomata.
  Investigations involve:
- liver function tests—features of cholestasis (raised alkaline phosphatase, cholesterol and bile acids)
- antimitochondrial antibodies
- liver biopsy—histological proof
- endoscopic retrograde cholangiopancreatography (ERCP)—rules out obstructive causes of cirrhosis.
  No specific therapy is available; liver transplantation is often necessary.

Complications are cholangitis (inflammation of the bile ducts, usually as a result of superimposed infection) and those of cirrhosis.

### Primary sclerosing cholangitis

Chronic inflammation and obliterative fibrosis of bile ducts with stricture formation causes progressive obstructive jaundice. The condition affects 1 per 100 000 with peak incidence between 25 and 40 years, males more so than females. Aetiology is unknown but is probably autoimmune in nature. However, unlike primary biliary cirrhosis, only 10% of patients have detectable autoantibodies.

Ulcerative colitis is also present in 60% of patients with primary sclerosing cholangitis.

The effects are:

- large intrahepatic and extrahepatic bile ducts—development of fibrous strictures with segmental dilatation causing the 'beaded' appearance on endoscopic retrograde cholangiopancreatography (ERCP)
- medium-sized ducts and ducts in portal tracts—inflammation with concentric fibrosis around ducts

- small bile ducts in portal tracts—replaced by collagenous scarring (vanishing bile ducts).

*Clinical features*—patients develop cholestatic jaundice (pale stools, dark urine and pruritus) with progression to cirrhosis over a period of about 10 years. There is an increased risk of developing cholangio-carcinomas.

Figure 8.24 summarizes disorders associated with biliary cirrhosis.

## Diseases of the gall bladder

### Gallstones (cholelithiasis)

Gallstones (stones formed in the gall bladder) are the most common cause of disease affecting the biliary tree. They occur in 10% of all adults in the UK, females more often than males by 2.5:1. The number of stones per patient has varied from 1 to 26 000.

However, despite the high incidence of gallstones, only about 1% of total patients with gallstones develop complications.

There are two types of gallstone—predominantly cholesterol stones (80% of all stones) and predominantly

**Fig. 8.24** Summary of disorders associated with biliary cirrhosis

| | Primary biliary cirrhosis | Secondary biliary cirrhosis | Primary sclerosing cholangitis |
|---|---|---|---|
| Prevalence | 5 per 100 000 | Unknown | 1 per 100 000 |
| Sex association | Females > males by 10:1; typically affecting middle-aged population | None | Males > females with peak incidence between 25 and 40 years |
| Aetiology | Unknown, probably autoimmune | Gallstones Tumours Strictures Congenital diseases Parasitic obstruction (rare) | Unknown |
| Bile duct changes | Progressive chronic granulomatous inflammatory damage with fibrosis Eventual cirrhosis | Development of bile infarcts and bile lakes Bile duct hyperplasia Eventual cirrhosis | Narrowing and obliteration of intra- and extrahepatic bile ducts Eventual cirrhosis |
| **Laboratory findings** | | | |
| Liver function tests | Features of cholestasis (increased alkaline phosphatase, cholesterol and bile acids) | Features of cholestasis (increased alkaline phosphatase, cholesterol and bile acids) | Features of cholestasis (increased alkaline phosphatase, cholesterol and bile acids) |
| Serology | Antimitochondrial antibodies | — | Hypergammaglobulinaemia |
| ERCP | Patent and non-dilated biliary tree | Dilation of large ducts | Fibrous strictures with segmental dilation → 'beaded' appearance |

*ERCP, endoscopic retrograde cholangiopancreatography*

pigment stones (20% of all stones). Both types also contain calcium salts, e.g. bilirubinate, carbonate, phosphate and palmitate.

### Cholesterol stones

The major constituent of the stone is cholesterol, which reaches levels beyond the solubilizing capacity of bile (supersaturation). This may occur because of:

- hypersecretion of cholesterol (most common mechanism)
- decreased secretion of bile salts, due to either defective bile synthesis or excessive intestinal loss of bile salts
- abnormal gall bladder function, usually hypomobility.

Risk factors for cholesterol stones are shown in Figure 8.25.

### Pigment stones

The major constituent of the stones is bile pigment (calcium bilirubinate). These stones are typically found in patients with chronic haemolysis due to increased bilirubin production, hence pigment stones are typically black.

### Complications, investigations and management

Gallstones may be asymptomatic (80% of cases), symptomatic (pain and other symptoms) or complicated.

Complications include:

- cholecystitis—inflammation of gall bladder caused by impaction of a stone in the neck of the gall bladder or cystic duct
- jaundice—impaction of stone in common bile duct (choledocholithiasis), leading to biliary obstruction and symptoms of biliary colic
- cholangitis—inflammation of bile duct usually as a result of biliary obstruction complicated with bacterial infection

- pancreatitis—impaction of stone distal to opening of pancreatic duct
- predisposition to carcinoma of the gall bladder.

Investigations are:

- ultrasound (most useful)
- abdominal X-ray—but stones are calcified in only 10–20% of cases
- oral cholecystography and CT scanning.

Management is by:

- surgery (cholecystectomy)
- bile acids (e.g. ursodeoxycholic acid)—can dissolve stones in some patients
- extracorporeal shock-wave lithotripsy—useful for those patients unsuitable for surgery.

## Cholecystitis

This is inflammation of the gall bladder. Aetiology is almost always associated with gallstones. There are two types, acute and chronic.

### Acute cholecystitis

This acute inflammation of the gall bladder is precipitated by the chemical effects of concentrated static bile. It is typically due to obstruction of outflow by stones at the gall bladder neck or cystic duct, and it may be exacerbated by secondary infection with enteric organisms such as *Escherichia coli*.

In severe cases, the lumen distends with pus causing increased risk of perforation and peritonitis.

Empyema may occur in an inflamed gall bladder greatly distended with pus.

### Chronic cholecystitis

Invariably associated with gallstones. The wall of the gall bladder is thickened and rigid from fibrosis, with variable chronic inflammatory infiltration of the mucosa and submucosa. The thickened wall may contain mucosal outpouches (Rokitansky–Aschoff sinuses).

Hartmann's pouch is a pathological dilatation in the neck of the gall bladder formed by increased intraluminal pressure or stone.

## Mucocele

This is sterile obstruction of the neck by a gallstone. A lack of inflammation permits the gall bladder to fill with mucus and distend.

## Carcinoma of the gall bladder

This is usually an adenocarcinoma, invariably associated with gallstones and chronic cholecystitis. Most cases are seen in women over the age of 70 years. There is a poor prognosis due to liver invasion.

| **Fig. 8.25** Risk factors for cholesterol stones | |
|---|---|
| Age | ↑Cholesterol secretion |
| Female | ↑Cholesterol secretion |
| Pregnancy | ↑ Cholesterol secretion ↓ Bile secretion Impaired gall bladder motility |
| Obesity | Cholesterol secretion |
| Rapid weight loss | Cholesterol secretion |
| Ethnic origin | May ↑ cholesterol secretion |
| Gallbladder stasis Brief fast Parental therapy Spinal cord injury | Impaired gall bladder motility |

# DISORDERS OF THE EXOCRINE PANCREAS

## Acute pancreatitis

This acute inflammation of the pancreas is caused by the destructive effect of enzymes released from pancreatic acini. It is relatively common, affecting 10–20 per 100 000 per year in Western communities. By far the most common causes of acute pancreatitis are gallstones (50% of cases) and alcohol ingestion (20%). These and other causes are classified in Figure 8.26.

## Pathogenesis

### Duct obstruction

Impaction of a gallstone distal to the site of union of a common bile duct and pancreatic duct results in:

- reflux of bile up pancreatic duct → toxic injury to pancreatic acini
- increased intraductal pressure → enzymatic leakage from pancreatic ducts.

Pancreatic proenzymes (zymogens) are inappropriately activated at some stage in this process, allowing autodigestion of pancreatic tissue. It is believed that the conversion of trypsinogen to trypsin is central to an activation cascade.

*Note*—chronic alcohol ingestion may also produce increased intraductal pressure due to production of a protein-rich pancreatic fluid, which can form solid plugs in smaller pancreatic ducts.

### Direct acinar injury

Less common causes of pancreatitis (e.g. viruses, drugs and trauma) may produce direct acinar damage.

| Fig. 8.26 Causes of acute pancreatitis | |
| --- | --- |
| **Cause** | **Example** |
| Mechanical obstruction of pancreatic ducts | Gallstones Trauma Postoperative |
| Metabolic/toxic causes | Alcohol Drugs, e.g. corticosteroids, thiazide diuretics, azathioprine Hypercalcaemia Hyperlipidaemia |
| Vascular/poor perfusion | Shock Atherosclerosis Hypothermia Polyarteritis nodosa |
| Infections | Mumps |

### Patterns of injury

Irrespective of the cause of pancreatitis, acinar damage leads to the liberation of lytic enzymes (proteases and lipases) causing necrosis of normal tissue. The three patterns of pancreatic necrosis are:

- periductal—necrosis of acinar cells adjacent to ducts. Typically caused by duct obstruction, particularly associated with gallstones and alcohol
- perilobular—necrosis of the periphery of lobules. Caused by poor vascular perfusion usually as a result of shock
- panlobular—necrosis affects all portions of the pancreatic lobule. This often develops from initial periductal or perilobular necrosis.

A vicious circle of necrosis occurs in which enzymatic release results in further acinar damage and further enzyme release:

- Lipases → fat necrosis
- Proteases → destruction of pancreatic parenchyma. Endocrine destruction results in hyperglycaemia
- Elastase and other enzymes → vascular damage with haemorrhage into pancreas or peritoneum. Extensive haemorrhage is known as acute haemorrhagic pancreatitis.

### Clinical features

Clinical features are:

- symptoms—severe central abdominal pain of sudden onset, often radiating into back. Nausea and vomiting
- signs—tachycardia, fever, jaundice, shock, ileus, rigid abdomen, discoloration around the umbilicus (Cullen's sign) or in the flanks (Grey Turner's sign).

### Complications, investigations and management

Complications may be:

- local affecting the pancreas—pancreatic pseudocyst, abscess formation
- gastrointestinal—gastric and duodenal erosions, bleeding, intestinal ileus

- systemic—shock, renal failure, acute respiratory distress syndrome (ARDS), hyperglycaemia, hypocalcaemia, peritonitis.

Diagnosis of acute pancreatitis is made by an elevated serum amylase (or lipase) alongside evidence of pancreatic swelling (on ultrasound or CT). Liver function tests tend to be deranged (↑ bilirubin, ↑ alkaline phosphatase, ↓ albumin).

Management is by physiological support and treatment of shock, respiratory failure and pain.

## Prognosis

Mortality is about 10–15% (negligible in mild cases, but up to 50% in cases with a severe haemorrhagic pancreatitis).

Death may be from shock, renal failure, sepsis or respiratory failure with contributory factors being protease-induced activation of complement, kinin and the fibrinolytic and coagulation cascades.

## Chronic pancreatitis

This is chronic inflammation and fibrosis of the pancreas with a relapsing and remitting course.

It is a relatively rare disease but with increasing incidence due to a rise in the incidence of alcoholism. Typically, it occurs between the ages of 35 and 45 years; males more so than females.

*Aetiology*—the main causes of chronic pancreatitis are outlined in Figure 8.27.

*Pathogenesis*—thought to be similar to the mechanisms involved in acute pancreatitis. However, there is permanent impairment of function.

*Morphological features*:

- Chronic inflammation with parenchymal fibrosis
- Loss of pancreatic parenchymal elements

- Duct strictures with formation of intrapancreatic calculi (stones).

*Clinical features*:

- Recurrent bouts of severe abdominal pain
- Malabsorption due to reduced exocrine function (decreased lipase and protease secretion)—steatorrhea (fat in faeces)
- Diabetes mellitus (destruction of pancreatic parenchyma)—this effect on the endocrine pancreas occurs in advanced disease.

Episodes of acute pancreatitis may complicate chronic pancreatitis.

Relevant investigations include imaging and function tests.

Imaging is by plain radiograph (for calcification of the pancreas), ultrasound, CT and ERCP.

Function tests are:

- secretin/CCK/stimulation test
- oral glucose tolerance test
- measurement of faecal pancreatic chymotrypsin or elastase.

Management is based on alcohol abstinence, pain relief, dietary fat restriction and surgery for correctable causes.

## Pseudocysts

A collection of fluid and necrotic inflammatory debris is localized either within the pancreas itself or, more commonly, in the adjacent tissue, particularly the lesser sac. They are not 'true' cysts (because they have no epithelial lining) but they are surrounded by a zone of inflammatory granulation tissue and they communicate into the pancreatic duct system. They occur in both acute and chronic forms of pancreatitis.

Although many pseudocysts spontaneously resolve, there is a risk of infection, compression or perforation.

| | Cause | Pathogenesis |
|---|---|---|
| Common | Chronic alcoholism (majority of cases) | Protein plugs form in ducts and become calculi; ducts are obstructed, inflamed and scarred |
| | Biliary tract disease | Gallstones or anatomical abnormalities of pancreatic ducts |
| | Idiopathic chronic pancreatitis | Pathogenesis uncertain |
| Rare | Cystic fibrosis | Protein plugs in ducts |
| | Familial pancreatitis | Autosomal dominant |
| | Tropical pancreatitis | Uncertain cause; prevalent in India and Africa |

**Fig. 8.27** Main causes of chronic pancreatitis

## Neoplasms of the pancreas

### Cystic tumours

These benign, well-circumscribed masses are composed of multiple cystic cavities lined by either serous or mucin-secreting epithelium.

### Carcinoma of the pancreas

This common tumour accounts for 3–5% of cancer deaths in the UK. Most tumours are adenocarcinomas arising from the pancreatic ducts. Incidence rises with age, and the cancer is twice as common in males as in females.

Associations include cigarette smoking, chronic pancreatitis, a diet high in fat and carbohydrate and diabetes in women. Around 10% of cases have a clear genetic association (e.g. hereditary pancreatitis, multiple endocrine neoplasia).

The development of pancreatic cancer follows an adenoma-adenocarcinoma sequence similar to that seen in colonic cancer (see Chapter 3). Precursor lesions with the potential to form adenocarcinomas are termed pancreatic intraepithelial neoplasias.

*Macroscopic appearance*—gritty, hard, grey nodules invading adjacent gland and local structures.

The tumour arises with different frequencies in different parts of the pancreas: 60% in the head, 15% in the body, 5% in the tail; 20% of pancreatic cancers exhibit a diffuse pattern.

Carcinoma in the head of the pancreas tends to present early with obstructive jaundice. As a result, tumours are on average smaller at diagnosis than in other sites.

*Microscopic appearance*—lesions are typically moderately differentiated adenocarcinomas composed of glandular spaces in a fibrous stroma.

*Routes of spread*:

* Local—causes obstructive jaundice, or invasion of the duodenum
* Lymphatic—spread to adjacent lymph nodes
* Blood—spread to the liver.

*Clinical features*:

* Weight loss, anorexia and chronic persistent pain in epigastrium radiating to the back
* Obstructive jaundice with painless palpable dilatation of gall bladder (Courvoisier's sign)
* Rarely, there may be vomiting (duodenal obstruction), venous thrombosis (migratory thrombophlebitis), acute pancreatitis or diabetes mellitus (destruction of islets of Langerhans with carcinoma).

*Management*:

* Curative resection (Whipple's procedure)—rarely possible due to extensive disease
* Palliative surgery—often performed to bypass obstruction of the bile duct (relieving jaundice) and obstruction of the duodenum.

Prognosis is extremely poor—5-year survival is just 5%.

## DISORDERS OF THE INTESTINE

## Congenital abnormalities

### Meckel's diverticulum

Diverticulum (outpouching) of the ileum is caused by incomplete regression of part of the yolk stalk (the vitelline duct) during the embryonic period.

Meckel's diverticulum occurs in 2% of the population and in males more than females by about 3:1.

> **HINTS AND TIPS**
>
> Rule of 2s for Meckel's diverticulum:
> * Prevalence—2% of the population
> * Site—usually 2 feet (60 cm) from the ileocaecal junction
> * Length—up to 2 inches (5 cm).

Macroscopically, it is up to 5 cm long and located around 60 cm from the ileocaecal junction.

Microscopically, it is true diverticulum, consisting of all three layers of bowel: mucosa, submucosa and muscularis propria. About half of cases also contain heterotopic gastric acid-secreting epithelium or pancreatic tissue.

*Complications*—the majority of these diverticula are asymptomatic; however, the complications include volvulus, inflammation, peptic ulceration and intussusception (telescoping of one portion of intestine into another).

### Congenital aganglionic megacolon (Hirschsprung's disease)

This congenital condition is characterized by dilatation of the colon due to the absence of the normal myenteric plexus distal to the dilatation. It results from the failure of neuroblast cells to migrate from the vagus into the developing gut. It occurs in 1 per 5000 live births.

This condition always involves the rectum, and it may be present in continuity for a variable distance along the bowel.

Macroscopically, there is a narrowing of an abnormally innervated bowel segment and dilatation and muscular hypertrophy of the bowel segment proximal to this.

Microscopically, there is an absence of normal myenteric and submucosal plexus ganglion cells, and hypertrophy of nerve fibres within submucosa and muscularis mucosae, with extension of abnormal axons up into the lamina propria.

*Clinical features*—the disease usually presents in early childhood with symptoms of colonic obstruction, i.e. constipation, abdominal distension and vomiting.

*Diagnosis*—barium enema reveals a small, empty rectum and dilatation above the narrowed segment. A biopsy of the rectal mucosa will confirm the diagnosis.

Treatment is by excision of the abnormal segments of colon and rectum.

### Acquired megacolon
Note that megacolon can also be a result of acquired disease. However, acquired megacolon differs macroscopically, from Hirschsprung's disease in that there is no narrowed segment, dilatation extends down to the anus, and the rectum is full of faeces.

Causes of acquired megacolon:

- Psychogenic megacolon—disregard for the urge to defaecate (usually in children or the depressed)
- Prolonged stimulant laxative abuse—degeneration of myenteric plexus
- Smooth muscle disorders—degeneration of colonic smooth muscle, e.g. scleroderma
- Chagas' disease—infection by *Trypanosoma cruzi* with destruction of myenteric plexus. Common in South America
- Obstruction—usually by neoplasm or inflammatory stricture
- Toxic megacolon—complication of ulcerative colitis (see below).

## Infections and enterocolitis
### Diarrhoea and dysentery
Diarrhoea is hard to define. Many consider it to mean frequent bowel evacuation or the passage of abnormally soft or liquid faeces, although it is clinically defined as the passage of more than 200 g of stool per day.

Dysentery is an inflammatory disorder of the intestinal tract causing severe diarrhoea with blood and mucus.

### Classification
Diarrhoea can be classified as:

- secretory—diarrhoea caused by a combined effect of excessive intestinal secretions and decreased absorption. Stool volumes may be very high and diarrhoea persists even when there is total fasting
- osmotic—diarrhoea caused by the presence of unabsorbed solute in the colon, which prevents the absorption of fluid. Ceases on fasting long enough to empty the small bowel

- exudative—diarrhoea due to inflammatory exudate consisting of extracellular fluid and pus mixed with blood
- deranged motility—diarrhoea as a result of either increased or decreased motility of the small intestine
- malabsorption—diarrhoea occurring as a result of malabsorption (see below).

The classification and causes of diarrhoea are described in Figure 8.28

## Infectious enterocolitis
Enterocolitis (inflammation of the colon and small intestine) is common and is often a result of infection.

### Viral gastroenteritis
Viruses are the most common cause of gastroenteritis in infants and young children; they account for 10% of all food poisoning outbreaks in the UK. Transmission is typically by a faecal–oral route. Symptoms are cramps, vomiting and fever but no blood in stools.

In children most cases are caused by three viruses:

- Rotavirus—causes 50% of infantile diarrhoea and accounts for some adult cases
- Adenovirus (especially types 40, 41)—second to rotavirus as cause of acute diarrhoea in young children
- Astrovirus—most infections occur in childhood and are mild.

In adults, the Norwalk virus accounts for 30% of cases of gastroenteritis. It is responsible for the 'winter vomiting disease'.

### Bacterial enterocolitis
The types of pathogenic mechanisms are as follows:

- Preformed toxin—ingestion of food contaminated with bacterial toxins, e.g. from *Staphylococcus aureus*, *Bacillus cereus*, *Clostridium perfringens*. Incubation period is very short (1–7 hours).
- Toxigenic organism—ingestion of bacteria that produce toxins in the gut, e.g. *Vibrio cholerae*, enterotoxigenic *Escherichia coli* (ETEC), and *Clostridium perfringens*. So-called 'traveller's diarrhoea' usually occurs by this mechanism and is extremely common.
- Enteroinvasive organism—ingestion of bacteria that invade the intestinal mucosa and may cause dysentery as a result of severe inflammation, e.g. *Salmonella typhi*, *Campylobacter jejuni*, *Shigella*, enterohaemorrhagic *Escherichia coli* (EHEC).
- Antibiotic-associated diarrhoea—occurs as a result of overgrowth of one type of bacteria because of disruption of normal gut flora following antibiotic treatment. Main culprit is *Clostridium difficile*, which causes necrosis of the colonic mucosa and pseudomembranous colitis (a false membrane in the colon). Patients develop fever, abdominal pain and

**Fig. 8.28** Classification and causes of diarrhoea

| Type | Causes |
|---|---|
| Secretory | Infections: bacteria producing enterotoxins, viral diarrhoea, *Giardia*<br>Irritants: laxatives, bile acids, hydroxyl fatty acids<br>Hormonal: VIP, glucagon, medullary carcinoma of the thyroid, Addison's disease<br>Mucosal infiltration: villous adenoma, lymphoma, collagen diseases<br>Congenital: chloridorrhea |
| Osmotic | Osmotic laxatives, e.g. lactulose, magnesium sulphate<br>Disaccharidase deficiency<br>Malabsorption syndromes<br>Congenital, e.g. chloridorrhea (secretory and osmotic), hexose malabsorption |
| Exudative | Inflammatory diseases, e.g. ulcerative colitis, Crohn's disease<br>Infections: bacteria causing invasion of the mucosa, i.e. enteroinvasive bacteria such as *Shigella*, *Campylobacter*, enterohaemorrhagic *Escherichia coli*; and *Entamoeba histolytica* |
| Deranged motility | Decreased motility:<br>• Systemic sclerosis and other collagen disorders<br>• Intestinal pseudo-obstruction<br>• Diabetic autonomic neuropathy<br>Increased motility:<br>• Carcinoid syndrome<br>• Postvagotomy state<br>• Thyrotoxicosis<br>• Unabsorbed bile salts entering colon |
| Malabsorption | May be a mixture of secretory, osmotic and exudative diarrhoea (see Fig. 8.33) |

VIP, vasoactive intestinal polypeptide.

diarrhoea. Clostridial overgrowth is also promoted by surgery, ischaemia, shock and burns. Other pathogens of antibiotic-associated diarrhoea are *Clostridium perfringens* and *Staphylococcus aureus*.

• Necrotizing enterocolitis—rare condition arising through a combination of ischaemia and infection. Ischaemia progresses to intestinal infarction and necrosis of the intestines. Infection of infarcted tissue results in gas gangrene (see Chapter 2), sepsis and shock with paralytic ileus. Most cases are seen in neonates. Adult cases are related to *Clostridium perfringens* infection.

Figure 8.29 provides a summary of common bacterial GI infections.

### Protozoa

Protozoal infection may result in:

• Chagas' disease—infection by *Trypanosoma cruzi* results in the destruction of the myenteric plexus over a period of years with resulting dilatation of various parts of the alimentary canal, especially the colon and oesophagus. Common in South America.
• Amoebic dysentery—this infection by *Entamoeba histolytica* is common throughout the tropics where it is spread by faecal–oral transmission of amoebic cysts. The condition follows a chronic course with abdominal pains. Periods of diarrhoea alternating with constipation are common.

• Giardiasis—This disease is caused by the parasitic protozoan *Giardia lamblia* in the small intestine. Infection occurs by eating food or water contaminated with parasitic cysts. Symptoms include diarrhoea, nausea, abdominal pain and flatulence, as well as the passage of pale, fatty stools. The disease occurs worldwide and it is particularly common in children.
• Other protozoal infections include balantidiasis (*Balantidium coli*), cryptosporidiosis (*Cryptosporidium*).

### Helminths (worms)

• Schistosomiasis (*Schistosoma mansoni* and *S. haematobium*) – eggs from these worms are laid in the mucosa of small and large bowel causing inflammation, ulceration and bleeding.
• Strongyloidiasis (*Strongyloides stercoralis*) – a chronic nematode infection that can become a hyperinfection and virulent if the patient's cellular immune status declines.

**Fig. 8.29** Summary of common bacterial GI infections

| Mechanism | Bacterium | Incubation period | Duration (days) | V | C | F | B |
|---|---|---|---|---|---|---|---|
| Preformed toxin | *Staphylococcus aureus* | 2–7 hours | 1 | + | + | ± | — |
| | *B. cereus* | 1–6 hours | 1 | + | + | — | — |
| Toxigenic organisms | *Vibrio cholerae* | 2–3 days | Up to 7 | + | — | — | — |
| | *Escherichia coli* (ETEC) | 12 hours–3 days | 2–4 | + | — | — | — |
| | *Clostridium perfringens* | 8 hours–1 day | 0.5–1 | — | + | — | — |
| Enteroinvasive bacteria | Non-typhoidal salmonella | 8–48 hours | 4–7 | + | ± | + | ± |
| | *Campylobacter jejuni* | 2–11 days | 3–21 | — | + | + | + |
| | *Shigella* | 1–4 days | 2–3 | — | + | + | + |
| | *Escherichia coli* (EHEC) | 1–5 days | 1–4 | + | + | + | + |
| Antibiotic-associated bacteria | *Clostridium difficile* | — | — | — | + | + | ± |

*B, blood in the stools; C, abdominal cramps; EHEC, enterohaemorrhagic Escherichia coli; ETEC, enterotoxigenic Escherichia coli; F, fever; V, vomiting.*

# Inflammatory disorders of the bowel

The most important of these are idiopathic in origin, namely Crohn's disease and ulcerative colitis (together termed 'inflammatory bowel disease'). These conditions are characterized by chronic, relapsing inflammation of the intestinal wall.

## Crohn's disease

A granulomatous inflammation of unknown cause that affects the full thickness of the bowel wall anywhere in the GI tract from mouth to anus, this disease is characterized by a relapsing and remitting course. Its incidence is about 5–7 per 100 000 in the UK, but this is increasing.

It usually presents in early adult life, with 90% of patients aged between 10 and 40 years, although a secondary peak occurs in the elderly. Females are affected slightly more than males. There is a higher incidence in northern Europe and the USA than elsewhere.

### Pathogenesis

Cause and pathogenesis are unknown, however there is a genetic predisposition with the *NOD2/CARD15* gene on chromosome 16. This gene codes for a protein which facilitates opsonization of gut bacteria; however, the putative infectious organism has not been confirmed.

### Macroscopic appearance

*Site*—most commonly affects the terminal ileum, but it may affect any part of the GI tract from the mouth to the anus in a discontinuous pattern. Two-thirds of cases affect only the terminal ileum, one-sixth affect only the colon, and one-sixth are in the terminal ileum and colon.

*Pattern*:

- 'Skip' lesions—normal bowel areas are present between diseased segments, with a sharp demarcation between the two
- Oedema of submucosa and mucosa
- Haemorrhagic ulcers—initially small and discrete, these progress to form deep, linear, fissured ulcers ('rose thorn' ulcers)
- Cobblestone pattern of bowel mucosa due to submucosal oedema and interconnecting deep fissured ulcers
- Thickened bowel wall due to oedema and fibrosis
- Fibrous strictures may cause partial obstruction
- Enlargement of mesenteric lymph nodes.

### Microscopic appearance

- Transmural inflammation—all layers of bowel wall are affected. Forms basis of fissures, adhesions, fistulae and sinuses
- Lymphoid aggregates develop deep in bowel wall
- Submucosal oedema
- Ulceration
- Non-caseating granulomas present in inflamed bowel wall and in mesenteric lymph nodes in about 60% of cases
- Evidence of persistent and inappropriate T-cell and macrophage activation with increased production of inflammatory cytokines.

### Clinical features

Clinical features are symptoms of abdominal pain, diarrhoea (possibly bloody) and weight loss, with signs of anaemia, clubbing, fever, mouth (aphthous) ulcers and abdominal mass (inflamed bowel loops, abscesses).

## Complications

The natural history of Crohn's disease is one of remissions and relapses of inflammation punctuated by complications.

Local complications are:

- severe inflammation—this may be life threatening, often with dilatation of the colon and passage of bacterial toxins into the bloodstream (toxic megacolon). There is a risk of bowel perforation
- fistulae and sinuses—inflammation of serosal layer leads to the formation of adhesions to other bowel loops, to parietal peritoneum of anterior abdominal wall, or to the bladder
- strictures and fibrous adhesions lead to intestinal obstruction
- carcinoma of bowel—increased incidence after many years
- haemorrhage—significant bleeding from areas of ulceration (rare).

Systemic complications, which develop in a minority of patients with Crohn's, are:

- malabsorption—due to diseased bowel or surgical resections
- skin disease—pyoderma gangrenosum, erythema nodosum
- eye disease—uveitis
- joint disease—polyarthropathy, sacroiliitis, ankylosing spondylitis
- chronic liver disease—pericholangitis, gallstones
- finger clubbing
- systemic amyloidosis (rare).

## Ulcerative colitis

This is a diffuse superficial inflammation of the colorectum of unknown cause, and characterized by relapses and remissions. It affects about 10 per 100 000 in the UK, with much lower rates in developing countries with warmer climates. Ulcerative colitis has a similar age distribution to Crohn's but the sex incidence is equal.

### Aetiopathogenesis

This is unknown, but the same hypotheses as for Crohn's have been proposed with the exception of smoking, which unusually is associated with a decreased risk. Again, inappropriate and persistent T-cell activation may play an important role in the pathogenesis.

### Macroscopic appearance

*Site*—ulcerative colitis usually begins distally as proctitis and then spreads proximally. It may affect the whole of the large bowel (pancolitis), and can, therefore, reach the terminal ileum ('backwash' ileitis).

The pattern is one of shallow ulceration (which may become confluent), with 'pseudopolyps', hyperaemia and haemorrhage. The diseased bowel is continuous, without gaps of normal tissue.

### Microscopic appearance

Inflammation is diffuse and is limited to mucosa and submucosa, with infiltration of both acute and chronic inflammatory cells. Other features are crypt abscesses with ulceration, crypt atrophy and Paneth cell metaplasia.

### Clinical features

Clinical features are symptoms of bloody diarrhoea, mucus, cramping discomfort and weight loss, signs of fever, tachycardia, pallor and abdominal tenderness.

### Complications

Acute local complications include perforation, dilatation, haemorrhage and dehydration (blood and fluid loss from extensive ulceration).

Chronic local complications include strictures, dysplasia and carcinoma (higher cancer risk than Crohn's).

Systemic complications are identical to those seen in Crohn's, except for an additional association with primary sclerosing cholangitis.

## A comparison of Crohn's and ulcerative colitis

Both Crohn's and ulcerative colitis are examples of inflammatory bowel disease and they have many features in common. However, in the majority of cases (about 90%), it is possible to distinguish between these two conditions (Figs 8.30, 8.31).

### Diagnosis

Diagnosis is by colonoscopy, barium and small bowel enema. Colonoscopy is the most sensitive test and biopsy specimens can be taken for histological examination (see Figure 8.32 for differences in microscopic appearance). This investigation is also important in

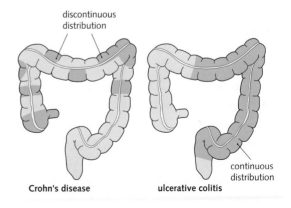

**Fig. 8.30** Comparisons of distribution along the bowel.

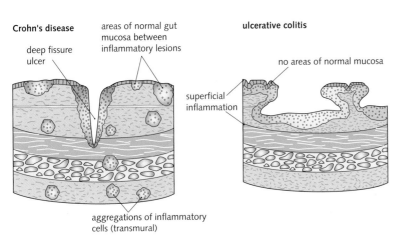

**Fig. 8.31**  Depth and distribution of lesions in the bowel wall.

Crohn's disease

deep fissure ulcer

areas of normal gut mucosa between inflammatory lesions

ulcerative colitis

no areas of normal mucosa

superficial inflammation

aggregations of inflammatory cells (transmural)

**Fig. 8.32** Comparison of the basic features of Crohn's disease and ulcerative colitis

|  | Crohn's disease | Ulcerative colitis |
|---|---|---|
| Incidence in UK | ~5–7 per 100 000 in UK | ~10 per 100 000 |
| Site | Any part of GI system but typically terminal ileum | Colon and rectum only |
| **Macroscopic** | | |
| Disease continuity | Discontinuous | Continuous |
| Bowel wall | Thickened with strictures and adhesions | Not thickened |
| Ulcers | Deep fissures form basis of fistulae | Flat based; do not extend to submucosa |
| **Microscopic** | | |
| Pattern of inflammation | Transmural Focal Granulomas (in 60% of cases) | Mucosal and submucosal Diffuse No granulomas |
| Crypt pattern | Little distortion | Distorted in long-standing disease; crypt abscesses |
| **Anal lesions** | | |
|  | Present in 75%; anal fistulae; ulceration or chronic fissure | Present in <25% |
| **Frequency of fistula** | | |
|  | 10–20% of cases | Uncommon |
| **Risk of developing cancer** | | |
|  | Slightly increased | Significantly increased |

the surveillance of patients with long-standing colitis as it allows severe dysplasia and early invasive cancer to be detected.

Rectal sparing, discrete patchy ulceration and peri-anal disease are classically seen on Crohn's colonoscopy. This contrasts with ulcerative colitis, with its confluent ulceration, which is most severe in the distal colon. Long-standing severe disease may show loss of haustral markings with a featureless, shortened hosepipe colon.

## Management
Management can be medical or surgical.

*Medical*:

• Corticosteroids—effective in inducing remission (local, i.e. topical steroid enemas used for

147

exacerbations of distal proctocolitis; systemic, i.e. oral prednisolone)

- 5-Aminosalicylic acid (5-ASA) compounds—can be used to maintain remission once remission has been induced by corticosteroids
- Azathioprine—immunosuppresant as a steriod-sparing agent
- TNFα blockers (infliximab)—used in active, fistulating Crohn's disease that is unresponsive to other treatments.

*Surgical*:

- Minimal resections for strictures, fistulae or perfo-rations (more common in Crohn's).
- Colectomy—indicated in cases of extensive disease affecting quality of life, failed medical therapy, fulminant colitis and severe dysplasia or cancer on colonoscopy surveillance. Pouch-forming opera-tions preserve sphincter function and avoid an ileostomy. This is suitable in ulcerative colitis but not in Crohn's, where recurrent disease may affect the pouch.

## Malabsorption syndromes

### General aspects of malabsorption syndromes

Malabsorption may be caused by disorders of:

- intraluminal digestion—assisted by, for example, gastric juices and pancreatic digestive enzymes (these are necessary for breakdown of macromolecules)
- intraluminal solubilization—liver secretes bile acids required for solubilization and absorption of fats
- terminal digestion—enzymes located on the brush border of the small intestinal mucosa hydrolyse large molecules for absorption, especially complex sugars (e.g. sucrase for sucrose and lactase for lactose)
- transepithelial transport—mucosa is specialized for absorption. Transverse mucosal folds and finger-like villi provide a vast surface area.

Systemic effects of the malabsorption syndromes:

- Weight loss and anorexia
- Abdominal distension and borborygmi (increased bowel sounds)
- Diarrhoea (loose, bulky stools)
- Steatorrhoea—malabsorption of fat, producing pale, foul-smelling stools that characteristically float in water
- Muscle wasting.

### Classification of malabsorption syndromes

This is described in Figure 8.33.

### Coeliac disease

This is caused by a chronic inflammatory response to the protein gliadin, a component of gluten (found in wheat, oats, barley and rye). Atrophy of small intestinal villi and crypt hyperplasia are the result. It affects about 1 per 1000 in most Caucasian populations of Western Europe; it is rare in other ethnic origins.

It can present at any age but it is an important cause of failure to thrive in infants and children.

Antigliadin antibodies are present in the majority of cases, although anti-endomyseal antibodies have a greater sensitivity and specificity as a diagnostic aid. Other tests that may be used are small-bowel biopsy and a gluten challenge, in which symptoms improve on a gluten-free diet, but relapse once this is stopped.

There is an increased incidence of disease in first-degree relatives of those affected. It sometimes occurs concurrently with dermatitis herpetiformis (itchy, blistering skin disease).

Macroscopically, the luminal surface becomes flat-tened, developing a mosaic-like pattern of crypt openings (Fig. 8.34).

Microscopically there is:

- mucosal inflammation with lymphocytic infil-tration
- loss of villous architecture ranging from blunting (partial villous atrophy) to complete flattening (to-tal villous atrophy) due to a high rate of cell loss
- increase in the depth of crypts with epithelial cell hyperplasia to compensate for those lost through damage.

Long-term complications are:

- chronic ulceration of the small intestine—may lead to strictures
- development of primary T-cell lymphoma of the small intestine
- development of adenocarcinoma (rare).

Management is by the complete withdrawal of glia-din from the diet (i.e. a gluten-free diet), which leads to gradual recovery of the villous structure. This may be partial or complete.

### Tropical sprue

This chronic and progressive malabsorption syndrome without a definable cause is seen in patients who live or have lived in the tropics, and in the absence of other intestinal disease or parasites. The disease occurs mainly in the West Indies and Asia.

Aetiology is unclear; however, the condition is thought to be infective, probably toxigenic *Escher-ichia coli*.

Clinical features and histological appearances resem-ble those of coeliac disease. However, a gluten-free diet has little beneficial effect.

**Fig. 8.33** Causes of malabsorption

| | |
|---|---|
| Defective intraluminal digestion or solubilization | Pancreatic insufficiency:<br>• Chronic pancreatitis<br>• Cystic fibrosis<br>• Carcinoma of the pancreas<br>Liver disease: failure of bile secretion into duct |
| Primary mucosal cell abnormalities | Lactase deficiency |
| Reduced surface area of small intestine | Conditions that cause villous atrophy:<br>• Coeliac disease<br>• Tropical sprue<br>• Crohn's disease<br>• Malnutrition<br>Iatrogenic:<br>• Extensive small intestine resection<br>• Jejunal ileal bypass procedures<br>• Postradiotherapy |
| Infection | Parasitic infestation of gut<br>Bacterial overgrowth in blind loops of diverticulae<br>Postinfective malabsorption<br>Giardiasis<br>Whipple's disease |
| Lymphatic obstruction | Primary lymphangiectasia<br>Lymphoma |
| Drug-induced | Cytotoxic drugs<br>Drugs that bind bile salts, e.g. cholestyramine and some antibiotics such as neomycin (which causes steatorrhoea) |
| Miscellaneous | Thyrotoxicosis®increased gastric emptying and motility<br>Zollinger–Ellison syndrome<br>Diabetes mellitus®bacterial overgrowth<br>Hypogammaglobulinaemia®infection |

## Whipple disease

Whipple disease is a multisystem disorder involving malabsorption, weight loss, lymphadenopathy and joint pain. The causative agent is the Gram-positive bacillus *Tropheryma whippelii*. This rare condition is characterized by tissue infiltration with foamy macrophages that are periodic acid-Schiff (PAS) reagent positive.

## Bacterial overgrowth syndrome

In this syndrome, there is malabsorption secondary to excessive bacteria in the small intestine, usually the jejunum.

Causes of small intestinal bacterial overgrowth are outlined in Figure 8.35.

Malabsorption is as a result of:

- deconjugation of bile salts by the bacteria, hence steatorrhoea
- damage to the small intestinal mucosa, probably by bacterial products

- binding of vitamin $B_{12}$ by bacteria, hence vitamin $B_{12}$ deficiency.

Diarrhoea is both secretory (due to bacterial products affecting mucosa) and osmotic (due to unabsorbed products and deficiency of disaccharidases because of mucosal damage).

Clinical features are weight loss, diarrhoea and anaemia (due to vitamin $B_{12}$ deficiency).

Management is by antibiotic therapy and surgical resection for a localized abnormality, e.g. stricture, fistula.

## Disaccharidase deficiency

The most important disaccharidase is lactase, which is essential for the digestion of milk sugar (lactose). All babies have lactase in their intestines but the enzyme disappears later in life in about 10% of northern Europeans, 40% of Greeks and Italians, and 80% of Africans and Asians. The presence of undigested lactose in the small intestine (following

**Fig. 8.34** Comparison of normal jejunal mucosa (A) and jejunal mucosa in coeliac disease with total villous atrophy (B).

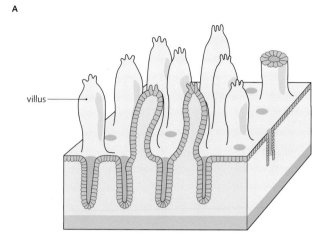

A

villus

B

absence of villi

**Fig. 8.35** Causes of small intestinal bacterial overgrowth

| Cause | Example |
|---|---|
| Excessive entry of bacteria | Achlorydria<br>Infected bile ducts<br>Gastrocolic fistula<br>Gastric surgery<br>Resection of ileocaecal valve |
| Defective immune mechanisms | Hypogammaglobulinaemia<br>Malnutrition<br>Old age |
| Stagnant region | Blind loops<br>Enterocolic fistulae<br>Jejunal diverticula<br>Strictures or other obstruction<br>Continent ileostomy |
| Disturbed motility | Systemic sclerosis<br>Intestinal pseudo-obstruction<br>Diabetic autonomic neuropathy |

consumption of raw milk) causes diarrhoea and abdominal pain.

## Obstruction of the bowel

### Major causes of bowel obstruction

Obstruction and pseudo-obstruction can be classified as follows:

- Simple mechanical obstruction—the bowel above the obstructing lesion becomes distended with fluid and gas.
- Strangulation obstruction—occlusion of the blood supply by constricting agents.
- Paralytic ileus—may arise as a consequence of peritonitis, pancreatitis or retroperitoneal bleeding.
- Pseudo-obstruction—abnormal gut motility rather than an organic obstructive lesion.

Examples of simple mechanical obstruction, strangulation obstruction and paralytic ileus types of obstructions are listed in Figure 8.36.

**Fig. 8.36** Major causes of bowel obstruction

| Cause | Example |
|---|---|
| Simple mechanism obstruction | Intraluminal:<br>• Foreign bodies<br>• Gallstone ileus<br>• Faecoliths<br>• Meconium in cystic fibrosis<br>Bowel wall:<br>• Adhesions<br>• Carcinoma<br>• Strictures<br>• Atresia<br>• Imperforate anus |
| Strangulation obstruction | Intussusception<br>Infarction<br>Volvulus<br>Internal/external hernias<br>Bands |
| Adynamic obstruction (paralytic ileus) | Abdominal causes: postoperative, peritonitis, vascular occlusion<br>Systemic causes: electrolyte disorders, uraemia, hypothyroidism<br>Drugs: anticholinergics, opiates |

## Hernias

This is the protrusion of the whole or part of a viscus from its normal position through a defect in the cavity wall in which it is contained. About 1 per 100 people has a hernia at some time. Hernias can be congenital or acquired. Acquired hernias are:

* secondary to increased intra-abdominal pressure—resulting from cough, straining at the stool, cysts, carcinoma, pregnancy
* iatrogenic—incisional hernias.

  *Classification*:

* Reducible—contents of sac can be completely returned to abdominal cavity
* Irreducible/incarcerated—content of sac cannot be completely returned to the abdominal cavity.

Common sites of abdominal hernias are inguinal (70%), femoral (20%) and umbilical (10%). Others are supraumbilical or linea alba, incisional hernias and hiatus hernia.

  *Complications*:

* Obstruction—constriction at the neck of the hernial sac causes obstruction of bowel loops within it.
* Strangulation—constriction at the neck of sac prevents venous return leading to venous congestion, arterial occlusion and gangrene. This may result in perforation leading to peritonitis/groin abscess.

Note that strangulation can occur without obstruction if only one wall of the viscus pouches into the sac (Richter's hernia).

Hernias must be repaired because of potential complications. The principles of surgical repair are identification of the sac and contents, mobilization of the sac, reduction of the contents, ligation of the sac and repairing the fascial defect.

### Inguinal hernia

The most common type of hernia, this is much more prevalent in men than in women. There are two types: indirect inguinal (85%) and direct inguinal (15%).

In indirect cases, the hernial sac enters the inguinal canal through the deep ring (lateral to the inferior epigastric artery) and then traverses through the canal to the superficial ring, where it may eventually reach the scrotum or labium major. It is the result of a congenital abnormality. Strangulation is a common complication due to the narrow neck of the hernial sac.

In direct cases, the hernial sac protrudes through a weakness in the fascia transversalis (medial to inferior epigastric artery) and it does not normally descend into the scrotum or labium major. It originates as a result of weakened abdominal muscles (usually acquired in the elderly). The neck of the sac is wide so strangulation is rare.

Clinically, it is difficult (often impossible) to distinguish between direct and indirect inguinal hernias.

### Femoral hernia

The hernial sac protrudes through the femoral canal inferior to the inguinal ligament (Fig. 8.37). There is an increasing incidence with age, and females are affected more than males by 2:1 (but inguinal hernia is still

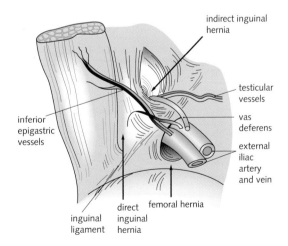

**Fig. 8.37** Sites of direct inguinal, indirect inguinal and femoral herniations. (Adapted with permission from Principles and Practice of Surgery, 3rd edn, by APM Forrest, PC Carter and IB Macleod, Churchill Livingstone, 1995.)

more common in both males and females). The most common complication is strangulation.

## Adhesions

Adhesions are by far the most common cause of mechanical obstruction in the small bowel, and they are defined as areas of fibrosis between adjacent membranes or organs resulting in their fusion. The causes can be congenital (e.g. bands in small children) or acquired.

Acquired causes are as follows:

- Inflammation, e.g. Crohn's disease, sclerosing peritonitis
- Infection, e.g. appendicitis, diverticulitis, tuberculosis, peritonitis
- Trauma, e.g. stab wounds
- Iatrogenic—postsurgery, irradiation
- Vascular—infarction/gangrene
- Malignancies.

## Intussusception

This is invagination of one part of the bowel into the adjoining segment (Fig. 8.38). The ileocaecal valve is the most common site, with the ileum invaginating into the caecum. It typically affects children under the age of 4 years.

Adult cases are extremely rare, and they are almost invariably precipitated by an intraluminal mass (e.g. tumour) or structural abnormality (e.g. Meckel's diverticulum).

As the contents of the intestine are pushed onwards by muscular contraction, more and more intestine is dragged into the adjoining bowel. The net effect is venous congestion of the invaginated portion, which may suffer infarction if mesenteric vessels are trapped.

Management is by barium reduction in children or by resection in adults because of the high incidence of organic causes.

## Volvulus

This is a twisting of part of the GI tract, usually leading to partial or complete obstruction (Fig. 8.39). It is most commonly seen in redundant loops of the sigmoid colon, but may also occur in the caecum, small intestine and stomach.

The most common complication is strangulation (causing infarction and possibly gangrene).

*Management*—may untwist spontaneously but surgical manipulation is usually performed.

## Colonic diverticulosis

### Definitions

A diverticulum is a sac or pouch formed at weak points in the wall of the alimentary tract; diverticulosis means that there is no evidence of inflammation. Diverticulitis is inflammation of a diverticulum, which commonly occurs in one or more colonic diverticula.

### Aetiopathogenesis of diverticula

Congenital diverticula are true diverticula containing all three coats of the bowel wall, e.g. Meckel's diverticulum.

Acquired diverticula may contain some (false diverticula) or all (true diverticula) coats of the bowel wall. They typically develop during adult life as a result of:

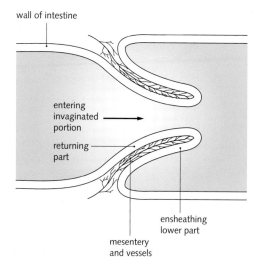

wall of intestine

entering
invaginated
portion

returning
part

ensheathing
lower part

mesentery
and vessels

**Fig. 8.38**  Intussusception.

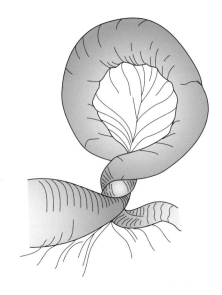

**Fig. 8.39**  Intestinal volvulus.

- pulsion from increased intraluminal pressure (e.g. straining at the stool) causing protrusion at points of focal weakness (e.g. at the sites of penetration of blood vessels)
- traction due to extrinsic disease.

Colonic diverticulosis is caused by a chronic lack of dietary fibre.

Although rare before 35 years of age, by 65 years of age at least one-third of the population of developed countries is affected. Rare in countries with high-fibre diets.

Diverticula are most common in the sigmoid colon emerging between mesenteric and antimesenteric taeniae.

Complications are:

- Inflammation (diverticulitis)—may cause severe pain and tenderness in left iliac fossa, alteration of bowel habit, fever, leucocytosis. There may be a palpable mass
- Perforation—results in peritonitis
- Obstruction—due to oedema or fibrosis in the inflamed segment of colon or to adherence of small bowel loops
- Stricture formation—long-standing diverticular disease may cause stricture formation and subacute intestinal obstruction
- Fistula—most common cause of colovesical fistula
- Bleeding—common complication.

---

### Clinical Note

The clinical course of colonic diverticular disease may be asymptomatic, but sometimes causes left-sided colicky abdominal pain and alteration of bowel habit (usually constipation) or rectal bleeding.

Diverticula can be visualized and diagnosed by barium enema and/or colonoscopy.

Treatment:

- Conservative—high-fibre diet results in improvement in most patients.
- Surgery—sigmoid colectomy with end-to-end anastomosis if there are persistent symptoms or when carcinoma cannot be excluded by radiology or colonoscopy.

---

## Vascular disorders of the bowel

### Ischaemic bowel disease

Ischaemic bowel disease may affect the small or large bowel, and it is most commonly seen in elderly patients with severe atherosclerosis. The causes are discussed below.

### Vessel disease

These are:

- vascular occlusion—emboli lodge in the superior mesenteric artery, which supplies all the small intestine except for the first part of the duodenum. Emboli are usually derived from cardiac mural thrombus
- vascular stenosis (less common)—occurs with thrombosis in a severely atherosclerotic mesenteric artery. Typically located near its origin from aorta. Resultant small bowel infarction is extensive and usually fatal
- vasculitic syndromes, e.g. polyarteritis nodosa, Henoch–Schönlein purpura, SLE.

### Strangulation

Thin-walled veins which drain blood from the small bowel become occluded by extrinsic pressure, e.g. from:

- loop of bowel in a narrow hernial sac
- intussusception
- volvulus
- adhesions.

Venous occlusion causes congestion and oedema of the bowel wall. Increased pressure prevents entry of oxygenated arterial blood leading to ischaemic necrosis.

### Classification of severity

Ischaemic infarcts are classified according to the depth of involvement:

- Mucosal infarction—transient or reversible infarction which may be followed by complete regeneration. However, increased permeability to toxic substances can cause gradual progression to a transmural infarct.
- Mural infarction—infarction of mucosa and submucosa up to the muscularis propria. The mucosa is ulcerated, oedematous and haemorrhagic. Healing occurs by granulation tissue formation. Mural infarction may lead to the development of fibrous strictures (occurs in about half of patients with ischaemic bowel disease).
- Transmural infarction—necrosis extends through the muscularis propria. The bowel is flaccid, dilated and liable to perforation. Surgical resection is an option, but many patients already have peritonitis, endotoxaemia and severe circulatory problems at the time of diagnosis, so the prognosis is poor.

The splenic flexure is a common and early site of ischaemic damage, as it is a watershed area between the distribution of superior and inferior mesenteric arteries.

## Angiodysplasia

In this condition, abnormal venous dilatations develop in the submucosa of the large intestine (typically the right side) often causing occult or massive intestinal bleeding. It occurs in the elderly and is associated with aortic valve disease.

It is thought to be a degenerative process resulting in increasing obstruction of the mucosal veins, which become tortuous and prone to bleeding.

## Haemorrhoids (piles)

These are dilated varicose veins forming in the anal canal. The most common of all anal conditions, they affect as much as 40% of the population at some time. Haemorrhoids develop as a result of increased intra-abdominal pressure, e.g. constipation and straining at the stool, pregnancy.

Rarely, raised portal hypertension can cause haemorrhoid formation.

Two anatomical areas are affected, although both are often involved at the same time:

1. Internal haemorrhoids—proximal to superior haemorrhoidal plexus, above the anorectal margin. These most commonly occur at three main points equidistant to the circumference of the anus (Fig. 8.40).
2. External haemorrhoids—below the anorectal margin.

Haemorrhoids are associated with bright red rectal bleeding after defaecation, pain and pruritus ani.

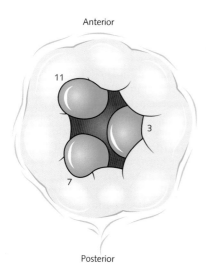

Anterior

11

3

7

Posterior

**Fig. 8.40** Diagram to illustrate the 3, 7, 11 distribution of haemorrhoids around the anus. (Adapted with permission from Lecture Notes in General Surgery, 12th edn, by H Ellis, Wiley-Blackwell, 2010.)

### Clinical classification

There are three degrees of haemorrhoid:

1. First degree—present in the lumen but do not prolapse; these tend to bleed
2. Second degree—prolapse on defaecation but return spontaneously
3. Third degree—remain prolapsed but can be digitally replaced.

Diagnosis is by proctoscopy (to visualize the haemorrhoids) or by sigmoidoscopy (to exclude coexisting rectal pathology).

Treatment involves reducing constipation and straining with a high fibre diet, or direct therapy to the haemorrhoid with injection sclerotherapy or band ligation. Surgical removal of the haemorrhoid (haemorrhoidectomy) is rarely required.

## Neoplastic disease of the intestine

Primary tumours of the small intestine are rare; those that do arise are outlined in Figure 8.41. In contrast, tumours of the large bowel are extremely common. The colon and rectum are frequently affected by both benign and malignant tumours.

## Classification of intestinal tumours

Intestinal tumours can be classified according to Figure 8.41.

## Neoplastic epithelial lesions

### Adenomas

These premalignant tumours are derived from the glandular epithelium of the large bowel. Common in older subjects, they are present in up to 50% of persons aged over 60, males more than females by 2:1.

Aetiology is probably multifactorial. Both genetic and environmental (dietary) factors have been implicated.

There are three types:

1. Tubular—rounded lesions (0.5–2 cm in size). Often pedunculated (i.e. have a stalk of normal mucosa). Microscopically composed of tube-shaped glands.
2. Villous—frond-like lesions about 0.6 cm thick, which occupy a broad area of mucosa (1–5 cm in diameter). Microscopically composed of fingerlike epithelial projections.
3. Tubulovillous—raised lesions (1–4 cm in size). Pedunculated but composed of both tube-shaped glands and finger-like epithelial projections.

Epithelium of all three types shows dysplastic features, which can be subjectively graded as mild, moderate or severe.

**Fig. 8.41** Types of intestinal tumours

| | Small intestine | Large bowel |
|---|---|---|
| Non-neoplastic polyps | Hamartomas<br>Juvenile polyps<br>Adenomatous polyps (in familial adenomatous polyposis and Gardner's syndrome)<br>Inflammatory fibroid polyps | Hyperplastic polyps: small, flat, pale lesions typically 5 mm in size, which occur most commonly in the rectum and sigmoid colon<br>Hamartomatous polyps: typically occur in childhood and in adolescence,eg. Peutz–Jeghers syndrome juvenile polyps (autosomal dominant), sporadic<br>Inflammatory 'pseudopolyps' (of ulcerative colitis) |
| Neoplastic epithelial lesions | Adenocarcinomas | Pre-malignant:<br>• Adenomas (dysplastic):<br>  Tubular adenoma<br>  Villous adenoma<br>  Tubulovillous adenoma<br>• Familial adenomatous polyposis<br>Malignant:<br>• Colorectal carcinoma |
| Mesenchymal lesions | Benign: lipoma, neurogenic tumours, leiomyoma and haemangioma<br>Malignant: some smooth muscle tumours (leiomyosaracomas) | Rare; usually incidental findings or at post-mortem; seldom responsible for symptoms; lipomas, leiomyomas, haemangiomas, neurofibromas |
| Lymphoma | Common site for primary lymphoma of the GI tract; coeliac disease is a major predisposing factor | Very uncommon in large bowel |
| Carcinoid tumours (neuroendocrine tumours) | Most common site for carcinoid tumours (especially appendix); lesions typically scattered singly throughout GI tract; may secrete gut hormones, e.g. somatostatin, cholecystokinin, pancreatic polypeptide and VIP | Rare; do not usually produce functioning hormones |

*Note: GI, gastrointestinal; VIP, vasoactive intestinal polypeptide*

## Progression from adenoma to carcinoma

Most carcinomas of the colon develop from previous adenomas. Progression from adenoma to carcinoma is the well-established basis of the polyp-cancer sequence for development of carcinoma of the colon.

Risk of malignant change is greatest where adenomas show the following features:

- Large—less than 1 cm (1% malignant); 1–2 cm (12% malignant); more than 2 cm (30% malignant)
- Villous—villous adenomas are more likely to undergo malignant transformation
- Severe dysplasia.

## Familial adenomatous polyposis

Familial adenomatous polyposis (FAP) is a rare autosomal dominant condition caused by a mutation in the APC gene located on the long arm of chromosome 5. It is characterized by the presence of innumerable adenomata of the large bowel from about the age of 25.

There is a 90% risk of developing a carcinoma of the colon by the age of 45.

## Hereditary non-polyposis colon cancer

This is an inherited form of colon cancer, without adenomas, which is due to mutation in DNA mismatch repair genes. This is associated with microsatellite instability.

## Colorectal carcinoma

This adenocarcinoma is derived from the glandular epithelium of the large bowel mucosa.

It is the second most common cause of death from neoplasia, with a peak incidence between 60 and 70 years of age; it is rare under the age of 40.

There is a high incidence in developed countries. 55 per 100 000 males and 35 per 100 000 females in the UK are diagnosed each year, with a higher incidence in Scotland for both sexes. Environmental factors are thought to play a large role in the aetiology of colorectal cancer. Risk factors are:

- high-fat, high-protein, low-fibre diets (effects on bowel transit time, bacterial flora and levels of cellulose, amino acids and bile acids in the bowel contents)
- presence of multiple sporadic adenomatous polyps
- long-standing and extensive ulcerative colitis
- familial adenomatous polyposis
- previous pelvic radiotherapy.

Macroscopically, the most common sites for colorectal carcinomas are illustrated in Figure 8.42.

Types of colorectal carcinomas are:

- polypoid—cauliflower-like growth
- annular—small, circumferential carcinomas that may cause stenosis
- ulcerated—tumours that present mainly with bleeding
- diffusely infiltrative—rare, but virtually identical to that seen in stomach. Often associated with carcinoma that develops in association with inflammatory bowel disease.

Right-sided carcinomas (ascending colon):

- Type of growth—polypoid
- Pathogenesis—faecal material is soft in ascending colon, and so lesions grow to large size before causing obstruction
- Presentation—later than for left-sided carcinomas.

Left-sided carcinomas (descending colon):

- Type of growth—annular, ulcerating
- Pathogenesis—lesions develop where faecal material is more solid
- Presentation—earlier due to mechanical obstruction to passage of faeces.

*Microscopic features*—98% of all cancers in the large intestine are adenocarcinomas; the majority of colorectal carcinomas are, therefore, moderately or well-differentiated adenocarcinomas forming recognizable glandular structures.

Poorly differentiated carcinomas have a poorer prognosis. Overall, 5-year survival is around 50%.

### Clinical Note

Spread of colorectal carcinoma:
- Local—adjacent bowel wall and adherent structures (e.g. bladder)
- Lymphatic—draining nodes
- Blood—to liver and then elsewhere
- Transcaelomic—along peritoneal cavity.

Prognosis relates to stage, which is assessed by the modified Dukes system (Fig. 8.43). Five-year survival is over 90% in Dukes A cancer, but less than 5% in Dukes D. Dukes C and D cancers (common presentations) require adjuvant chemotherapy and/or radiotherapy after surgical resection.

## DISORDERS OF THE PERITONEUM

## Inflammation: peritonitis

### Peritoneal infection

This can either be of primary or secondary infection. Primary infection (less common) is seen in patients with nephrotic syndrome (peritoneal dialysis), cirrhosis with ascites or abdominal trauma.

Secondary infection (most common) is typically an extension of inflammatory processes from the abdominal cavity. For example:

- appendicitis
- ruptured ulcers—peptic, ulcerative colitis, typhoid ulcers, ulcerated neoplasms
- cholecystitis, pancreatitis, salpingitis
- diverticulitis
- chlamydial infection—a complication of female pelvic inflammatory disease that is increasing in incidence
- strangulated bowel.

Organisms involved are typically a mixture of normal gut commensals with a predominance of anaerobic bacteria and coliforms.

Irritation of the peritoneum by leaking bile, gastric juice, pancreatic enzymes or urine produces an exudate that is initially sterile but which usually becomes infected within 6–12 hours.

As peritonitis develops, inflammation of visceral and parietal peritoneum produces a purulent exudate; the intestine becomes flaccid, dilated and covered with fibrinous plaques that form adhesions between bowel loops.

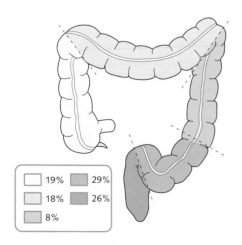

| | |
|---|---|
| 19% | 29% |
| 18% | 26% |
| 8% | |

**Fig. 8.42**   Site and incidence of carcinomas of the large intestine.

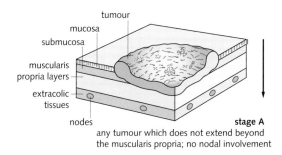

stage A
any tumour which does not extend beyond
the muscularis propria; no nodal involvement

stage B
tumour extends beyond the muscularis
propria; no nodal involvement

stage C
any depth of tumour;
tumour present in nodes

stage D
distant metastases

**Fig. 8.43**   Staging of carcinoma of the colon using the Dukes system.

Clinical features are:

- tenderness, guarding, and rebound tenderness
- board-like abdominal rigidity
- absent bowel sounds (paralytic ileus)
- increased pulse and temperature.

**Complications and management**
Complications are:

- hypovolaemic shock

- severe toxaemia from absorbed bacterial products
- paralytic ileus—paralysis of gut motility as a result of inflammation of the serosa of the small bowel
- fibrous adhesions as a result of organization of fibrinous adhesion by granulation tissue
- abscesses, particularly in the paracolic gutters and beneath the diaphragm (subphrenic recesses)
- portal pyophlebitis—spread via the portal vein to the liver.

Diagnosis is by clinical examination and erect abdominal X-ray, which may show air under the diaphragm from perforated viscus. Blood cultures may reveal the organism responsible.

Management is by:

- treatment of shock
- antibiotic therapy
- surgery—removal of contaminating source, e.g. appendicitis or perforated bowel
- peritoneal toilet and lavage.

See Figure 8.44 for a summary of peritoneal infection.

## Retroperitoneal fibrosis

This dense progressive fibrosis of the peritoneum particularly affects the visceral peritoneum of the small intestine. In most cases no cause is found, although there are rare associations with some medications (practolol and methysergide). It is also seen in patients undergoing long term continuous ambulatory peritoneal dialysis.

## Mesenteric cysts

These are cysts found within the mesenteries of the abdominal cavity, or attached to the peritoneal lining.

### Sequestered lymphatic channels (cystic lymphangiomas)
These cystic developmental abnormalities of lymphoid type are typically asymptomatic and discovered incidentally at laparotomy or autopsy.

### Pinched-off enteric diverticula (enterogenous cysts)
These common lesions are found either incorporated in the bowel wall or in mesentery detached and separated from the tract.

### 'Walled-off' infections
This localized peritonitis is due to the capacity of omentum to wall-off infection (pseudocysts).

## Neoplasms

## Primary mesothelioma

A rare condition, this is associated with exposure to asbestos. It corresponds to the much more common pleural mesothelioma (see Chapter 7).

**Fig. 8.44** Summary of peritoneal infection

| | |
|---|---|
| Aetiology | Primary infection (less common): nephrotic syndrome, peritoneal dialysis, cirrhosis with ascites, abdominal trauma<br>Secondary infection (most common): typically an extension of inflammatory processes from abdominal cavity, e.g. appendicitis, ruptured ulcers (peptic, ulcerative colitis, typhoid ulcers, ulcerated neoplasms), cholecystitis, pancreatitis, salpingitis, diverticulitis, strangulated bowel |
| Organisms involved | Normal gut commensals with anaerobic bacteria and coliforms predominating |
| Pathogenesis | Leaking bile, gastric juice, pancreatic enzymes or urine cause irritation and inflammation of peritoneum producing an exudate that typically becomes infected; intestine becomes flaccid, dilated and covered with fibrinous plaques forming adhesions between bowel loops |
| Clinical features | Guarding and rebound tenderness<br>Board-like abdominal rigidity<br>Absent bowel sounds (paralytic ileus)<br>Increased pulse and temperature |
| Complications | Local: ileus, fibrinous adhesions, abscesses, portal pyophlebitis<br>Systemic: hypovolaemic shock, severe toxaemia |

**HINTS AND TIPS**

The peritoneal cavity is a common site of metastases; malignancy of any organ within the peritoneal cavity may lead to peritonitis.

Metastases result in the effusion of protein-rich fluid into the cavity (i.e. an exudate) containing neoplastic cells, which also grow as tiny white nodules on the mesothelial surface of the cavity. Nodules eventually coalesce to form tumour sheets over the surface of the viscera.

## Secondary

These most common tumours metastasize to the peritoneal cavity of the stomach, ovary, pancreas and colon.

In this chapter, you will learn to:
- Describe abnormalities of kidney structure, notably the common cystic diseases.
- Understand the patterns of glomerular disease and common mechanisms of injury.
- Describe common glomerular diseases and how pathology relates to clinical presentation.
- Recognize that glomerular lesions occur in systemic diseases, giving common examples.
- Recall the pathology of renal tubular and interstitial diseases.
- Describe disorders of renal blood vessels.
- Understand the neoplasms commonly encountered within the kidney and urinary tract.
- Describe disorders of the urinary tract, focusing on causes of obstruction.

## ABNORMALITIES OF KIDNEY STRUCTURE

### Congenital abnormalities of the kidney

Congenital anomalies of kidneys are common, affecting 3–4% of newborn infants.

#### Agenesis of the kidney

##### Unilateral
Unilateral agenesis occurs in 1 in 1000 births. It may occur alongside other congenital disease such as spina bifida. The solitary kidney undergoes marked hypertrophy and is susceptible to infections, trauma and progressive glomerulosclerosis. It affects males more than females by 2:1; the left kidney is usually the absent one.

##### Bilateral
Occurrence of bilateral agenesis is 1 in 3000 births, as part of Potter's syndrome. Affected infants have abnormal facies, and they often have abnormalities of the lower urinary tract, lungs and nervous system.

Characteristically, there is oligohydramnios in pregnancy as the kidneys are not present to contribute to amniotic fluid (absence of fetal urine). The disorder is not compatible with postnatal life.

#### Hypoplasia

Kidneys fail to reach the normal adult size either as a result of a congenital maldevelopment or due to shrinkage, which may have occurred as a result of chronic infection in early life.

### Horseshoe kidney

The poles of the kidneys are fused, usually inferiorly, to form a large U-shaped (horseshoe) kidney. This affects about 1 in 500 people, but it is typically asymptomatic as the collecting system develops normally. However, Wilms' tumours are 2 to 8 times more frequent in children with horseshoe kidneys than in the general population.

### Cystic diseases of the kidney

#### Overview of cystic kidney disease

This heterogeneous group of diseases comprises:
- Hereditary disorders
- Developmental (but not hereditary) disorders
- Acquired disorders.

Each disease is distinguished by a characteristic distribution of cysts, illustrated in Figure 9.1.

Figure 9.2 provides a summary of cystic diseases of the kidney.

**HINTS AND TIPS**

Accurate diagnosis of cystic diseases is important for two reasons:
1. Appropriate patient management to delay onset of renal failure
2. Appropriate genetic counselling in the case of hereditary cystic diseases.

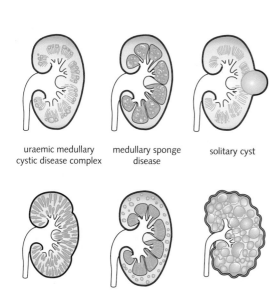

uraemic medullary cystic disease complex

medullary sponge disease

solitary cyst

childhood cystic disease

congenital nephrotic syndrome

adult polycystic disease

**Fig. 9.1** Macroscopic features of cystic diseases of the kidney.

## Cystic renal dysplasia

The failure of differentiation of metanephric tissues affects the whole or just one segment of a kidney, either unilaterally or bilaterally. Affected areas are replaced by solid or cystic masses, in which cartilage is usually prominent.

The condition often presents in childhood as an abdominal mass and it requires surgical excision to exclude a malignant tumour (e.g. nephroblastoma). Prognosis is good for unilateral lesions.

## Adult polycystic kidney disease

Adult polycystic kidney disease (APKD) is a hereditary disease. Both kidneys are progressively replaced by fluid-filled cysts, which develop and enlarge over a period of years.

Incidence is 1 per 1250 live births, accounting for 8% of all end-stage renal disease, with the sexes equally affected.

It is inherited as an autosomal dominant disorder; 85% of cases are linked to the $\alpha$-globin cluster located on the small arm of chromosome 16 (autosomal dominant polycystic kidney disease-1; ADPKD-1). ADPKD-2 gene mutations (15% of cases) have a slower disease onset. Both mutations are associated with berry aneurysms of the cerebral arteries and with cysts of the liver, pancreas and lung.

The condition is asymptomatic at first but—eventually—replacement and compression of the functioning renal parenchyma by the enlarging cysts leads to slowly progressive impairment of renal function.

Macroscopically, in fully developed APKD, the kidneys are asymmetrically enlarged and are composed of numerous large cysts (each up to 5 cm in diameter). Haemorrhage into the cysts is common, leading to bloodstained contents.

Microscopically, the cysts are lined by flattened cuboidal epithelium and communicate both with calyces and with each other. Surrounding parenchyma often shows extensive fibrosis and arteriosclerosis.

Complications are as follows:

- Chronic renal failure and uraemia
- Hypertension—often preceding development of cardiac failure

**Fig. 9.2** Summary of cystic diseases of the kidney

| Type of cystic disease | Clinical features |
|---|---|
| **Hereditary** | |
| Adult polycystic disease (autosomal dominant) Infantile polycystic disease (autosomal recessive) | Chronic renal failure and hypertension |
| Medullary cystic disease (autosomal dominant) Juvenile nephronophthisis (autosomal recessive) | Early-onset chronic renal failure |
| Medullary sponge kidney (occasionally familial) | Renal stones predispose to renal colic and infection |
| **Developmental** | |
| Cystic renal dysplasia | Typically asymptomatic |
| **Acquired** | |
| Simple renal cysts Dialysis-associated cystic disease | Typically asymptomatic |

- subarachnoid haemorrhage (10% of cases)—predisposed by the combination of berry aneurysms and hypertension.

### Clinical Note

APKD typically presents in the fourth decade or later, often with a large lobulated abdominal mass, pain or haematuria.

Diagnosis is by ultrasound, which shows multiple bilateral cysts. Screening susceptible 18-year-olds has a 95% successful diagnosis rate. Genetic analysis is sometimes used to exclude disease.

Management is by:
- Blood pressure control—uncontrolled hypertension accelerates renal failure
- Treating urinary infections and cardiac failure
- Eventual dialysis or transplantation.

## Infantile (childhood) polycystic disease

This is a less common autosomal recessive disorder, in which there is cystic replacement of both kidneys present at birth. Cysts are composed of dilated tubules and collecting ducts.

This is a rare condition (at 1 per 10 000 live births), and is associated with cysts of the liver, pancreas, and lungs.

It presents in stillborn or neonates with enlarged kidneys (12–16 times normal size) containing a radiating cystic pattern in the medulla and cortex ('sunburst' pattern; see Fig. 9.1). Rarely, it may present in childhood with renal insufficiency.

*Prognosis*—affected infants often die within the first 2 months of life; those that survive tend to develop a form of hepatic fibrosis.

## Cystic diseases of the renal medulla

### Medullary sponge kidney (tubular ectasia)

Multiple cysts develop in renal papillae, with an incidence of 1 in 20 000. Renal function is not usually impaired and the main clinical problem is the development of renal stones that predispose to renal colic and infection.

### Nephronophthisis complex (uraemic medullary cystic disease complex)

This describes a group of hereditary diseases characterized by development of cysts at the corticomedullary junction of the kidney. These diseases are associated with tubular atrophy and interstitial fibrosis. Important examples are:

- juvenile nephronophthisis—autosomal recessive disease presenting at about 11 years of age
- medullary cystic disease—autosomal dominant trait presenting at about 20 years of age.

Clinically, these conditions are characterized by thirst (polydipsia) and polyuria (due to nephrogenic diabetes insipidus; see Chapter 10) and eventually result in early-onset chronic renal failure. Together, they account for about 20–25% of cases of end-stage renal failure in the first three decades of life.

## Simple cysts

These common lesions occur as solitary or occasionally multiple cystic spaces in otherwise normal kidneys. Incidence increases with age.

The abnormality is widely believed to be acquired, but the cause is unknown.

Macroscopically, cysts are of variable size (generally smaller than 5 cm), and they contain clear watery fluid.

Microscopically, they are lined by flattened cuboidal epithelium and surrounded by a thin fibrous capsule. Clinically, cysts may cause renal enlargement, but they have no effect on renal function. However, they require clinical differentiation from tumours and other cystic disorders.

## DISEASES OF THE GLOMERULUS

## Overview of glomerular disease

Glomerular diseases are typically caused by disturbances of structure. Four significant components of the glomerulus may be damaged:

1. Endothelial cells lining the capillary
2. Glomerular basement membrane
3. Mesangium, i.e. the supporting mesentery to the capillary, which comprises mesangial cells (phagocytic support cells) and associated extracellular material (mesangial matrix)
4. Epithelial cells or podocytes, which form an outer coating to the capillary. These cells are in contact with the outer surface of the basement membrane via a series of foot processes.

## Patterns of glomerular disease

Many forms of glomerulonephritis are idiopathic and so are often classified according to their histological changes:

1. Global—affecting the whole glomerulus uniformly
2. Segmental—affecting one glomerular segment while sparing the others within that glomerulus
3. Diffuse—affecting all glomeruli in both kidneys
4. Focal—affecting a proportion of glomeruli, sparing others.

Thus a glomerular disease may be described as one of 'diffuse global', 'diffuse segmental', 'focal global' or 'focal segmental'. The vast majority are either 'diffuse global' or 'focal segmental'.

This explains how some glomerular diseases cause sudden acute renal failure (diffuse global diseases), whereas others cause a selective partial renal failure (focal segmental diseases).

## Aetiology of glomerular diseases

Glomerular diseases may be classified as (Figs 9.3, 9.4):

- primary (majority)—idiopathic
- secondary—disease process is secondary to systemic disease
- hereditary—Alport's syndrome, Fabry's syndrome and congenital nephrotic syndrome.

# Clinical manifestations of glomerular disease

Glomerular pathology produces a spectrum of presentations from pure proteinuria (reflects injury to podocytes and architecture) to pure haematuria (inflammatory proliferative changes). Many diseases lie somewhere along this spectrum with a mixture of proteinuria and haematuria to differing degrees.

Five key syndromes cover most presentations. These are described below.

## 1. Asymptomatic haematuria

This is haematuria without significant proteinuria, which may be continuous or intermittent, varying in severity from macroscopic to microscopic.

---

**Fig. 9.3** Aetiology of glomerular disorders

| Aetiology | Example |
| --- | --- |
| **Primary disorders** | |
| Antiglomerular basement membrane disease: proliferative | Goodpasture's syndrome |
| Immune complex-mediated lesions | |
| Proliferative | Diffuse proliferative glomerulonephritis<br>Focal proliferative glomerulonephritis<br>Membranoproliferative glomerulonephritis<br>Crescentic glomerulonephritis |
| Membranous | Membranous glomerulopathy |
| Glomerulosclerosis | Focal segmental glomerulosclerosis |
| Minimal change | Minimal change disease |
| **Secondary disorders** | |
| Immune complex-mediated conditions | Systemic lupus erythematosus<br>Henoch–Schönlein purpura<br>Infective endocarditis |
| Metabolic conditions | Diabetes mellitus<br>Renal amyloidosis<br>Multiple myeloma |
| Vascular conditions | Polyarteritis nodosa<br>Wegener's granulomatosis<br>Haemolytic uraemic syndrome<br>Idiopathic thrombocytopenic purpura<br>Disseminated intravascular coagulation |
| **Hereditary disorders** | |
| | Alport's and Fabry's syndromes |

**Fig. 9.4** Clinical manifestations of glomerular disease and the conditions that cause them

| Clinical manifestations | Causative renal disease |
| --- | --- |
| Asymptomatic haematuria | Exercise haematuria<br>IgA nephropathy<br>Henoch–Schönlein purpura<br>Bacterial endocarditis<br>Systemic lupus erythematosus<br>Polyarteritis nodosa |
| Asymptomatic proteinuria | Primary:<br>• Focal segmental glomerulosclerosis<br>• Membranoproliferative glomerulonephritis<br>Secondary:<br>• Henoch–Schönlein purpura<br>• Systemic lupus erythematosus<br>• Polyarteritis nodosa<br>• Bacterial endocarditis |
| Acute nephritic syndrome | Primary:<br>• Poststreptococcal glomerulonephritis<br>• Rapidly progressive glomerulonephritis<br>• Goodpasture's syndrome<br>Secondary:<br>• Systemic lupus erythematosus<br>• Polyarteritis nodosa<br>• Wegener's granulomatosis<br>• Henoch–Schönlein purpura<br>• Essential cryoglobulinaemia |
| Nephrotic syndrome | Primary:<br>• Minimal change disease<br>• Membranous glomerulopathy<br>• Membranoproliferative glomerulonephritis<br>• Focal proliferative glomerulonephritis<br>• Focal glomerulosclerosis<br>Secondary:<br>• Immune complex-mediated conditions<br>  Systemic lupus erythematosus<br>  Henoch–Schönlein purpura<br>  Infective endocarditis<br>• Metabolic conditions<br>  Diabetes mellitus<br>  Renal amyloidosis<br>• Vascular conditions<br>  Polyarteritis nodosa<br>  Wegener's granulomatosis<br>  Haemolytic uraemic syndrome<br>• Infections<br>  Malaria, syphilis, hepatitis B |
| Chronic renal failure | All of the above except minimal change disease |

## 2. Asymptomatic proteinuria

This proteinuria (> 0.3 g every 24 hours) without haematuria may be continuous, orthostatic (postural) or transient. It is typically detected at a routine medical examination.

## 3. Acute nephritic syndrome

This presents with a sudden onset of haematuria, proteinuria (often with urinary casts) and hypertension. Loin pain and headache may be present and the patient will often feel unwell.

## 4. Nephrotic syndrome

Here, there is proteinuria (usually > 3 g every 24 hours) with hypoproteinemia and oedema. There is also hypercholesterolaemia, an increased tendency to clotting and greater risk of infection. It may be due to primary or secondary glomerular disease.

## 5. Chronic renal failure

This is an irreversible deterioration in renal function caused by the destruction of more and more individual nephrons over a long period of time. Impairment of excretory metabolic and endocrine functions of the kidney leads to the clinical syndrome of uraemia.

Figure 9.5 lists the symptoms and signs of renal failure.

*Management*—excretory function of the kidney can be partially replaced by dialysis. However, replacement of the endocrine and metabolic functions can only be achieved by successful renal transplantation.

Unless some form of supportive therapy—such as dialysis or transplantation—is available, chronic renal failure is eventually fatal.

# The mechanism of glomerular injury

Many glomerular diseases are caused by immune-mediated damage (listed below). Different patterns of immune-mediated damage point to different diagnoses. It is therefore important to identify the site, type and pattern of immune complexes and complement within the glomerulus by immunohistochemistry and electron microscopy.

The four main mechanisms of immune-mediated damage are as follows:

## 1. Circulating immune complex nephritis

This is the most common pattern of immunological disease.

**Mechanism**
Soluble antigen–antibody complexes circulating in the blood are trapped at the basement membrane, the mesangium or both. Complexes activate the complement cascade via the classical pathway. Activated components of complement bring about the characteristic acute inflammation of glomerulonephritis by attracting neutrophil polymorphs, increasing vascular permeability and causing membrane damage (see Fig. 2.7).

| Condition | Features |
|---|---|
| Mesangial IgA disease | A focal proliferative glomerulonephritis Serum IgA levels are raised and IgA is deposited in the mesangium and basement membrane |
| Goodpasture's syndrome | A focal proliferative glomerulonephritis. The Goodpasture antigen is a domain of type IV collagen in the basement membrane; this is a target for the autoantibodies |
| Type I MPGN | An immune complex disease thought to involve a disorder of complement, characterized by subendothelial deposits There is a persistently low serum C3 |
| Type II MPGN | An autoimmune-mediated abnormality of complement. There is marked thickening of the capillary walls due to deposition of C3 (dense deposit disease) |

**Fig. 9.5** Examples of proliferative glomerulonephritis disease

*MPGN, membranoproliferative glomerulonephritis.*

## Example

SLE: depending on the size and charge of the immune complexes, they may get trapped at the endothelial, intramembranous or subepithelial region of the GBM or mesangium.

## 2. In-situ immune complex formation

### Mechanism

Circulating antigens become 'planted' or trapped in the glomerulus, where they are targeted by circulating antibodies such that immune complexes are formed within the glomerulus itself. This in-situ formation explains why, unlike circulating immune complex nephritis described above, there is little complement and no inflammatory or proliferative responses.

### Example

Post-streptococcal glomerulonephritis: streptococcal antigens are implanted into the GBM during infection and are implanted into the glomerulus

## 3. Cytotoxic antibodies

### Mechanism

Autoantibodies to the glomerular basement membrane (anti-GBM antibodies).

### Example

This is the basis of Goodpasture's syndrome, in which autoantibodies target a domain on the α3 type IV collagen chain. These antibodies may cross-react with collagen of the lung, producing simultaneous lung and kidney disease.

## 4. Activation of the alternative complement pathway

### Mechanism

The alternative complement pathway is normally activated by the presence of bacterial cell walls, and it is independent of immune complex formation (see Fig. 2.6). However, in certain disease conditions, the alternative pathway can be activated by different mechanisms.

### Example

In type II membranoproliferative glomerulonephritis, a circulating autoantibody (termed 'C3 nephritic factor') activates complement via the alternative pathway by stabilizing the enzyme C3-convertase. This enzyme normally activates C3 but has a very short half-life. Thus, stabilization of C3-convertase prolongs the activation of C3.

# Proliferative glomerulonephritis

This group of disorders is characterized histologically by varying degrees of proliferation of mesangial and epithelial (and sometimes endothelial) cells within the glomerulus.

The majority of cases of glomerulonephritis (over 70%) belong to this group.

Proliferative glomerulonephritis can be divided according to histological appearance into:

* diffuse proliferative
* rapidly progressive
* focal proliferative
* membranoproliferative.

However, it must be emphasized that these subdivisions are not diagnoses but rather describe a pattern of reaction caused by glomerular insult.

## Diffuse proliferative glomerulonephritis

Diffuse, global, acute inflammation of glomeruli is caused by the deposition of immune complexes in the glomeruli, stimulated by a preceding infection.

Aetiology is as follows:

* Poststreptococcal (most common)—onset is 1–2 weeks after a primary pharyngeal or skin infection with group A β-haemolytic streptococci.
* Non-streptococcal (less common)—a range of bacterial, viral and protozoal infections can also stimulate this pattern of disease.

Those antibodies produced to combat initial infection cross-react with cellular antigens producing immune complexes. These complexes circulate in the blood and are filtered-out in the glomerulus, producing four main histological changes:

1. Immune complex deposition—in lumps on the epithelial side of the glomerular basement membrane.
2. Neutrophil infiltration—activation of complement attracts neutrophils into the glomerulus.
3. Endothelial cell proliferation—degranulation of neutrophils damages endothelial cells, stimulating their proliferation.
4. Mild mesangial cell proliferation—mediated by factors derived from complement and platelets.

## Rapidly progressive glomerulonephritis (crescentic glomerulonephritis)

Rapidly progressive glomerulonephritis (RPGN) is a manifestation of severe glomerular injury characterized by the formation of cellular crescent-shaped masses within the Bowman's space. It occurs in a small percentage of patients with poststreptococcal glomerulonephritis (see above) but it can also be associated with many other forms of glomerular damage.

If damage to the glomerular capillaries is severe, fibrin and blood leak into Bowman's space stimulating epithelial cell proliferation, and entry of inflammatory infiltrate. Crescent-shaped cellular masses composed of epithelial cells, macrophages and monocytes are formed within the Bowman's space. These crescents are associated with glomerular ischaemia and ultimately they result in permanent glomerular damage.

## Focal proliferative glomerulonephritis

Here, there is an acute inflammation with cellular proliferation occurring in only a proportion of all glomeruli (focal) and usually affecting only one segment of the glomerular tufts (segmental). Therefore, the condition is more accurately described as focal segmental proliferative glomerulonephritis.

Several diseases can cause this pattern of response. These can be classified into two groups:

1. Primary—mainly mesangial IgA disease and Goodpasture's syndrome (Fig. 9.5)
2. Secondary—associated with other systemic diseases including infective endocarditis, vasculitis and connective tissue diseases.

Immunohistochemistry and electron microscopy are required to distinguish them.

## Membranoproliferative glomerulonephritis

Membranoproliferative glomerulonephritis (MPGN) is a diffuse, global pattern of glomerulonephritis with features of both proliferation and membrane thickening (hence the name). It is also known as mesangiocapillary glomerulonephritis.

Diseases causing MPGN can be classified into two groups:

1. Primary (majority)—idiopathic. Subdivided according to clinical and pathological features into type I (90% of cases) and type II (10% of cases) (see Table 9.5)
2. Secondary—a few are secondary to systemic disorders such as SLE, infective endocarditis, malaria and infected ventricular cerebrospinal fluid (CSF) shunts.

## Membranous nephropathy

There is a pattern of reaction in which the glomerular capillary basement membrane is uniformly thickened, partly due to immunoglobulin-based deposits. Unlike the proliferative types of glomerulonephritis, membranous nephropathy has no associated inflammation or endothelial/epithelial proliferation, although the mesangial cell population may be slightly increased.

**Fig. 9.6** Conditions associated with membranous nephropathy

| Type | Example |
|---|---|
| Infections | Malaria<br>Syphilis<br>Hepatitis B |
| Malignancy | Carcinoma (lung, breast, gastrointestinal tract)<br>Lymphoma |
| Drugs | Gold, mercury, penicillamine, captopril |
| Systemic disease | Systemic lupus erythematosus (10% of renal involvement is of the membranous pattern) |

It affects all age groups, but the highest incidence is between fifth and seventh decades. Males are affected more than females.

Aetiology is as follows:

- Primary—80–90% of cases have no apparent reason for development of immune complexes, and are classed as primary or idiopathic membranous nephropathy.
- Secondary—membranous nephropathy is found in association with a number of conditions which are listed in Figure 9.6.

There are four pathological stages:

1. In-situ formation of immune complexes on the epithelial side of the basement membrane (diffuse, global pattern)
2. Mild mesangial increase
3. New basement membrane is deposited around immune complex deposits
4. Immune complex deposits disappear, leaving thickened 'lacy' basement membrane.

Over many years, the abnormal glomeruli develop increased mesangial matrix produced by the mesangial cells. This, together with membrane thickening, causes gradual hyalinization of the glomeruli (glomerulosclerosis) and death of individual nephrons.

Abnormality of the basement membrane renders it unusually permeable resulting in heavy proteinuria.

### Clinical Note

Membranous nephropathy is the most common cause of nephrotic syndrome in adults.

Prognosis is variable and related to cause but in crude figures: one-third of patients undergo spontaneous remission without treatment, one-third are stabilized with persisting proteinuria and one-third progress to develop chronic renal failure.

Long-term prognosis may be improved by treatment with high-dose corticosteroids and alkylating agents (e.g. cyclophosphamide), although there are significant side effects.

## Minimal change disease (lipoid nephrosis)

The characteristic feature in this nephropathy is that no significant abnormalities can be detected by light microscopy.

It is the most common cause of nephrotic syndrome in children. Males are affected more than females, however it is less common in adults, but still accounts for 25% of cases of nephrotic syndrome.

Aetiology is unknown, although in some cases an association with respiratory infection has been noted.

Pathogenesis is postulated to be immunologically related (cell-mediated damage to the basement membrane) because of the near universal response to corticosteroid therapy. Ultimately, polyanionic charges of the glomerular basement membrane are depleted, leading to failure of protein retention.

*Morphological features*—with electron microscopy, there is a diagnostic loss of epithelial foot processes. Tubules may show accumulation of lipid in lining cells, giving rise to the alternative name of 'lipoid nephrosis'.

Prognosis in children is good, with no permanent renal damage. In adults, the outlook is variable.

## Focal segmental glomerulosclerosis

The glomerulus is partially replaced by hyaline material, which, in most cases, is excess mesangial matrix.

Aetiology and pathology is variable and related to age:

- Primary (most common)—idiopathic disease affecting children and young adults. Focal deposition of IgM are seen at biopsy.
- Secondary—in later adult life the condition is usually secondary to other disorders, especially HIV.

Focal glomerulosclerosis initially affects the juxtamedullary glomeruli, causing an increase in mesangial matrix, which gradually expands to destroy the surrounding lobule, until global sclerosis occurs. In time, similar lesions appear in glomeruli throughout the cortex.

### HINTS AND TIPS

It is useful to remember that the clinical syndromes of glomerulonephritis broadly relate to histological findings:

- Asymptomatic proteinuria and nephrotic syndrome are associated with basement membrane thickening as a result of either structural change or deposition of excessive mesangial matrix, e.g. membranous nephropathy, glomerulosclerosis.
- Asymptomatic haematuria and nephritic syndrome are associated with proliferation of the endothelial or mesangial cells, e.g. diffuse, global glomerulonephritis.
- Mixed nephritic/nephrotic syndrome is associated with combined damage to the basement membrane and cell proliferation, e.g. membranoproliferative glomerulonephritis.

## Hereditary glomerulonephritis

### Alport's syndrome

This syndrome is characterized by the clinical triad of deafness, glomerulonephritis and ocular lesions. Inheritance is complex; it is X-linked in most families (a mutation of the *COLIVα5* gene), with an autosomal recessive pattern in the rest. Both types of disease are clinically indistinguishable. The genes affected encode basement membrane collagens that are found in the glomerulus and elsewhere in the body, e.g. the cochlea.

The clinical features are:

- glomerulonephritis—usually presents as microscopic haematuria and proteinuria in childhood. There is subsequent development of nephrotic syndrome with progression to renal failure, occurring by the second decade in males, but often not until the fifth decade in females, as they are only carriers of the disease in the X-linked form
- Ocular disease—occurs in only severely affected patients
- Deafness—only for high-pitched sounds; this may be difficult to demonstrate.

### Fabry's syndrome

A rare, X-linked recessive syndrome of glycosphingolipid metabolism resulting in painful extremities, red hyperkeratotic papules on skin, proteinuria and renal failure.

## Chronic glomerulonephritis

Chronic renal failure associated with small, contracted kidneys, in which all the glomeruli are hyalinized (end-stage kidneys). It may be caused by many diseases, particularly proliferative types of acute glomerulonephritis.

In patients who present for the first time with chronic glomerulonephritis, it is often not possible to ascertain the cause because of diffuse global glomerular destruction. However, it is likely that many patients presenting for the first time have had IgA nephropathy

Macroscopically, affected kidneys are small and there is granularity of the external surface, reflecting fine scarring due to nephron hyalinization. However, the pelvicalyceal system is normal, an important distinction from cases of end-stage kidney disease due to chronic pyelonephritis.

Microscopically, there is hyalinization of the glomeruli, tubular atrophy and interstitial fibrosis.

### Clinical Note

Transplantation is the only method of fully correcting the loss of renal function in chronic renal failure. Renal replacement therapy (e.g. haemodialysis) maintains low levels of blood purification, but cannot fully replace the metabolic functions of a kidney. It is also time consuming, so affecting quality of life. Renal transplantation has become increasingly successful, with 3-year graft survival now reaching 80% due to better matching of donors (ABO and HLA matching) and improved post-transplantation immunosuppression.

## GLOMERULAR LESIONS IN SYSTEMIC DISEASE

### Systemic lupus erythematosus

Around half of all SLE patients will display renal involvement within 5 years of diagnosis. The majority of these cases are glomerular lesions, which may be of numerous histological patterns. Clinically, there is a potential spectrum from minor abnormalities such as asymptomatic proteinuria to severe glomerular disease leading to renal failure.

The basis of glomerular damage is immune-complex deposition in the basement membrane (leading to basement membrane thickening) or in the mesangium (leading to mesangial expansion).

Patterns of glomerular damage that may occur include:

- diffuse MPGN—associated with a mixed nephritic/nephrotic syndrome and rapid progression to renal failure
- focal segmental proliferative glomerulonephritis—associated with haematuria, proteinuria and slow progression
- diffuse membranous nephropathy—associated with nephrotic syndrome and slow progression to chronic renal failure.

### Immune complexes

The immune complexes of SLE are characterized by the presence of IgG, IgA, IgM, C3 and C1q (known as a 'full-house' of deposits). The detection of this pattern of immunoglobulins and complement factors, together with the particular location of the immune complexes in relation to the glomerular basement membrane, is an important factor in distinguishing lupus glomerulonephritis from non-lupus patterns.

Note that, although glomerular lesions are the main abnormalities of renal involvement in SLE, there may also be extraglomerular vascular abnormalities and tubular damage, particularly interstitial nephritis.

### Henoch–Schönlein purpura

This immune complex-mediated systemic vasculitis affects small arteries in the skin, joints, intestine, and kidneys (see Chapters 6 and 13). Light microscopy reveals mesangial IgA deposits.

Significant renal damage occurs in over one-third of cases, ranging from proteinuria, possibly with nephrotic syndrome, to RPGN.

### Diabetic glomerulosclerosis

Diabetic glomerular damage causes an increase in the permeability of the glomerular capillary basement membrane, leading to proteinuria and occasionally nephrotic syndrome.

The pathogenesis of basement membrane changes is probably related to the persistent insulin deficiency and/or hyperglycaemia of the diabetic state. This stimulates biochemical alterations in the composition of the basement membrane, most notably a deficiency of proteoglycans with an excess of collagen IV and fibronectin. Glomerular hypertrophy may occur in response to hyperfiltration (increased glomerular blood flow in diabetes). It is likely that the increased glycosylation of proteins also contributes to glomerular damage.

Histologically, three types of glomerular lesion occur, representing a continuous spectrum of increasing severity:

1. Capillary wall thickening—diabetic microangiopathy occurring in renal blood vessels to produce a mild proteinuria
2. Diffuse glomerulosclerosis—excess mesangial matrix formation in an even pattern throughout the glomerulus combined with capillary thickening eventually encroaches on the capillaries
3. Nodular glomerulosclerosis (Kimmelstiel–Wilson nodules)—nodular expansion of the mesangium at the tips of the glomerular lobules is very characteristic of diabetes.

Diabetic sclerosis causes progressive hyalinization of glomeruli with obliteration of capillary loops and death of individual nephrons. Over a period of years this leads to chronic renal failure.

*Prognosis*—approximately 10% of all diabetics die in renal failure. This rises to 50% if patients developing diabetes in childhood are considered separately.

## Amyloidosis

This is a condition in which amyloid—an extracellular fibrillar protein—is deposited in a variety of tissues (see Chapter 13). Amyloidosis is an important cause of the nephrotic syndrome in adults.

Amyloid is deposited as fibrils in the glomerular basement membrane and in the mesangium of the kidney, resulting in membrane thickening and increased mesangial matrix formation. The net result is the development of:

- proteinuria—membrane thickening leads to an increase in membrane permeability
- nephrotic syndrome—increased deposition of amyloid causes progression of protein loss
- chronic renal failure—combined effect of amyloid deposition and increased mesangial matrix formation eventually leads to expansion of the mesangium causing compression of the glomerular capillary system and transition into chronic renal failure.

Amyloid is also deposited in the walls of intrarenal vessels, particularly the afferent arterioles.

## Polyarteritis nodosa

Polyarteritis nodosa is a systemic disease characterized by inflammatory necrosis of the walls of small and medium-sized arteries (see Chapter 6). Necrosis of medium-sized arteries causes small infarcts in the kidney; necrosis of arterioles and the glomerular tuft produces infarction of entire glomeruli or segments. This is visible as fibrinoid necrosis.

## Wegener's granulomatosis

This immune complex-mediated systemic necrotizing vasculitis primarily affects the nose, upper respiratory tract and kidneys. Renal involvement is of variable severity causing one of the following:

- Focal segmental glomerulonephritis (asymptomatic haematuria or nephritic syndrome)
- Rapidly progressive glomerulonephritis (rapidly progressive acute renal failure).

This condition usually responds to immunosuppressive therapy.

## DISEASES OF THE TUBULES AND INTERSTITIUM

### Acute tubular necrosis

This acute, but usually reversible, renal failure is caused by necrosis of renal tubular epithelial cells resulting from ischaemic, metabolic or toxic disturbances. The causes of acute tubular necrosis (ATN) are shown in Figure 9.7.

The aetiology is:

- ischaemic (most common)—caused by failure of renal perfusion, typically the result of hypotension and hypovolaemia in shock
- toxic—uncommon (heavy metals, organic solvents).

There are three phases to ATN (oliguric, polyuric and recovery) as follows:

1. Oliguric phase—necrosis of renal tubular cells and interstitial oedema causes tubule blockage and reduced glomerular blood flow and filtration.
2. Polyuric phase—tubules slowly open as phagocytic cells begin to remove necrotic material. Polyuria is caused by the temporary loss of the medullary concentration gradient. Regenerated renal tubule cells are undifferentiated.
3. Recovery phase—differentiated tubular cells restore renal function.

The morphologic features are:

- Ischaemic ATN—kidneys are pale and swollen. Histology reveals flattened, vacuolated epithelial cells along the entire length of the tubules.
- Necrotic ATN—kidneys are red and swollen. Histology reveals flattened, vacuolated epithelial cells

**Fig. 9.7** Causes of acute tubular necrosis

| Type of ATN | Causes |
|---|---|
| Ischaemic | Major surgery<br>Extensive acute blood loss<br>Severe burns<br>Haemorrhage |
| Toxic | Endogenous products:<br>haemoglobinuria and myoglobinuria<br>Heavy metals: lead, mercury<br>Organic solvents: chloroform,<br>carbon tetrachloride<br>Drugs: antibiotics, NSAIDs, ciclosporin<br>Others: paraquat, phenol,<br>ethylene glycol, poisonous fungi |

**Fig. 9.8** Symptoms and signs of renal failure

| Symptoms | Signs |
|---|---|
| General malaise | Uraemia |
| Breathlessness on exertion | Anaemia |
| Nausea and vomiting | Metabolic bone disease (renal osteodystrophy) |
| Disordered gastrointestinal motility | Hypertension |
| Headaches | Acidosis |
| Pruritus | Neuropathy |
| Pigmentation | Generalized myopathy |
| | Endocrine abnormalities |

restricted to proximal tubular cells, those of the distal tubule being spared.

Clinical features are oliguria (less than 500 mL urine output per day) with features of renal failure (see Fig. 9.8). As mentioned, some patients develop polyuria during recovery.

### HINTS AND TIPS

A knowledge of the aetiology (ischaemic versus toxic) and an understanding of the pathogenesis (oliguric and polyuric phases) of ATN make the morphological and clinical features easy to remember.

Treatment:

- Oliguric phase—supportive measures to prevent hyperkalaemia and fluid overload
- Polyuric phase—replacement of fluid and electrolytes to compensate for excessive loss from urine.

The prognosis depends on the speed and efficiency with which corrective measures are put into operation, and the severity of the causal disorder.

## Tubulointerstitial nephritis

### Acute pyelonephritis

This is acute suppurative inflammation of the tubules and interstitium caused by bacterial infection. There are three age peaks: childhood, pregnancy and in the elderly.

Most cases of infection are caused by enterobacteria from the patient's faecal flora (e.g. *Escherichia coli*, *Proteus* and *Klebsiella* species) or by staphylococci from skin

(perineal) flora. The organism may enter the kidney by one of two routes: ascending infection from the lower urinary tract (promoted by pregnancy, glycosuria in diabetes, stasis of urine) or via the blood in bacteraemia/septicaemia.

Macroscopically, the condition is characterized by numerous abscesses throughout the kidney:

- Cortical abscesses—small, yellowish-white abscesses, usually spherical, less than 2 mm in diameter and sometimes surrounded by a zone of hyperaemia. Most prominent on subcapsular surface.
- Medullary abscesses—yellowish-white linear streaks that converge on the papilla. Pelvicalyceal mucosa is hyperaemic or covered with a fibrinopurulent exudate.

Microscopically, there is focal inflammation with infiltration of tubules by neutrophils, interstitial oedema and tubular necrosis.

Clinical features are fever, rigors and pain in the back.

This condition is often associated with dysuria and urgency of micturition—signs of a lower urinary tract infection.

Acute pyelonephritis may resolve with or without scarring or chronic infection. In severe cases, pyonephrosis (pus-filled kidney associated with obstruction), renal papillary necrosis, perinephric abscess or death may occur.

Diagnosis is by examination of midstream urine, especially cultured to demonstrate responsible organisms:

- Significant bacteriuria is defined as $>10^5$ culture-forming units per mL (to eliminate cases of extraneous bacterial contamination).
- Significant pyuria is defined as $>10$ neutrophil polymorphs per high power field.

Treatment is by oral antibiotic therapy (e.g. trimethoprim, ampicillin or amoxicillin, which are active against *Escherichia coli*). Intravenous antibiotic therapy is used for more severe or septicaemic cases.

Untreated, infection may spread to cause Gram-negative septicaemia with shock.

## Chronic pyelonephritis

Chronic inflammation of the tubules and interstitium is associated with nephron destruction and coarse scarring of the kidneys. The two forms—obstructive and reflux-associated—are described below.

### Reflux-associated chronic pyelonephritis

Reflux of urine from the bladder into the ureter predisposes to recurrent bouts of inflammation. It is most common in childhood and early adult life, with males affected more than females.

Normally, the ureter enters the bladder obliquely so that contraction of the bladder wall during micturition closes the ureteric orifice. In patients with vesicoureteric reflux, the terminal portion of the ureter is short and oriented at approximately 90° to the mucosal surface. Contraction of the bladder tends to hold the ureteric orifice open, thus facilitating reflux of urine, enabling organisms to gain access to the kidney from the bladder.

Macroscopically, the kidneys have irregular areas of scarring seen as depressed areas, 1–2 cm in size, most commonly sited in the renal calyces at the poles of the kidney but often associated with fibrous scarring of the renal papilla. Involvement may be either bilateral or unilateral.

Microscopically, kidneys have irregular areas of interstitial fibrosis with chronic inflammatory cell infiltration (chronic interstitial nephritis). Tubules are atrophic, or they may be dilated and contain proteinaceous casts. Glomeruli show periglomerular fibrosis and many demonstrate complete hyalinization.

Clinical features are symptoms of urinary tract infection and of uraemia.

Diagnosis is by:

- intravenous urography—reveals reduction in kidney size and focal scarring associated with clubbing of the adjacent calyces
- urine culture– for identification of infecting organism.

Treatment is by antibiotic therapy, control of hypertension, and removal of the source of obstruction.

*Prognosis*—the course is usually long and punctuated by acute exacerbations.

Other diseases of the tubules and interstitium are illustrated in Figure 9.9.

## DISEASES OF THE RENAL BLOOD VESSELS

### Benign nephrosclerosis

This hyaline sclerosis of the arterioles and small arteries of the kidney is associated with benign hypertension and worsened by diabetes mellitus.

The condition is an important complication of long-standing benign hypertension, chronic renal failure being one of its major sequelae.

This is the most common form of nephropathy found in approximately 75% of autopsies over the age of 60 years.

In long-standing benign hypertension, there is reduced flow of blood to the glomeruli caused by vascular changes that affect:

- branches of the renal artery—thickening of arterial walls due to fibroelastic intimal proliferation, elastic lamina reduplication and muscular hypertrophy of the media. Results in focal areas of ischaemia with scarring.
- afferent arterioles—undergo hyalinization (arteriolosclerosis), their muscular walls being replaced by a rigid and inelastic amorphous material.

A progressive reduction in blood flow to the nephrons leads to chronic ischaemia with slow conversion of individual glomeruli into a mass of hyaline tissue devoid of capillary lumina (Fig. 9.10).

Blood supply to the tubules is also derived from glomerular blood flow. There is, therefore, eventual ischaemic destruction of the associated tubule.

The process gradually destroys individual nephrons over a period of many years.

*Clinical features*—no clinical symptoms initially, although a gradual increase in blood levels of urea and a reduction in glomerular filtration rate occur.

| Fig. 9.9 Diseases of the tubules and interstitium | |
|---|---|
| **Condition** | **Features** |
| Toxic and drug induced | Inflammation of the renal interstitium and tubules (tubulointerstitial nephritis) due to exposure to toxic agents. Two types: acute and chronic |
| Urate nephrophathy | Affects a small group of patients with hyperuricaemia |
| Hypercalcaemia and nephrocalcinosis | Hypercalcaemia causes calcification of the renal parenchyma and tubular damage |
| Multiple myeloma | Some types of myeloma are characterized by proliferating plasma cells, which produce monoclonal free light chains (Bence Jones proteins). These cause physical obstruction and damage to the tubules |

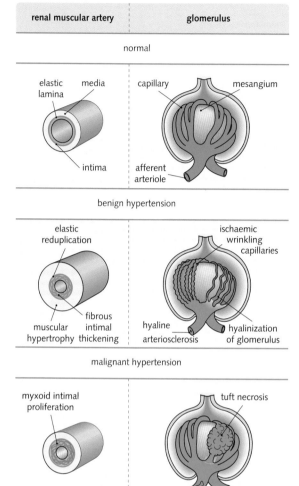

| renal muscular artery | glomerulus |
|---|---|

normal

elastic lamina | media
capillary | mesangium
intima
afferent arteriole

benign hypertension

elastic reduplication
ischaemic wrinkling capillaries
muscular hypertrophy | fibrous intimal thickening
hyaline arteriosclerosis | hyalinization of glomerulus

malignant hypertension

myxoid intimal proliferation
tuft necrosis
fibrinoid necrosis

**Fig. 9.10** Vascular changes associated with hypertensive renal disease.

Eventually, critical numbers of nephrons become dysfunctional and the patient develops manifestations of chronic renal failure.

*Prognosis*—less than 5% of patients with well-developed benign nephrosclerosis die from renal failure. Death in the great majority of cases of benign hypertension occurs from congestive heart failure, coronary insufficiency, cerebrovascular accidents, or the development of malignant hypertension.

## Malignant nephrosclerosis

Renal disease is associated with malignant, accelerated hypertension. This form of hypertension usually develops in individuals with pre-existing benign hypertension.

*Pathogenesis*—in accelerated hypertension, the rise in blood pressure is very rapid, causing a pattern of renal damage that differs from that seen in benign hypertension:

- Larger muscular vessels undergo fibroelastic proliferation of the intima, but no muscular hypertrophy. This is stimulated by factors such as platelet-derived growth factor.
- Afferent arterioles frequently undergo necrosis, often with fibrin in their damaged walls (fibrinoid necrosis) following exposure to the sudden high pressures.
- Glomerular capillary network—segmental fibrinoid necrosis of glomerular tuft.

The patient develops acute renal failure when sufficient nephrons are rendered non-functional. Afferent arteriole necrosis stimulates the renin-angiotensin system, which contributes to ischaemia by promoting intrarenal vasoconstriction.

The renal changes seen in benign and accelerated hypertensive nephrosclerosis are summarized in Figure 9.2.

Untreated accelerated hypertension causes death from renal failure in 90% of cases, usually with marked rapidity. However, if hypertension is treated adequately, before there is evidence of impairment of renal function by a raised blood urea, then prognosis is good and subsequent renal failure unusual.

## Renal artery stenosis

This narrowing of the renal arteries is typically caused by generalized atherosclerosis but rarely by arterial fibromuscular dysplasia.

Atherosclerotic occlusion of the renal artery is usually most severe at its origin from the aorta. Renal artery stenosis at this point can lead to two main pathological processes:

1. Chronic ischaemia of the affected kidney—reduction in function of all nephrons on that side produces an end-stage shrunken kidney. However, the contralateral kidney undergoes compensatory hypertrophy so that renal function is largely unaffected.
2. Renovascular hypertension—inadequate perfusion of the kidney caused by renal artery stenosis may lead to hyper-reninism and subsequent abnormal activation of the renin-angiotensin system. This condition is important in that it is one of the rare recognized causes of hypertension that is amenable to surgical correction.

**HINTS AND TIPS**

A useful diagnostic pointer for renal artery stenosis is to look for associated features of:
- vascular disease elsewhere
- severe or drug-resistant hypertension
- abdominal bruits (over the kidneys).

# Thrombotic microangiopathies

## Haemolytic uraemic syndrome

Haemolytic uraemic syndrome (HUS) is a complex syndrome of disordered platelet function that is characterized by the triad of thrombocytopenia, haemolysis and acute renal failure.

There are three subtypes of HUS: childhood, adult and secondary.

### Childhood HUS

This usually affects children under 4 years of age. Many cases are associated with intestinal infection by verocytotoxin-producing *Escherichia coli* (notably type 0157). The immediate prognosis is better than for adult and secondary types, but future risk of renal disease is increased.

### Adult HUS

This is more frequently fatal than childhood HUS and is associated with the following conditions:

- Pregnancy—occurring postpartum even several months after delivery
- Oestrogen therapy—contraceptive pills or oestrogen therapy for men with prostatic carcinoma
- Infections, e.g. typhoid, viruses and shigellosis
- Chemotherapeutic and immunosuppressive therapy, e.g. ciclosporin.

### Secondary HUS

This occurs as a complication of:

- malignant hypertension
- progressive systemic sclerosis
- SLE (often as a result of antiphospholipid syndrome)
- transplant rejection.

### Pathogenesis

Platelets adhere to damaged endothelium of small vessels, including the glomerular capillaries, where they undergo aggregation and trigger fibrin deposition. Reduced prostaglandin and nitric oxide production from the damaged endothelium promotes platelet aggregation. Fibrin strands form a tight mesh that deforms the erythrocytes as they are forced through the obstruction (microangiopathic haemolysis).

Morphological features are:

- endocapillary proliferation—in response to fibrin and platelet deposition in glomerular tufts
- luminal narrowing—arterioles and small arteries show fibrin and erythrocytes in the walls, often with thrombosis which, when extensive, can result in cortical necrosis.

### Clinical features and prognosis

Clinical features are:

- sudden onset of oliguria with haematuria and occasionally melaena

- jaundice
- anaemia with schistocytes (fragmented erythrocytes) and thrombocytopenia
- hypertension in 50% of cases.

In childhood HUS, symptoms are often preceded by a prodromal episode of diarrhoea or flu-like illness lasting for 5–15 days.

Prognosis depends on the severity of attack, but mortality may be as high as 40%.

## Thrombotic thrombocytopenic purpura

Thrombotic thrombocytopenic purpura (TTP) and HUS are thought to represent the same disease process, but with a different distribution of thrombotic lesions. In TTP, occlusive plugs lead to widespread ischaemic organ damage, often affecting the brain more than the kidney, resulting in early neurological abnormalities and progressive renal impairment.

## Renal infarcts

There are two mechanisms of renal infarction: embolic infarction and diffuse cortical necrosis.

### Embolic renal disease

Renal infarcts are usually due to the passage of emboli down renal arterial branches. The most common causes are:

- embolization of atheromatous material
- 'cholesterol emboli'—these are showers of cholesterol microemboli that may occur as a complication of arterial interventions (e.g. arteriography) in those with severe atheromatous disease
- mural thrombotic material arising from the left side of the heart, most commonly after myocardial infarction
- bacterial vegetation from infective endocarditis.

Resultant infarcts may be clinically silent or may result in haematuria and loin pain. Macroscopically, infarcts are pale or white and they have a characteristic wedge shape with the apex directed towards the hilum.

### Diffuse cortical necrosis

This rare pattern of renal infarction is associated with conditions resulting in severe hypotension, the most common of which are hypovolaemic shock, severe sepsis and eclampsia of pregnancy.

The pathogenesis is uncertain, but diffuse spasm of renal blood vessels is thought to play a major part in precipitating ischaemic damage.

Macroscopically, necrosis is confined to the outer part of the renal cortex, which in the acute stages is pale and focally haemorrhagic.

This condition results in acute renal failure, and prognosis depends on the extent of the damage.

# NEOPLASTIC DISEASE OF THE KIDNEY

## Benign tumours of the kidney

These are common incidental findings at post mortem examination in about 20% of all patients; however, they rarely cause clinical problems.

### Cortical adenoma

These are benign epithelial tumours derived from renal tubular epithelium.

Macroscopically, they are discrete nodules, usually less than 20 mm in diameter, situated in the cortex of the kidney.

Microscopically, appearances are similar to those of renal cell carcinomas, both being composed of well-differentiated large clear cells with small nuclei.

Difficulty in differentiating between these tumours had prompted the adoption of an arbitrary cut-off of 3 cm in size to distinguish between the smaller adenomas and the typically larger carcinomas. However, the distinction has proved unreliable and it is now considered that all adenomas should be treated.

### Renal fibroma or hamartoma (renomedullary interstitial cell tumour)

This is the most common benign tumour of the kidney. It is composed of renal interstitial cells.

Macroscopically, there are firm white nodules situated in the medulla, typically 3–10 mm in size.

Microscopically, it is composed of spindle cells that surround the adjacent tubules.

These tumours are of no functional or clinical significance and do not undergo malignant transformation.

## Malignant tumours of the kidney

### Renal cell carcinoma (renal adenocarcinoma; hypernephroma)

An adenocarcinoma derived from the renal tubular epithelium in adults, this tumour accounts for about 3% of all carcinomas and about 90% of primary malignant renal tumours. It is usually seen after the age of 50 years. Males are more often affected than females by 3:1.

There is an increased incidence in those who smoke tobacco (double the relative risk of non-smokers) and also in patients with von Hippel–Lindau syndrome, a rare hereditary condition (this suggests a genetic predisposition).

*Associations*—paraneoplastic syndromes of hypercalcaemia, hypertension and polycythaemia.

Macroscopically, tumours occur most commonly at the upper pole of a kidney. They are usually rounded masses, with a yellowish cut surface marked with areas of haemorrhage and necrosis.

Microscopically, they are composed of either clear or granular cell types. The most common is the 'clear cell pattern', in which tumour cells have clear cytoplasm because of the high content of glycogen and lipid. Granular cell types are derived from tubular and papillary carcinomas.

Route of spread is:

- local—eroding through renal capsule into perinephric fat
- lymphatic—to para-aortic and other nodes
- blood-borne metastasis—involving the lungs, bone, brain and other sites as a result of tumour invasion of the renal vein. A characteristic feature is that large tumours may grow as a solid core along the main renal vein even entering the inferior vena cava.

Clinical features are:

- common presenting symptoms—haematuria (60%), loin pain (40%), loin mass (25%)
- occasional presenting symptoms—bone metastasis, brain metastasis or polycythaemia.

Prognosis depends on the stage at presentation. If the tumour is confined within a renal capsule there is a 75% 5-year survival. However, prognosis is very poor if metastases are present at diagnosis.

---

**Clinical Note**

Differential diagnosis of unilateral enlargement of the kidney is:

- hydronephrosis
- tumour
- renal vein thrombosis.

---

### Urothelial carcinoma of the renal pelvis

This malignant tumour of the renal pelvis is derived from the transitional cells of the urothelium, and it is histologically identical to transitional cell carcinoma of the bladder. Indeed, coexistence with bladder cancer occurs in half of cases. It is associated with analgesic abuse and exposure to aniline dyes used in the dye, rubber and plastics industries. Some cases have also been reported to develop many years after the use of 'Thorotrast', an α-particle-emitting contrast agent used in retrograde pyelography.

Tumours generally present early with haematuria or obstruction.

## Wilms' tumour (nephroblastoma)

This malignant embryonal tumour is derived from the primitive metanephros. It is the most common childhood urological malignancy, with a peak incidence between the ages of 1 and 4 years. Males and females are equally affected.

At least three different types of genes are important in the formation of Wilm's tumour. The most characterized of these is the tumour suppressor gene WT1, located on chromosome 11.

Macroscopically, large amounts of kidney are replaced by rounded masses of solid, fleshy, white lesions with frequent areas of necrosis. The tumour is aggressive and grows rapidly; extension beyond the capsule into perinephric fat and even into the root of mesentery is frequent. Spread to lungs occurs early and is identified in a high proportion of cases at the time of diagnosis.

Microscopically, it is composed of up to four elements:

1. Primitive, small cell, blastaematous tissue—resembles developing metanephric blastaema
2. Immature-looking glomerular structures
3. Epithelial tubules
4. Stroma composed of spindle cells and striated muscle.

*Clinical presentation*—large abdominal mass, abdominal pain, haematuria and hypertension are all recognized presentations.

Prognosis is related to the spread of the tumour at diagnosis. Treatment is by surgical nephrectomy with adjuvant chemotherapy (and potentially radiotherapy). Survival rates 5 years after diagnosis have increased to 80%.

## DISORDERS OF THE URINARY TRACT

## Congenital abnormalities of the urinary tract

### Ureteric abnormalities

These occur in up to 3% of people, although they have no clinical significance in most cases.

### Double and bifid ureters

The most common ureteric abnormality. These often occur in association with the duplication of the renal pelvis. They may be associated with vesicoureteric reflux and are predisposed to recurrent infections.

### Ureteropelvic junction obstruction

This is most commonly caused by a stricture that may be either intrinsic (within the wall of the ureter) or extrinsic (associated with external factors such as an aberrant vessel). This appears to provide a barrier to the conduction of a wave of contraction of the ureter, and is the most common cause of hydronephrosis in children.

## Bladder abnormalities

### Diverticula

Congenital diverticula are rare and are more often acquired as a result of bladder outlet obstruction. Symptoms are due to stasis and the resultant infection.

## Urethral abnormalities

### Hypospadias

The urethra opens on to the underside of the penis, either on the glans (glandular hypospadias), at the junction of the glans with the shaft (coronal hypospadias) or on the shaft itself (penile hypospadias).

### Epispadias

The urethra opens on to the dorsal (upper) surface of the penis.

All varieties can be corrected surgically.

## Urinary tract obstruction

This is obstruction of urine drainage from the kidney occurring at any level within the urinary tract. Obstruction may be caused by either a structural lesion (majority) or congenital neuromuscular defects that prevent contraction waves, and thus the flow of urine.

Structural lesions can be classified into:

- intrinsic lesions—within the urinary tract, e.g. stones, caseous or necrotic debris, fibrosis following trauma or infection, tumour
- extrinsic lesions—cause pressure from without, e.g. tumours of the rectum, prostate and the bladder, aberrant renal arteries, retroperitoneal fibrosis, pregnancy.

Causes vary according to the site of the obstruction (Fig. 9.11). In the list below, * indicates the most common sites of obstruction:

- Renal pelvis—calculi, tumours
- Pelviureteric junction*—stricture, calculi, extrinsic compression
- Ureter—calculi, extrinsic compression (pregnancy, tumour, fibrosis)
- Bladder neck*—tumour, calculi
- Urethra*—prostatic hyperplasia or carcinoma, urethral valves, urethral stricture.

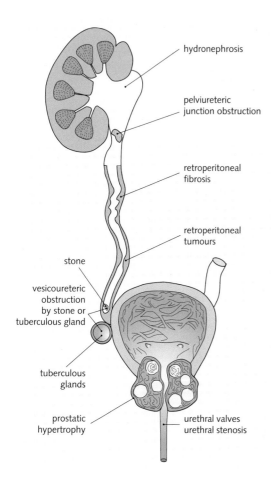

**Fig. 9.11** Urinary tract showing common sites of obstruction.

*Pathogenesis*—obstruction at any point in the urinary tract causes increased pressure superior to the blockage, with dilatation of the renal pelvis and calyces (hydronephrosis):

- Obstruction at the pelviureteric junction → hydronephrosis
- Obstruction of the ureter → hydroureter with subsequent development of hydronephrosis
- Obstruction of the bladder neck or urethra → bladder distension with hypertrophy of its muscle (seen on cystoscopic examination as trabeculation). Subsequently leads to hydroureter and hydronephrosis.

## Hydronephrosis

Hydronephrosis may be:

- unilateral—caused by unilateral obstruction anywhere above the bladder. It is typically detected late, because renal function is maintained by the non-obstructed kidney. Renal parenchyma becomes severely atrophic and renal function is permanently impaired (end-stage hydronephrosis)
- bilateral—caused by obstruction at the level of the bladder or urethra. Obstruction is typically detected at an earlier stage, as renal failure develops before severe atrophy of both kidneys.

In both forms, urinary tract obstruction predisposes to cystitis and pyelonephritis as well as stone formation.

### Effects of hydronephrosis

The net result of hydronephrosis is that fluid entering the collecting ducts cannot empty into the renal pelvis and intrarenal resorption of fluid occurs.

If the obstruction is removed at this stage then renal function returns to normal. However, persistence of obstruction leads to atrophy of the renal tubules and promotes interstitial inflammation, which leads to glomerular hyalinization and fibrosis.

Clinical features depend on the cause and site of the lesion.

Obstruction above the bladder will cause either an acute onset of renal colic or a gradual onset of aching pain in the loins, sometimes aggravated by drinking.

The clinical feature of obstruction below the bladder is difficulty in micturition, occasionally with distension of the bladder; it may progress to bilateral loin pain.

Superimposed infection causes malaise, fever, dysuria and sometimes septicaemia.

Management is by removal of the obstruction and treatment of the infection.

## Urolithiasis (urinary calculi)

This is the formation of stones in the urinary tract. It affects 1–5% of the population in the UK and onset is typically after 30 years of age, with males affected more than females.

Stones can form anywhere in the urinary tract but the most common site is within the renal pelvis.

Composition of stones:

- Calcium oxalate (70–75%)
- Triple phosphates (15%)—magnesium ammonium phosphate stones
- Uric acid (5–10%)
- Calculi in cystinuria and oxalosis.

Aetiology is:

- Acquired—as a result of obstruction, persistent infection, or reduced urine volume
- Inherited—primary metabolic disturbances, e.g. cystinuria.

The mechanism of stone formation is not well understood, but it is thought to involve an excess of solute in the urine (due to either a primary increase in metabolite or to stasis) or reduced solubility of solute in the urine (due to persistently abnormal urinary pH).

Calculi vary greatly in size, from sand-like particles to large round stones.

The condition may present with:

- renal colic often with nausea and vomiting—caused by the passage of small stones along the ureter
- dull ache in the loins—due to the presence of stones in the kidney
- recurrent and intractable urinary tract infection, haematuria or renal failure.

Occasionally, the condition is asymptomatic and discovered only during radiological examination for another disease.

Management is by bed rest, application of warmth to the site of pain and administration of analgesia.

Small stones (< 0.5 cm) in diameter are usually passed naturally. Larger stones may require lithotripsy or endoscopic surgery.

## Inflammation of the urinary tract

### Cystitis

This is inflammation of the bladder and it is extremely common—most women will have one or more episodes of cystitis. Females are affected more often than males because they have a shorter urethra (i.e. less travelling distance for bacteria).

#### Aetiology

The condition is most commonly due to infection but it is occasionally caused by physical agents, e.g. radiation or mechanical irritants. Infective causes are:

- Bacterial infection (most common)—usually Gram-negative coliform bacilli, e.g. *Escherichia coli* and *Proteus* species, but *Streptococcus faecalis*, *Pseudomonas aeruginosa* and staphylococci are also common
- Viral infection—adenovirus may cause haemorrhagic cystitis in children
- Parasites—*Schistosoma haematobium*, which is common in Africa
- Fungi—*Candida*.

Risk factors are:

- urinary retention—due to obstruction, bladder paralysis, diverticula, calculi, foreign bodies, tumours, uterine prolapse
- infection of adjacent structures, e.g. prostatitis, urethritis and diverticular disease of the colon
- diabetes mellitus—glycosuria favours infection
- pregnancy
- trauma, e.g. catheterization.

Infection normally ascends from the urethra but may descend from the kidney in some cases of renal infection (e.g. renal tuberculosis). Direct spread from adjacent organs (e.g. diverticulitis) may occur but haematogenous and lymphatic spread are rare.

Macroscopically, there is acute inflammation with oedema, erythema and later ulceration of bladder mucosa.

Microscopically, there is infiltration of mucosa with acute inflammatory cells.

*Clinical features*—the classic triad of increased urinary frequency, lower abdominal pain and dysuria are common. Systemic effects of inflammation (e.g. fever) may also occur.

#### Investigation, treatment and sequelae

*Investigations*—examination of midstream urine.

*Treatment*—with antibiotics (e.g. trimethoprim), high fluid intake and addressing underlying causes such as obstruction.

*Sequelae*:

- Resolution (common)
- Chronicity if the underlying cause is untreatable
- Development of pyelonephritis and associated complications.

### Ureteritis

This inflammation of the ureter is usually due to an ascending urinary tract infection.

Causative organisms are the same as for cystitis; an acute bacterial cystitis may lead to an ascending ureteritis.

*Complications*—organisms may gain access to the renal parenchyma to produce acute pyelonephritis, with the formation of abscesses in the renal medulla and cortex.

## Neoplastic disease of the urinary tract

### Bladder metaplasia

#### Glandular metaplasia (cystitis glandularis)

These small, rounded collections of urothelial cells are found just below the urothelial surface (Brunn's nests). They develop a central lumen surrounded by cuboidal or columnar cells. They are quite common and often seen in the normal bladder.

Occasionally, there is metaplasia to an intestinal variant of cystitis glandularis, lined by colonic, mucin-secreting epithelium.

#### Adenomatous metaplasia (nephrogenic adenoma)

This benign condition is characterized by metaplasia of the urothelium to cuboidal epithelium. Metaplastic areas resemble collecting tubules of the kidney. It is associated with chronic infections, e.g. tuberculosis.

#### Squamous metaplasia

There are two types:

1. Keratinizing squamous metaplasia (leucoplakia)— the bladder mucosa develops white plaques, which

are often secondary to chronic irritation, e.g. calculi. A significant proportion progresses to squamous carcinoma of the bladder.

2. Non-keratinizing squamous metaplasia (vaginal metaplasia)—white plaques are seen on the trigone. This only occurs in women and it has no pathological significance.

## Tumours of the bladder

### Transitional cell papilloma
These are rare, benign tumours of the bladder that may represent the first stage of transitional cell carcinoma. A fibrovascular stalk attaches their branched structure to the mucosa.

### Transitional cell carcinoma
These are tumours of the urothelium, affecting 1 in 5000 in the UK and accounting for 3% of all cancer deaths. They are most commonly found in those aged 60–70 years, with males affected more than females by 3:1. Cigarette smoking is an important cause.

Aetiology is as follows:

- Chemicals—exposure to environmental agents excreted in high concentrations in the urine. Known carcinogens are associated with cigarette smoking, aniline dyes and the rubber industry.
- Leucoplakia (see above)—associated with bladder stones.
- Bladder diverticula—about 3% are complicated with tumour.

Most tumours are at the base of trigone and around the ureteric orifices.

Morphological types:

- Papillary (most common)—warty masses projecting into the lumen with little or no invasion of the bladder wall. Only a small percentage evolves into invasive carcinoma.
- Solid—tumours grow directly into the bladder wall and are often ulcerated or encrusted. Most are invasive from the outset.
- Mixed papillary and solid.
- Flat in-situ carcinoma—reddened mucosal surface due to underlying telangiectatic blood vessels. May become invasive.

### HINTS AND TIPS

The majority of urothelial cancers are caused by exposure to environmental agents. Therefore, bladder

tumours are usually multiple, and they are often found in conjunction with urothelial tumours at other sites of the lower urinary tract, e.g. renal pelvis, ureters or urethra.

### Other tumours of the bladder
Only a small proportion of bladder cancers are of squamous origin (squamous cell carcinoma). They are most often associated with schistosomiasis infection. Adenocarcinomas and mesenchymal tumours are rare. Secondary tumours usually occur following direct invasion from the cervix, prostate or rectum.

### Grading and staging of bladder carcinomas
The degree of differentiation (grade) and extent of spread (stage) are important indicators for prognosis.

Transitional cell carcinomas are graded I–III:

- Grade I (well differentiated)—vast majority are papillary growths with no evidence of invasion.
- Grade II (moderately well differentiated)—usually papillary but many are either invasive at presentation or become so. Cells show significant atypicality and an increase in mitotic figures.
- Grade III (poorly differentiated)—mainly solid lesions which are extensively invasive. Cells are pleomorphic with numerous mitoses.

TNM staging follows the same principles as other cancers.

Spread is as follows:

- Local—to pelvic structures
- Lymphatic—to iliac and para-aortic lymph nodes
- Haematogenous—to liver and lung.

Clinically, the disease classically presents with painless haematuria, but symptoms of recurrent urinary tract infections may occur. Rarely, it may present with hydronephrosis (from ureteric obstruction), pneumaturia from vesicocolic fistula, or incontinence from vesicovaginal fistula.

Treatment usually involves transurethral resection of tumour, with the potential for intravesical chemotherapy in multiple tumours. Radical cystectomy may be considered for patients with invasive disease.

Prognosis depends on the histological type of the tumour and extent of spread. Papillary, non-invasive tumours have an excellent prognosis, whereas solid, invasive, urothelial tumours have an overall 5-year survival rate of only 35%.

# Pathology of the endocrine system

## Objectives

In this chapter, you will learn to:
- Describe disorders of the pituitary gland leading to hyperpituitarism and hypopituitarism.
- Describe the causes and patterns of thyroid dysfunction.
- Describe the causes and patterns of parathyroid dysfunction.
- Understand Cushing's syndrome and other disorders of adrenal hyperfunction.
- Understand the importance of adrenal hypofunction and crisis.
- Recall the pathology and complications associated with diabetes mellitus.
- Briefly describe endocrine tumours including the important multiple endocrine neoplasia syndromes.

## DISORDERS OF THE PITUITARY

The pituitary (hypophysis) is a small (500–1000 mg), bean-shaped gland lying in the sella turcica in the base of the skull. It is composed of two parts:

1. Anterior lobe (adenohypophysis)—synthesizes and secretes a number of hormones (Fig. 10.1), most of which act on other endocrine glands.
2. Posterior lobe (neurohypophysis)—stores and secretes two hormones synthesized in the hypothalamus: antidiuretic hormone (ADH; vasopressin) and oxytocin. This lobe is in direct continuity with the hypothalamus, to which it is connected via the pituitary stalk.

Secretion of the pituitary hormones is regulated by neural and chemical stimuli from the hypothalamus, diseases of which cause secondary abnormalities in pituitary function.

This cooperation between the nervous system and endocrine apparatus is referred to as neuroendocrine signalling. Figure 10.2 shows the integration of signals between the hypothalamus, pituitary and thyroid gland in the release of thyroid hormones, with feedback loops acting at each level.

Neuroendocrine cells are defined as those that release a hormone in response to a neural stimulus. Important examples include:

- neurons of the supra-optic nucleus (projecting into the posterior pituitary), which release ADH
- chromaffin cells of the adrenal medulla, which release epinephrine (adrenaline).

## The anterior pituitary: hyperpituitarism

Hyperpituitarism is defined as excessive secretion of one or more of the pituitary hormones. Its most common causes are functioning (hormone-secreting) adenomas of the anterior lobe.

### Anterior lobe adenomas

Anterior lobe adenomas comprise about 10% of all intracranial tumours (posterior lobe adenomas do not occur). These tumours do not usually metastasize, but they are often life threatening because of their position and ability to secrete excess hormone.

### Effects of pituitary adenomas

Pituitary adenomas cause problems because of a combination of endocrine effects (excessive secretion of a particular hormone) and compressive effects, caused by an increase in local pressure of the following:

- Remainder of the pituitary → hypopituitarism
- Optic chiasm → visual field defects, notably bi-temporal haemianopia
- Brain (large tumours) → distortion of the midbrain with raised intracranial pressure and hydrocephalus
- Dura → headaches
- Cavernous sinus → CN III, IV or VI nerve palsies.

The endocrine effects depend on which hormone is being excessively secreted (see below).

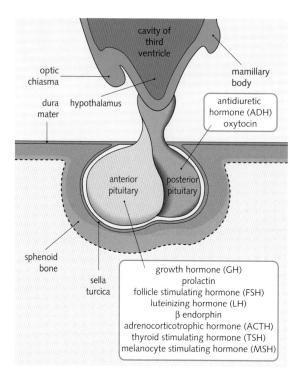

**Fig. 10.1** Pituitary and hypothalamus, with the hormones released.

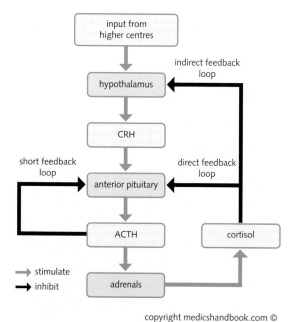

copyright medicshandbook.com ©

**Fig. 10.2** Schematic representation of the integration between the higher centre, hypothalamus, pituitary and target organ signalling. The example is for cortisol, highlighting the feedback loops that control hormone release at each level. (CRH; corticotropin-releasing hormone, ACTH; adrencorticotropic hormone). (Redrawn with permission from medicshandbook.com).

*Investigations:*

- Imaging—plain X-ray (can detect enlargement of sella turcica and erosion of the clinoid processes) and MRI (for visualization and sizing of the tumour; this is superior to CT scanning).
- Hormone assays (e.g. growth hormone, prolactin).
- Functional testing of the pituitaryadrenal axis, e.g. ACTH stimulation test in which a dose of adreno-corticotrophic hormone (ACTH) is given and the plasma cortisol response measured.
- Visual field assessment.

## Types of functioning adenomas

Functioning adenomas may produce any of the anterior lobe (adenophyseal) hormones but the majority produce prolactin (prolactinomas-lactotroph adenomas), growth hormone (somatotroph adenomas) or ACTH (corticotroph adenomas).

### Prolactinomas

This most common pituitary tumour (30% of all pituitary tumours) has abnormally raised serum prolactin levels associated with amenorrhea and galactorrhea, and with ejaculatory failure or impotence in men. Mild prolactin increases are seen with compression of the hypothalamus by any pituitary adenoma (the 'stalk effect').

### Somatotroph adenoma

The second most common pituitary tumour, it results in hypersecretion of growth hormone, the effects of which depend on the developmental stage of the affected individual:

- Pre-epiphyseal union (prepubertal) leads to gigantism, i.e. excessive growth in a regular and initially well-proportioned manner.
- Postepiphyseal union (adults) leads to acromegaly, which is characterized by enlargement of the hands, feet and head. They may also present with secondary diabetes (growth hormone is an insulin antagonist) or cardiovascular effects (Fig. 10.3).

### Corticotrophin adenoma

Overproduction of ACTH by the pituitary gland (Cushing's disease) causes adrenal hyperplasia, resulting in the excessive secretion of glucocorticoids causing Cushing's syndrome, the effects of which are described later (see page 182).

## Other functioning adenomas

Other endocrine secreting adenomas, e.g. of thyroid-stimulating hormone (TSH), luteinizing hormone (LH) and follicle-stimulating hormone (FSH), are extremely rare.

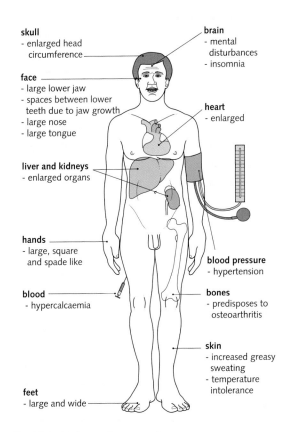

**Fig. 10.3** Features of acromegaly.

skull
- enlarged head circumference

face
- large lower jaw
- spaces between lower teeth due to jaw growth
- large nose
- large tongue

liver and kidneys
- enlarged organs

hands
- large, square and spade like

blood
- hypercalcaemia

feet
- large and wide

brain
- mental disturbances
- insomnia

heart
- enlarged

blood pressure
- hypertension

bones
- predisposes to osteoarthritis

skin
- increased greasy sweating
- temperature intolerance

# The anterior pituitary: hypopituitarism

Hypopituitarism is defined as insufficient secretion of the pituitary hormones. The clinical features depend on the patient's age and on the type and severity of the hormone deficiencies (Fig. 10.4).

Hypopituitarism can be caused by either hypothalamic lesions or pituitary lesions.

Hypothalamic lesions are:

- idiopathic deficiency of one or more of the releasing factors, e.g. gonadotrophin-releasing hormone (GnRH; Kallmann's syndrome), growth-hormone releasing factor (GHRH) or, more rarely, thyrotrophin-releasing hormone (TRH) or corticotrophin-releasing factor (CRF)
- infarction
- inflammation, e.g. sarcoidosis, tuberculous meningitis.
- suprasellar tumours, e.g. craniopharyngioma or, more rarely, pinealoma, teratoma or a secondary tumour from another site.

Pituitary lesions are:

- idiopathic deficiency of one or more of the pituitary hormones

- sheehan's syndrome—ischaemic necrosis of the anterior pituitary due to hypotensive shock occurring as a result of obstetric haemorrhage. Initially there is a loss of gonadotrophins, then subsequent loss of TSH and ACTH
- empty sella syndrome—an enlarged, empty sella turcica that is not filled with pituitary tissue. This may be a primary anatomical variant or it may follow spontaneous infarction, surgery, or radiotherapy of a tumour
- trauma, including surgery and radiotherapy.
- granulomatous lesions—sarcoidosis, tuberculosis, histiocytosis.

## Management

Management is by substitution therapy according to the deficiencies demonstrated, e.g. cortisol replacement for ACTH deficiency, thyroid hormone replacement for TSH deficiency.

## The posterior pituitary

Diseases of the posterior pituitary are much less common than those of the anterior pituitary and are usually the result of damage to the hypothalamus by tumour invasion or infarction. Posterior pituitary diseases typically cause disorders of abnormal ADH secretion. There are no known effects of abnormal oxytocin secretion.

## Diabetes insipidus

Diabetes insipidus (DI) is a rare condition characterized by the persistent excretion of excessive quantities of dilute urine (polyuria) and by constant thirst (polydipsia).

There are two types (Fig. 10.5):

1. Cranial DI—caused by the failure of ADH production
2. Nephrogenic DI—distal tubules are refractory to the water reabsorptive action of ADH.

*Clinical features*—irrespective of aetiology, reabsorption of water from the glomerular filtrate in the renal collecting ducts does not occur, resulting in polyuria (up to 20 L per day is possible) and high risk of body water depletion. DI is potentially lethal without appropriate therapy.

*Investigations*—there is high clinical suspicion if a patient has a high plasma osmolality with low or immeasurable plasma ADH, and a non-maximally concentrated urine. A water deprivation test is run for 8 hours or until 3% of the body weight is lost. Demonstration of continued polyuria and increased haemoconcentration indicates DI. This test serves to differentiate DI from

**Fig. 10.4** Clinical features associated with specific forms of hypopituitarism

| Hormone deficiency | Clinical features | Tests to exclude hypofunction of anterior pituitary |
|---|---|---|
| Gonadotrophin deficiency | Prepubertal:<br>• Failure to enter puberty<br>• Undescended testes<br>• Obesity<br>• Eunuchoidism<br>Postpubertal:<br>• Infertility<br>• Amenorrhoea<br>• Oligospermia<br>• Progressive loss of secondary sex characteristics (hypogonadism)<br>• Osteoporotic collapse of spine→ loss of stature | LH reserves adequate if:<br>• Males have a normal testosterone<br>• Females are ovulating<br>FSH reserves adequate if:<br>• Males have a normal spermatogenesis<br>• Females are ovulating |
| GH deficiency | Children: failure of longitudinal growth<br>Adults: tendency to hypoglycaemia | GH reserves adequate if: random plasma level >20 mU/L stress or otherwise elevated GH peak >20 mU/L |
| TSH deficiency | Fetus or newborn: cretinism<br>Adults: hypothyroidism | TSH reserves adequate if serum thyroxine within normal range |
| ACTH deficiency | Features of primary hypoadrenalism but with decreased pigmentation (rather than an increase) | ACTH reserves adequate if: random plasma cortisol >550 nmol/L stress-induced cortisol rise >550 nmol/L |

Note: ACTH, adrenocorticotrophic hormone; FSH, follicle-stimulating hormone; GH, growth hormone; LH, luteinizing hormone; TSH, thyroid-stimulating hormone.

psychogenic polydipsia. The test is then followed by ADH administration to differentiate between cranial DI (kidneys are responsive to ADH) or nephrogenic DI (kidneys are unresponsive to ADH).

*Treatment of mild DI*—the effects of dehydration can be counteracted by greatly increasing water intake (polydipsia).

*Treatment of moderate to severe DI*:

• Cranial DI—treatment with desmopressin (ADH analogue but without vasoactive effects).
• Nephrogenic DI—treatment with thiazide diuretics, producing a decrease in urine volume by approximately 50%.

**HINTS AND TIPS**

Diabetes insipidus and diabetes mellitus are two distinct conditions that both feature polyuria.

# Syndrome of inappropriate antidiuretic hormone secretion

Increased secretion of ADH occurs as a complication of other diseases (primary hypersecretion of ADH is not recognized). The condition is characterized by water retention with haemodilution and by inappropriately concentrated urine. In severe cases, cerebral oedema supervenes with impaired consciousness, but body oedema is not usually seen as free water is evenly distributed to all body compartments.

The causes are:

• idiopathic
• tumours—ectopic secretion of ADH, especially by small cell carcinomas of the lung and some other neuroendocrine tumours
• trauma—skull fracture, head injury or surgery may produce transiently increased secretion of ADH
• intracranial inflammation—meningitis, tuberculosis, syphilis

**Fig. 10.5** Causes of cranial and nephrogenic diabetes insipidus (DI)

| | Cause | Features |
|---|---|---|
| Cranial DI | Hypothalamic or pituitary stalk damage | Surgical damage, usually in the course of tumour removal<br>Head injury, usually transient<br>Hypothalamic tumour (either primary or secondary)<br>Hypothalamic inflammatory lesions, e.g. sarcoidosis, encephalitis, meningitis |
| | Genetic defect | Dominant<br>Recessive: DIDMOAD syndrome-association of DI with diabetes mellitus (DM), optic atrophy (OA) and deafness (D) |
| | Idiopathic | About 30% of cases have no known cause |
| Nephrogenic DI | Hereditary | Abnormal ADH receptors |
| | Metabolic abnormalities | Hypokalaemia<br>Hypercalcaemia |
| | Drug therapy | Lithium<br>Demethylchlortetracycline |
| | Poisoning | Heavy metals |

Note: ADH, antidiuretic hormone.

- non-neoplastic lung disease (e.g. pneumonia, pulmonary embolus) probably due to involvement of intrathoracic baroreceptors.

Figure 10.6 shows a comparison table of features of DI with those of inappropriate ADH secretion.

## THYROID DISORDERS

## Congenital disorders of the thyroid

### Thyroglossal cysts

As the embryo grows, the thyroid descends into the neck, during migration; the gland remains connected to the tongue by a narrow canal, the thyroglossal duct, which later becomes solid and finally disappears.

Cystic remnants of parts of the thyroglossal duct are known as thyroglossal cysts (Fig. 10.7). These cysts may form anywhere along the course of descent but are always located near or in the midline of the neck. Cysts usually develop as painless, progressively enlarging and movable masses. It does not lead to any alterations in thyroid function.

## Thyrotoxicosis (hyperthyroidism)

This syndrome is caused by the excessive secretion of thyroid hormones—typically both thyroxine ($T_4$) and tri-iodothyronine ($T_3$)—in the bloodstream. Symptoms include tachycardia, sweating, tremor, anxiety, increased appetite, loss of weight and intolerance of heat.

Hyperthyroidism can be classified on the basis of aetiology into:

- primary hyperthyroidism ($\uparrow$ thyroid hormones, $\downarrow$ TSH)—hypersecretion of thyroid hormones, which is not secondary to increased levels of TSH (the rise in thyroid hormones actually suppresses TSH)
- secondary hyperthyroidism ($\uparrow$ thyroid hormones, $\uparrow$ TSH)—overstimulation of the thyroid gland caused by excess TSH produced by a tumour in the pituitary or elsewhere (rare).

Primary hyperthyroidism is caused by:

- Graves' disease (exophthalmic goitre)—the most common cause of thyrotoxicosis, characterized by a diffusely enlarged thyroid gland that is stimulated to produce excess hormone by an IgG autoantibody
- toxic multinodular goitre (Plummer's disease)—second most common cause of hyperthyroidism

**Fig. 10.6** Comparison of features of diabetes insipidus with those of inappropriate ADH secretion

| Condition | Imbalance | Urinary and plasma osmolality | Symptoms |
|---|---|---|---|
| Diabetes insipidus | ↓ ADH | Low urinary osmolality<br>High plasma osmolality | Polyuria (5–20 L/day)<br>Thirst<br>Polydipsia (may lead to severe dehydration, exhaustion, coma) |
| Syndrome of inappropriate ADH secretion | ↑ ADH | High urinary osmolality<br>Low plasma osmolality<br>(dilutional hyponatraemia) | Oliguria<br>Water intoxication (may lead to confusion, neurological disturbances, coma) |

Note: ADH, antidiuretic hormone.

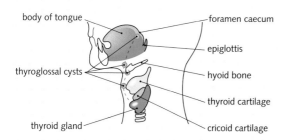

**Fig. 10.7** Path of descent of thyroid gland (broken line) and localization of thyroglossal cysts.

- toxic adenoma—solitary thyroid nodule producing excess hormone with remainder of the thyroid gland being suppressed
- thyroiditis—inflammation of the thyroid causing hyperthyroidism (e.g. De Quervain's thyroiditis). Note that thyroiditis is more commonly associated with hypothyroidism (see below)
- drugs—either direct ingestion of large doses of thyroid hormone (thyrotoxicosis factitia) or through iodide-inducing drugs (e.g. amiodarone).

## Effects of thyrotoxicosis

Signs and symptoms of thyrotoxicosis are a consequence of an increase in the body's metabolism, which occurs as a direct result of increased concentrations of the thyroid hormones.

The most important symptoms diagnostically are:

- heat intolerance and excessive sweating (hyperhidrosis)
- nervousness and irritability
- weight loss with normal or increased appetite
- goitre (an enlargement of the thyroid gland).

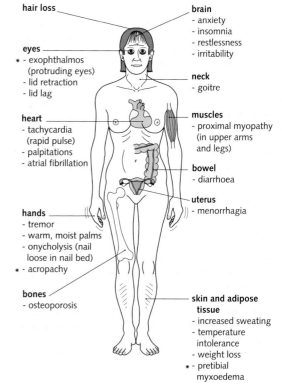

**Fig. 10.8** Summary diagram illustrating features of thyrotoxicosis. (* = additional features seen only in Graves' disease.)

Other symptoms are summarised in Figure 10.8.

**Investigations**—hyperthyroidism is confirmed by raised serum thyroxine and/or lowered serum TSH.

**Management**—options in thyrotoxicosis are:

- surgery—reduces the amount of functioning thyroid tissue

- radioactive iodine—to destroy part of the gland
- drugs (such as carbimazole or propylthiouracil)—interfere with the production of thyroid hormones.

## Graves' disease

Graves' disease is an autoimmune disorder that results in thyrotoxicosis due to over-stimulation of the thyroid gland by autoantibodies. It is the most common form of thyrotoxicosis, females being affected more than males by 8:1. It is usually associated with a diffuse enlargement of the thyroid.

*Pathogenesis*—IgG-type immunoglobulins bind to TSH membrane receptors and cause prolonged stimulation of the thyroid, lasting for as long as 12 hours (cf. 1 hour for TSH). The autoantibody binds at a site different to the hormone-binding locus and is termed the TSH-receptor autoantibody (TRAb); 95% of Graves' disease patients are positive for TRAbs.

Histologically, the gland shows diffuse hypertrophy and hyperplasia of acinar epithelium, reduction of stored colloid and local accumulations of lymphocytes with lymphoid follicle formation.

The clinical features of Graves' disease are similar to those of general thyrotoxicosis but with some additional features (see Fig. 10.8), namely:

- exophthalmos (protrusion of the eyeballs in their sockets)—due to the infiltration of orbital tissues by fat, mucopolysaccharides and lymphocytes. May cause compression of the optic nerve, hence blindness. However, only about 5% of Graves' patients show signs of exophthalmos
- thyroid acropachy—enlargement of fingernails
- pretibial myxoedema—accumulation of mucoproteins in the deep dermis of the skin.

Treatment is as for thyrotoxicosis.

## Hypothyroidism

Decreased activity of the thyroid gland results in decreased production of thyroid hormones. There are two forms:

1. Hypothyroidism present at birth → cretinism or congenital hypothyroidism
2. Hypothyroidism in adults → myxoedema.

## Cretinism (congenital hypothyroidism)

This condition occurs as a result of extreme hypothyroidism during fetal life, infancy or childhood. It has the following types and aetiology:

- endemic cretinism—occurs in iodine-deficient countries where goitre is common

- sporadic cretinism—caused by congenital hypoplasia or absence of the thyroid gland and often associated with deaf mutism
- dyshormonogenesis—a congenital familial recessive enzyme defect causing an inability to complete the formation of thyroid hormones. TSH is increased, and the thyroid gland is enlarged and shows epithelial hyperplasia.

The clinical features of cretinism are:

- severe mental retardation
- impaired growth—skeletal growth is inhibited more than soft tissue growth
- coarse, dry skin
- lack of hair and teeth
- protuberant abdomen (often with umbilical hernia)
- protruding tongue.

Management is by early detection and treatment with thyroxine, which can prevent an irreversible mental defect and cerebellar damage. Many countries now have screening programmes to measure serum TSH and/or thyroxine levels on heel-prick blood samples taken on the fourth or fifth day of life.

## Hypothyroidism in adults (myxoedema)

This common clinical condition is associated with decreased function of the thyroid gland and a decrease in the circulating level of thyroid hormones. It affects 1% of people in the UK, with females more than males by 6:1. It can present at any age but most commonly between 30 and 50 years of age.

Note that, strictly speaking, myxoedema describes a non-pitting, oedematous reaction characteristic of hypothyroidism caused by the deposition of a mucoid substance (*myxa*-is a Greek prefix denoting mucus) in the skin and elsewhere in the body. However, the terms 'myxoedema' and 'hypothyroidism of adults' are now frequently used interchangeably.

Hypothyroidism can be classified according to aetiology:

- Primary (↓ thyroid hormones, ↑ TSH)—failure of the thyroid gland itself. This is much more common than secondary hypothyroidism. Note that subclinical hypothyroidism describes an increase in TSH but with normal thyroid hormone levels, and is increasingly being treated with the aim of reducing progression to full disease.
- Secondary (↓ thyroid hormones, ↑TSH)—failure of TSH production due to pituitary disease.

The causes of primary hypothyroidism are:

- autoimmune thyroiditis—atrophic form, e.g. primary atrophic thyroiditis and goitrous form (such as Hashimoto's thyroiditis)

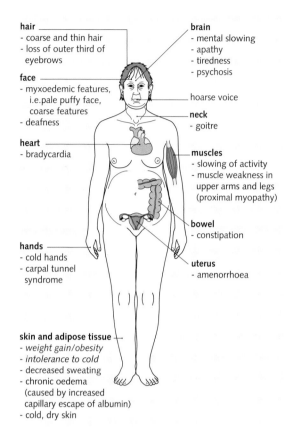

hair
- coarse and thin hair
- loss of outer third of eyebrows

face
- myxoedemic features, i.e. pale puffy face, coarse features
- deafness

heart
- bradycardia

hands
- cold hands
- carpal tunnel syndrome

skin and adipose tissue
- *weight gain/obesity*
- *intolerance to cold*
- decreased sweating
- chronic oedema (caused by increased capillary escape of albumin)
- cold, dry skin

brain
- mental slowing
- apathy
- tiredness
- psychosis

hoarse voice

neck
- goitre

muscles
- slowing of activity
- muscle weakness in upper arms and legs (proximal myopathy)

bowel
- constipation

uterus
- amenorrhoea

**Fig. 10.9** Summary diagram illustrating features of hypothyroidism in the adult (myxoedema).

- Graves' disease—approximately 5% of patients with thyrotoxicosis develop hypothyroidism in later years, unrelated to treatment. Probably caused by a spectrum of antithyroid antibodies, some of which stimulate TSH receptor and some of which are destructive
- treatment of hyperthyroidism—surgical ablation, radioiodine or drug treatment
- severe iodine deficiency (rare in the UK)—iodine must be virtually absent from the diet before myxoedema develops.

The effects of hypothyroidism are shown in Figure 10.9.

### Clinical Note

Signs and symptoms of hypothyroidism are both widespread (due to reduced body metabolism) and localized (myxoedema due to the accumulation of mucoproteins). The most important symptoms diagnostically are:
• mental and physical slowness
• tiredness

- cold intolerance
- dryness of skin and hair.
  Investigations are:
- serum thyroxine concentration (decreased)
- serum TSH concentration (reduced in secondary hypothyroidism but increased in primary hypothyroidism).
  The treatment is oral thyroxine daily for life.

## Thyroiditis

This inflammation of the thyroid gland can have a viral or autoimmune aetiology.

## Hashimoto's thyroiditis (most common cause of hypothyroidism)

This autoimmune disease results in destructive thyroiditis. It can occur at any age, but typically affects the middle-aged, and females more than males by 12:1.

Thyroid peroxidase antibodies are most commonly found in the serum of affected individuals (90% of cases). The disease is associated with the HLA-DR5 and HLA-B8 haplotypes, and patients with Hashimoto's disease (and Graves' disease) show a high incidence of other autoimmune diseases.

Macroscopically, the thyroid gland is usually:

- diffusely enlarged (typically 2–5 times normal size)
- firm in consistency
- white or grey on a cut surface as a result of the disappearance of brown (iodine-rich) colloid (thyroglobulin), and its replacement by lymphocytes.

Microscopically, the thyroid gland shows:

- small thyroid follicles infiltrated by lymphocytes and plasma cells
- lymphoid follicle formation and increased fibrous tissue stroma
- acini lined with abnormal, highly eosinophilic epithelial cells (proliferation of mitochondria) known as Askanazy or Hürthle cells
- reduced colloid content of disrupted acini.

The condition may present due to goitre formation or because of the symptoms of hypothyroidism. The hypothyroid state tends to develop slowly. However, damage to thyroid follicles may lead to the release of thyroglobulin into the circulation causing transient thyrotoxicosis. Some cases proceed to primary atrophic thyroiditis. Furthermore, there is an increased incidence of non-Hodgkin's lymphoma originating in the thyroid of patients with Hashimoto's thyroiditis.

Treatment is by oral thyroxine, which overcomes hypothyroidism and reduces the size of the goitre.

# De Quervain's thyroiditis

A rare, viral thyroiditis seen in young and middle-aged women as a slightly diffuse tender swelling of the thyroid; this is also known as subacute, giant cell or granulomatous thyroiditis. The condition usually occurs in association with a transient febrile illness, often during various viral epidemics.

The most commonly associated viruses are Coxsackie, mumps and adenovirus.

Characteristic features are:

- painful enlargement of the thyroid (about twice normal size; normal weight is 20–30 g)
- history of usually short duration
- preceding general malaise, pyrexia or upper respiratory infection.

Histological examination shows:

- inflammation with a giant cell granulomatous reaction engulfing leaked colloid (hence the synonyms giant cell or granulomatous thyroiditis)
- degeneration of follicles with inflammatory cell infiltration (neutrophils, plasma cells, lymphocytes and histiocytes)
- fibrous scarring (late).

The illness is usually self-limiting and settles in a few weeks. Transient hyperthyroidism can result from the release of thyroglobulin and excessive amounts of thyroid hormone.

Severe thyroiditis may be fatal in the elderly and debilitated.

# Subacute lymphocytic thyroiditis

This form of autoimmune thyroiditis is characterized by focal lymphocytic infiltration of the thyroid (also known as focal lymphocytic thyroiditis).

Histological changes are similar to those in Hashimoto's thyroiditis, but they are focal rather than diffuse. The disease is less severe than Hashimoto's thyroiditis, and it is often asymptomatic. It may also present with the symptoms of hyperthyroidism.

A comparison of the main types of thyroiditis is provided in Figure 10.10.

# Thyroid goitres

## Definitions

A goitre is any enlargement of the thyroid gland. There are two types:

1. Toxic goitre, i.e. goitre associated with thyrotoxicosis
2. Non-toxic goitre, i.e. goitre associated with normal or reduced levels of thyroid hormones.

## Toxic goitre

### Graves' disease
This is the most common cause of toxic goitre (described above).

### Toxic multinodular goitre
This results from the development of hyperthyroidism in a multinodular goitre (see below).

## Non-toxic goitres

### Diffuse non-toxic goitre (simple goitre)
This diffuse enlargement of the thyroid gland is classified into:

- endemic goitre—due to iodine deficiency.
- sporadic goitre—caused by goitrogenic agents (substances that induce goitre formation) or familial in origin. Examples of goitrogenic agents include certain cabbage species, because of their thiourea content, and specific drugs or chemicals, such as iodide, para-minosalicylic acid and drugs used in the treatment of thyrotoxicosis. Familial cases show inherited autosomal recessive traits, which interfere with hormone synthesis via various enzyme pathways
- physiological goitre—enlargement of the thyroid gland in females during puberty or pregnancy.

**Fig. 10.10** Summary of features of thyroiditis

|  | Hashimoto's thyroiditis | De Quervain's thyroiditis | Subacute lymphocytic thyroiditis |
|---|---|---|---|
| Aetiology | Autoimmune | Viral | Autoimmune |
| Histological features | Diffuse lymphocytic infiltration of thyroid | Giant cell granulomatous inflammatory reaction | Focal lymphocytic infiltration of thyroid |
| Hypothyroidism | Common | Rare | Rare |

## Multinodular goitre

This is the most common cause of thyroid enlargement and is seen particularly in the elderly (nearly all simple goitres eventually become multinodular). The exact aetiology is uncertain but it may represent an uneven responsiveness of various parts of the thyroid to fluctuating TSH levels over a period of many years.

Morphological features are:

- irregular hyperplastic enlargement of the entire thyroid gland due to the development of well-circumscribed nodules of varying size
- larger nodules filled with brown, gelatinous colloid; consequently, it is often termed multinodular colloid goitres.

Most patients have normal thyroid function and generally seek treatment for cosmetic reasons (an unsightly swelling in the neck) or compression symptoms, e.g. pressure on the trachea producing stridor or pressure on the recurrent laryngeal nerve producing hoarseness.

However, toxic changes occasionally occur in a multinodular goitre resulting in hyperthyroidism, when it is termed a toxic multinodular goitre.

## Neoplasms of the thyroid

Tumours of the thyroid are generally benign. Carcinomas are rare and lymphomas are rarer still.

## Benign tumours

### Thyroid adenomas

These are solitary, or multiple, encapsulated solid nodules. Compression of the adjacent gland is a common feature, and the centre may show areas of haemorrhage and cystic changes. The most common type is follicular adenoma, which consists of colloid-containing microfollicles and columns of larger cells of alveolar arrangement.

### HINTS AND TIPS

A reminder of the differences between primary and secondary hyperthyroidism and hypothyroidism:
- Primary hyperthyroidism—↑ thyroid hormones, ↓ TSH
- Secondary hyperthyroidism—↑ thyroid hormones, ↑ TSH (excess TSH production due to pituitary tumour)
- Primary hypothyroidism—↓ thyroid hormones, ↑ TSH
- Secondary hypothyroidism—↓ thyroid hormones, ↓ TSH (failure of TSH production due to pituitary disease).

Rarely, follicular adenomas may synthesize excess thyroid hormones ('toxic adenomas'), causing thyrotoxicosis.

## Malignant tumours

These rare tumours account for less than 1% of total cancer deaths in the UK, with females affected more than males by 3:1. Types of malignant thyroid tumours and their basic features are outlined in Figure 10.11.

### Papillary adenocarcinoma

This is the most common thyroid cancer. It is a well-differentiated tumour most commonly found in younger patients. It presents as a non-encapsulated infiltrative mass. It is a slow growing tumour with an excellent prognosis.

Histologically it consists of epithelial papillary projections into gland-like spaces and calcified spherules

Fig. 10.11 Types and features of malignant thyroid tumours

| | Tumour type | Origin of tumour | Frequency (%) | Typical age range (years) | Spread | Prognosis (% for 10-year survival) |
|---|---|---|---|---|---|---|
| Differentiated carcinoma | Papillary | Follicular cells | 70 | 20–40 | Lymph nodes | 95 |
| | Follicular | Follicular cells | 10 | 40–60 | Bloodstream | 60 |
| Undifferentiated carcinoma | Anaplastic | Follicular cells | 5 | >60 | Aggressive local invasion; bloodstream | 1 |
| Medullary carcinoma | — | Parafollicular C cells | 5–10 | >40 | Local, lymphatic and blood | 50 (but very variable) |
| Lymphoma | — | Lymphocytes | 5–10 | >60 | Lymphatic | 10 |

may be present (psoammoma bodies). Epithelial cell nuclei are large with clear areas centrally (described as 'Orphan Annie nuclei').

### Follicular adenocarcinoma
Characterized histologically by uniform follicles, spread is usually to bones, lungs and brain via the bloodstream.

Many of these tumours retain the ability to take up radioactive iodine ($^{131}I$), which may be used as a highly effective targeted form of radiotherapy, usually after surgical thyroidectomy. The prognosis, therefore, is good.

### Anaplastic carcinoma
This highly malignant, poorly differentiated adenocarcinoma usually presents in the elderly as a diffusely infiltrative mass. In about half of cases there is a history of multinodular goitre.

Histologically, the dominant features are those of a spindle cell tumour with or without giant cell areas, or a small cell pattern.

The prognosis is very poor due to the rapid local invasion of structures such as the trachea, producing respiratory obstruction.

### Medullary carcinoma
This rare neuroendocrine tumour arises from parafollicular C cells, which commonly synthesize and secrete calcitonin but which may also secrete 5-hydroxytryptamine (serotonin), various peptides of the tachykinin family, ACTH and prostaglandins.

High levels of serum calcitonin are useful diagnostically but produce no clinical effects.

Although medullary carcinoma is most common in the elderly, it also occurs in younger individuals, where it is commonly associated with other endocrine tumours, such as phaeochromocytoma as part of the multiple endocrine neoplasia (MEN) syndromes IIa and IIb (see p. 201).

### Lymphomas
Most thyroid lymphomas are regarded as tumours of mucosa-associated lymphoma tissue. Interestingly, non-Hodgkin's B cell lymphomas occasionally arise in long-standing, autoimmune thyroiditis, especially Hashimoto's disease.

## PARATHYROID DISORDERS

## Parathyroid hormone

Parathyroid hormone (PTH) is a polypeptide (84 amino acid residues) secreted by the chief cells of the parathyroid glands. The main action of PTH is to increase serum calcium and decrease serum phosphate.

In bone, PTH stimulates osteoclastic bone resorption and inhibits osteoblastic bone deposition. The net effect is the release of calcium from bone.

In the kidney, PTH has the following effects:

- Increases calcium reabsorption
- Decreases phosphate reabsorption
- Increases 1-hydroxylation of 25-hydroxyvitamin D (i.e. activates vitamin D).

PTH also increases gastrointestinal calcium absorption.

## Hyperparathyroidism

Hyperparathyroidism is defined as an elevated secretion of PTH, of which there are three main types:

1. Primary—hypersecretion of PTH by adenoma or hyperplasia of the gland
2. Secondary—physiological increase in PTH secretions in response to hypocalcaemia of any cause
3. Tertiary—supervention of an autonomous hypersecreting adenoma in long-standing secondary hyperparathyroidism.

---

**HINTS AND TIPS**

Understanding the physiological functions of PTH is essential to an understanding of the clinical effects produced by its hypo- or hypersecretion.

---

## Primary hyperparathyroidism

This is the most common of the parathyroid disorders, and is an important cause of hypercalcaemia. More than 90% of patients are over 50 years of age and the condition affects females more than males by nearly 3:1. The aetiology of primary hyperparathyroidism is outlined in Figure 10.12.

### Effects of hyperparathyroidism
The clinical effects are the result of hypercalcaemia and bone resorption.

Effects of hypercalcaemia:

- Renal stones due to hypercalcuria
- Excessive calcification of blood vessels
- General muscle weakness and tiredness
- Exacerbation of hypertension and potential shortening of the QT interval
- Thirst and polyuria (may be dehydrated due to impaired concentrating ability of kidney)
- Anorexia and constipation.

**Fig. 10.12** Aetiology of primary hyperparathyroidism

| Type | Frequency | Features |
|---|---|---|
| Adenoma | 75% | Orange–brown, well-encapsulated tumour of various size but seldom >1 cm diameter Tumours are usually solitary, affecting only one of the parathyroids, the others often showing atrophy; they are deep seated and rarely palpable |
| Primary hyperplasia | 20% | Diffuse enlargement of all the parathyroid glands |
| Parathyroid carcinoma | 5% | Usually resembles adenoma but is poorly encapsulated and invasive locally |

Effects of bone resorption:

- 'Brown tumours'—haemorrhagic and cystic tumour-like areas in the bone, containing large masses of giant osteoclastic cells.
- Osteitis fibrosa cystica (von Recklinghausen disease of bone)—multiple brown tumours combined with fibrous replacement of resorbed bone.
- Changes may present clinically as bone pain, fracture or deformity.

However, about 50% of patients with biochemical evidence of primary hyperparathyroidism are asymptomatic. Investigations are:

- biochemical—increased patients with biochemical evidence of primary hyperparathyroidism and $Ca^{2+}$, and decreased $PO_4^{3-}$
- radiological—90% normal; 10% show evidence of bone resorption, particularly phalangeal erosions.

Management is by rehydration, medical reduction in plasma calcium using bisphosphonates and eventual surgical removal of abnormal parathyroid glands.

## Secondary hyperparathyroidism

This is compensatory hyperplasia of the parathyroid glands, occurring in response to diseases of chronic low serum calcium or increased serum phosphate.

Its causes are:

- chronic renal failure and some renal tubular disorders (most common cause)
- steatorrhoea and other malabsorption syndromes.

Morphological changes of the parathyroid glands are:

- hyperplastic enlargement of all parathyroid glands, but to a lesser degree than in primary hyperplasia
- increase in 'water clear' cells and chief cells of the parathyroid glands, with loss of stromal fat cells.

*Clinical manifestations*—symptoms of bone resorption are dominant.

## Renal osteodystrophy

Skeletal abnormalities, arising as a result of raised PTH secondary to chronic renal disease, are known as renal osteodystrophy.

The pathogenesis of renal osteodystrophy is shown in Figure 10.13.

Abnormalities vary widely according to the nature of the renal lesion, its duration and the age of the patient, but include:

- osteitis fibrosa cystica (see above)
- rickets or osteomalacia due to reduced activation of vitamin D
- osteosclerosis—increased radiodensity of certain bones, particularly the parts of vertebrae adjacent to the intervertebral discs.

Note that the symptoms of hypercalcaemia are not a feature of secondary hyperparathyroidism; calcium levels are likely to be decreased as this is driving the compensatory PTH secretion.

The investigations are both biochemical (raised PTH and normal or lowered $Ca^{2+}$) and radiological (bone changes).

## Tertiary hyperparathyroidism

This condition, resulting from chronic overstimulation of the parathyroid glands in renal failure, causes one or more of the glands to become an autonomous hypersecreting adenoma with resultant hypercalcaemia.

Figure 10.14 gives a comparison of primary, secondary and tertiary hyperparathyroidism.

**Fig. 10.13** Pathogenesis of renal osteodystrophy.

$\downarrow$ vit. D activation

Renal disease $\rightarrow$      +      $\rightarrow \downarrow$ serum $Ca^{2+} \rightarrow \uparrow$PTH $\rightarrow \uparrow$ bone resorption

$\downarrow Ca^{2+}$ reabsorption

**Fig. 10.14** Comparison of primary, secondary and tertiary hyperparathyroidism

|  | Primary | Secondary | Tertiary |
|---|---|---|---|
| Serum PTH and Ca$^{2+}$ | ↑PTH; ↑Ca$^{2+}$ | ↑PTH; normal or ↑Ca$^{2+}$ | ↑PTH; ↑Ca$^{2+}$ |
| Aetiology | Adenoma<br>Hyperplasia<br>Carcinoma | Chronic renal failure<br>Malabsorption<br>Osteomalacia and rickets<br>Pregnancy and lactation | Adenoma resulting from overstimulation of glands in secondary hyperparathyroidism |
| Predominant effects | Hyper-calcaemia | Increased bone absorption | Hypercalcaemia and increased bone resorption |

Note: PTH, parathyroid hormone.

## Hypoparathyroidism

Hypoparathyroidism is a condition of reduced or absent PTH secretion, resulting in hypocalcaemia and hyperphosphataemia. It is far less common than hyperparathyroidism.

The causes of hypoparathyroidism are:

- removal or damage of the parathyroid glands during thyroidectomy—most common
- autoimmune parathyroid disease—usually occurs in patients who have another autoimmune endocrine disease, e.g. Addison's disease
- congenital deficiency (DiGeorge syndrome)—rare, congenital disorder caused by arrested development of the third and fourth branchial arches, resulting in an almost complete absence of the thymus (see Chapter 13) and parathyroid gland.

The effects of hypoparathyroidism are:

- ↓ release of Ca$^{2+}$ from bones
- ↓ Ca$^{2+}$ reabsorption but ↑ PO$_4^{3-}$ reabsorption by kidney
- ↓ 1-hydroxylation of 25-hydroxyvitamin D by kidney.

Most symptoms of hypoparathyroidism are those of hypocalcaemia:

- Tetany—muscular spasm provoked by lowered plasma Ca$^{2+}$
- Convulsions
- Paraesthesiae
- Psychiatric disturbances, e.g. depression, confusional state and even psychosis
- Rarely—cataracts, parkinsonian-like movement disorders, alopecia, brittle nails.

Management is by treatment with large doses of oral vitamin D; the acute phase requires intravenous calcium and calcitriol (1,25-dihydroxycholecalciferol, i.e. activated vitamin D).

# DISORDERS OF THE ADRENAL GLAND

## Hormones of the adrenal gland

The adrenal gland has two structurally and functionally distinct endocrine components derived from different embryonic tissue: the cortex and the medulla.

### Cortex

This is the outer part of the gland, which is derived from the mesoderm. It synthesizes, stores, and secretes various cholesterol-derived hormones, namely:

- glucocorticoid hormones, e.g. cortisol—primarily from the zona fasciculata
- mineralocorticoid hormones, e.g. aldosterone—from the zona glomerulosa
- sex steroids, i.e. oestrogens and androgens—from the zona reticularis.

### Medulla

This is the inner part of the gland, which is derived from the neuroectoderm, forming part of the sympathetic nervous system. Chromaffin cells synthesize and secrete the vasoactive amines epinephrine (adrenaline) and norepinephrine (noradrenaline).

## Hyperfunction of the adrenal cortex

### Cushing's syndrome

The symptoms and signs of Cushing's syndrome are associated with prolonged inappropriate elevation of free corticosteroid levels (Fig. 10.15).

**Fig. 10.15** Systemic effects of Cushing's syndrome.

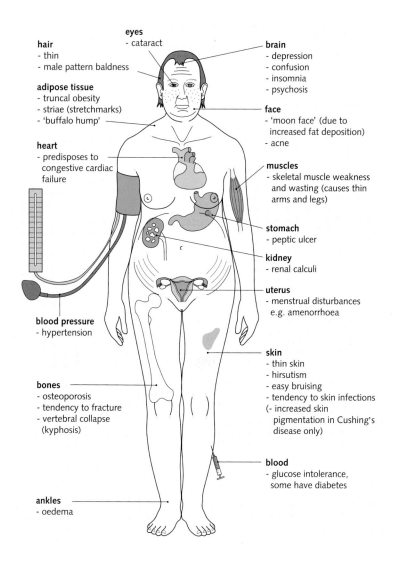

*Clinical features*—the main effects of sustained elevation of glucocorticoid secretion are:

- central obesity and moon face
- plethora and acne
- menstrual irregularity
- hirsutism and hair thinning
- hypertension
- diabetes
- osteoporosis—may cause collapse of vertebrae, rib fractures
- muscle wasting and weakness
- atrophy of skin and dermis—paper thin skin with bruising tendency, purple striae.

*Aetiopathogenesis*—patients with Cushing's syndrome can be classified into two groups on the basis of whether the aetiology of the condition is ACTH-dependent or independent (Fig. 10.16).

ACTH-dependent aetiology:

- Pituitary hypersecretion of ACTH (Cushing's disease)—bilateral adrenal hyperplasia secondary

| **Fig. 10.16** Classification of Cushing's syndrome | |
|---|---|
| **Type** | **Cause** |
| ACTH dependent | Iatrogenic (ACTH therapy) Pituitary hypersecretion of ACTH Ectopic ACTH syndrome (benign or malignant non-endocrine tumour) |
| Non-ACTH dependent | Iatrogenic, e.g. prednisolone Adrenal cortical adenoma Adrenal cortical carcinoma |

to excessive secretion of ACTH by a corticotroph adenoma of the pituitary gland (see p. 182).

- Production of ectopic ACTH or corticotrophin-releasing hormone (CRH) by non-endocrine neoplasm, e.g. small cell lung cancer and some carcinoid tumours. In cases of malignant bronchial tumour, the patient rarely survives long enough to develop any physical features of Cushing's syndrome.

Non-ACTH-dependent aetiology:

- Iatrogenic steroid therapy—most common cause of Cushing's syndrome.
- Adrenal cortical adenoma—extremely common as an incidental finding in up to 30% of all post-mortem examinations. The yellow colour is due to stored lipid (mainly cholesterol) from which the hormones are synthesized. The vast majority have no clinical effects (i.e. they are non-functioning adenomas), with only a small percentage producing Cushing's syndrome.
- Adrenal cortical carcinoma—rare and almost always associated with the overproduction of hormones, usually glucocorticoids and sex steroids. Patients usually have features of Cushing's syndrome mixed with androgenic effects which are particularly noticeable in women. Local invasion and metastatic spread are common.

### HINTS AND TIPS

The therapeutic administration of glucocorticosteroids (e.g. prednisolone) is a common cause of the features of Cushing's syndrome. Avoid confusing the disease and the syndrome. *Remember:* Cushing's disease is used specifically to describe Cushing's syndrome secondary to excessive pituitary ACTH secretion.

Irrespective of the aetiology, the diagnosis is based on clinical features and the demonstration of a raised plasma cortisol level.

The aetiology of the disorder is elucidated through:

- raised urinary cortisol in the first instance, but further testing is required.
- low-dose dexamethasone suppression test (suppression of cortisol levels in Cushing's disease due to suppression of pituitary ACTH secretion, but a lack of suppression suggests ACTH-independent Cushing's syndrome).
- MRI and CT scan visualization of pituitary and adrenal glands.
- analysis of blood ACTH (high = pituitary adenoma or ectopic ACTH source; low = primary adrenal tumour due to feedback suppression).

Treatment of the underlying cause is essential as untreated Cushing's syndrome has a 50% 5-year mortality rate.

## Hyperaldosteronism

Excessive production of aldosterone by the zona glomerulosa of the adrenal cortex results in increased $Na^+$ retention and increased $K^+$ loss.

The aetiology is as follows:

- Primary hyperaldosteronism—autonomous hypersecretion of aldosterone, usually caused by adrenal cortical adenomas (Conn's syndrome).
- Secondary hyperaldosteronism—hypersecretion of aldosterone secondary to increased serum renin. May be precipitated by renal tumours and oedema (congestive cardiac failure, cirrhosis or nephrotic syndrome). This is more common than the primary form of the disorder.

The effects of hyperaldosteronism are shown in Figure 10.17.

Clinical features are:

- Hypertension—often the only presenting feature. Commonly occurs in the younger age group.
- Hypokalaemia—usually accompanies hypertension and may give rise to polyuria, nocturia, polydipsia, paraesthesia, cardiac arrhythmias, muscle weakness or paralysis.

Secondary hyperaldosteronism also has additional features of underlying disease. Biochemical diagnosis:

- $\uparrow Na^+$, $\downarrow K^+$
- $\uparrow$ aldosterone
- plasma renin—$\downarrow$ in Conn's syndrome but $\uparrow$ in secondary hyperaldosteronism.

Radiological diagnosis is by visualization of adrenal cortical adenoma by CT scan or MRI.

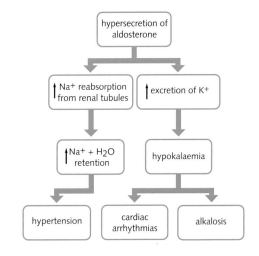

**Fig. 10.17**   Effects of hyperaldosteronism.

*Management*:

- Primary hyperaldosteronism—medical aldosterone antagonism (e.g. spironolactone) or surgical removal of the affected adrenal.
- Secondary hyperaldosteronism—treatment of the underlying cause.

## Congenital adrenal hyperplasia

This autosomal recessive disorder is usually caused by a deficiency of the enzyme 21-hydroxylase, required for the synthesis of both cortisol and aldosterone. 21-Hydroxylase acts on 17OH-progesterone and, consequently, raised levels of 17OH-progesterone are measured in the blood of affected individuals; this is routinely tested in the first week of life. Failure of cortisol production produces an increase in ACTH secretion by the pituitary and hyperplasia of the adrenal cortex.

Production of androgens by the adrenal cortex does not require 21-hydroxylase. Consequently adrenal hyperplasia causes excessive secretion of androgens resulting in masculinization of females and precocious puberty in males. Aldosterone deficiency is serious, causing a life-threatening salt loss ('salt wasting syndrome') unless replacement therapy is given.

## Hypofunction of the adrenal cortex

### Addison's disease

This rare condition of chronic adrenal insufficiency is due to a lack of glucocorticoids and mineralocorticoids.

The clinical features outlined in Figure 10.18 are a result of glucocorticoid and mineralocorticoid insufficiency, loss of adrenal androgen production and increased ACTH secretion.

*Aetiology*—autoimmune destruction of the cortex of both adrenals is the most common cause of Addison's disease, commonly associated with other autoimmune diseases. Addison's disease can also be caused by tuberculosis (previously most common cause) and metastatic cancers.

Biochemical features:

- Measurement of plasma ACTH and cortisol—$\uparrow$ ACTH, $\downarrow$ cortisol
- ACTH stimulation test—ACTH is administered and plasma cortisol levels are monitored. Failure of cortisol levels to rise indicates Addison's disease
- Plasma electrolytes—$\downarrow$ Na$^+$, normal or $\uparrow$ K$^+$, $\uparrow$ urea
- Blood glucose—usually low
- $\uparrow$ Plasma renin activity and normal or $\downarrow$ aldosterone.

Management is by glucocorticoid replacement therapy and usually mineralocorticoid therapy.

## Primary acute adrenocortical insufficiency (adrenal crisis)

This may occur as a result of:

- iatrogenic—abrupt cessation of prolonged high-dose therapeutic corticosteroids (prolonged corticosteroid therapy produces lowered endogenous steroid production, leading to atrophy of the adrenal cortex)
- bilateral massive adrenal haemorrhage—caused by Gram-negative (usually meningococcal) septicaemia (Waterhouse–Friderichsen syndrome) producing haemorrhage and disseminated intravascular coagulation. Adrenal haemorrhage is also seen in neonates following traumatic birth.

**Fig. 10.18** Clinical features of Addison's disease

| Hormonal abnormality | Clinical features |
| --- | --- |
| Glucocorticoid insufficiency | Vomiting and loss of appetite<br>Weight loss<br>Lethargy and weakness<br>Postural hypotension<br>Hypoglycaemia |
| Mineralocorticoid insufficiency | $\downarrow$serum Na$^+$, $\uparrow$serum K$^+$<br>Chronic dehydration<br>Hypotension |
| Increased ACTH secretion | Brownish pigmentation of skin and buccal mucosa |
| Loss of adrenal androgen | Decreased body hair, especially in females |
| *Note: ACTH, adrenocorticotrophic hormone* | |

**Clinical Note**

Clinical features of an adrenal crisis are:
- profound hypotension and cardiovascular collapse (shock)
- vomiting
- diarrhoea
- abdominal pain
- pyrexia.

An adrenal crisis is a medical emergency and requires intravenous hydrocortisone and fluid replacement. The precipitating cause should be sought and if possible treated.

## Secondary adrenocortical insufficiency

This adrenocortical insufficiency is caused by adrenal atrophy secondary to:

- hypothalamic or pituitary disease (tumours, infection, infarction, surgical destruction), which produces lowered ACTH, hence lowered endogenous glucocorticoids and aldosterone
- glucocorticoid therapy, which produces lowered ACTH (suppression), hence lowered endogenous glucocorticoids and aldosterone.

## The adrenal medulla

### Phaeochromocytoma

This is a rare tumour of the chromaffin cells—the cells that secrete epinephrine (adrenaline) and norepinephrine (noradrenaline) in the adrenal medulla (see p. 193).

### Tumours of extra-adrenal paraganglia

#### Neuroblastomas

These rare catecholamine producing tumours are derived from neuroblasts. They originate from the adrenal medulla and can present with an abdominal mass.

Neuroblastomas are almost exclusively tumours of children, occurring very rarely over the age of 5 years. They are highly malignant and usually inoperable.

## DISORDERS OF THE ENDOCRINE PANCREAS

## Diabetes mellitus

Diabetes mellitus (DM) is a multisystem disease of an abnormal metabolic state characterized by hyperglycaemia due to inadequate insulin action/production. It can be classified into primary and secondary.

Primary DM is a disorder of insulin production/action. It accounts for 95% of diabetic cases.

In 5% of cases, diabetes may be secondary to:

- pancreatic diseases, e.g. chronic pancreatitis
- hypersecretion of hormones that antagonize the effects of insulin, e.g. glucocorticoids in Cushing's syndrome, growth hormone in acromegaly, epinephrine (adrenaline) in pheochromocytomas.

Primary DM is by far the most important cause of diabetes and it is further classified into:

- Type I, also known as insulin-dependent DM (IDDM) or juvenile-onset diabetes.
- Type II, also known as non-insulin-dependent DM (NIDDM) or mature-onset diabetes.

The basic features of these two types of diabetes are described in Figure 10.19.

## Type I diabetes mellitus

*Aetiology and pathogenesis*—type I diabetes mellitus is an organ specific, autoimmune-induced disorder characterized by antibody-mediated destruction of the β-cell population of the islet of Langerhans.

Two main factors are thought to predispose to autoimmunity:

1. Genetic predisposition—90–95% of patients with type I diabetes are HLA-DR3 or HLA-DR4 positive, a feature that is also seen in other organ-specific autoimmune diseases. However, identical twins show a 40% concordance in the development of the disease, indicating the additional importance of environmental factors.
2. Viral infection—viral infection may trigger the autoimmune reaction; viruses implicated include mumps, measles and Coxsackie B.

One postulated mechanism is that viruses induce mild structural damage to the islet cells, thereby releasing previously shielded β-cell antigens and leading to the recruitment and activation of lymphocytes in the pancreatic tissue.

Histologically, the pancreas shows lymphocytic infiltration and destruction of insulin-secreting cells of islets of Langerhans (β-cells). This results in insulin deficiency with hyperglycaemia and other secondary metabolic complications.

## Type II diabetes mellitus

*Aetiology and pathogenesis*—the precise aetiopathogenesis of type II diabetes is unclear but the following factors are thought to be involved:

- Genetic factors—familial tendency with up to 90% concordance rate amongst identical twins. However, there are no HLA associations and inheritance is considered to be polygenic.

**Fig. 10.19** Table comparing type I and type II diabetes mellitus (DM)

| Type I | Type II |
|---|---|
| Childhood/adolescent onset | Middle-aged/elderly onset |
| 1/3 of primary diabetes | 2/3 of primary diabetes |
| Females = males | Females = males |
| Acute/subacute onset | Gradual onset |
| Thin | Obese |
| Ketoacidosis common | Ketoacidosis rare |
| Plasma insulin absent or low | Plasma insulin normal or raised |
| Insulin sensitive | Insulin insensitive (end-organ resistance) |
| Autoimmune mechanism (islet cell antibodies present) | Non-autoimmune mechanism (no islet cell antibodies) |
| Genetic predisposition associated with HLA-DR genotype | Polygenic inheritance |

- Insulin resistance—tissues are unable to respond to insulin because of an impairment in the function of insulin receptors on the surface of target cells. This is associated with obesity, sedentary lifestyle and poor diet; it is increasingly being seen in younger (even adolescent) individuals.
- Relative insulin deficiency—reduced secretion compared with the amounts required, possibly related to islet cell ageing.

## Diagnosis of diabetes mellitus

Irrespective of aetiology, the diagnosis of DM depends on the finding of hyperglycaemia. However, the distribution curve of blood glucose concentration for whole populations is unimodal, with no clear division between normal and abnormal values.

Diagnostic criteria (Fig. 10.20) are, therefore, arbitrary and, in general, diabetes mellitus is indicated by either:

- fasting venous plasma glucose level of > 7.0 mmol/L
- random venous plasma glucose level of > 11.1 mmol/L.

A distinction is made between diabetes mellitus and impaired glucose tolerance in cases where fasting or random blood sugar level is borderline; in this case, the response to an oral load of glucose can be assessed via a glucose tolerance test.

## Complications of diabetes mellitus

### Acute complications

Individuals with diabetes are particularly prone to several types of coma. These result from (in decreasing order of frequency):

**Fig. 10.20** Diagnostic criteria for diabetes mellitus using an oral glucose tolerance test

| Diagnosis | Venous plasma blood glucose | |
|---|---|---|
| | *Fasting sample* | *2 hours after 75g glucose load* |
| Normal | <5.6 mmol/L | <7.8 mmol/L |
| Impaired glucose tolerance | 5.6–6.9 mmol/L | 7.8–11.0 mmol/L |
| Diabetes mellitus | ≥7.0 mmol/L | ≥11.1 mmol/L |

- hypoglycaemia—complication of overtreatment with insulin
- diabetic ketoacidosis (DKA)—common in type I diabetes due to ↑ breakdown of triglycerides → ↓ production of ketone bodies → ketoacidosis → impaired consciousness
- hyperosmolar non-ketotic (HONK) state—↑ plasma glucose concentration → ↑ plasma osmolarity → cerebral dehydration → coma. More common in type II diabetes
- lactic acidosis—increased concentrations of lactic acid (produced as an end product of glycolysis instead of pyruvate) may cause coma.

## Chronic complications

In recent years, with the advent of insulin therapy and various oral hypoglycaemic agents, morbidity and mortality associated with DM are more commonly the result of the chronic rather than the acute complications of the disorder (Fig. 10.21).

The complications of diabetes are macrovascular (affecting large and medium-sized muscular arteries) and microvascular (small vessel microangiopathy).

Macrovascular changes involve accelerated atherosclerosis. In diabetic microangiopathy, small arterioles and capillaries show a characteristic pattern of wall thickening, which is due to a marked expansion of the basement membrane (termed hyaline arteriolosclerosis).

Therefore, the most important chronic complications of diabetes are:

- macrovascular accelerated atherosclerosis increasing stroke and myocardial infarction risk
- renal disease—diabetic nephropathy (mainly microvascular)
- eye disease—diabetic retinopathy (microvascular)

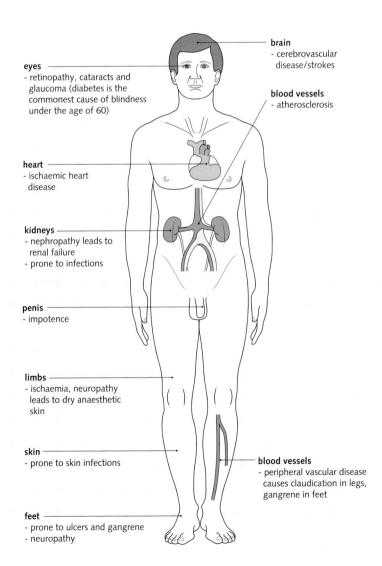

**Fig. 10.21**  Chronic complications of diabetes mellitus.

**brain**
- cerebrovascular disease/strokes

**eyes**
- retinopathy, cataracts and glaucoma (diabetes is the commonest cause of blindness under the age of 60)

**blood vessels**
- atherosclerosis

**heart**
- ischaemic heart disease

**kidneys**
- nephropathy leads to renal failure
- prone to infections

**penis**
- impotence

**limbs**
- ischaemia, neuropathy leads to dry anaesthetic skin

**skin**
- prone to skin infections

**blood vessels**
- peripheral vascular disease causes claudication in legs, gangrene in feet

**feet**
- prone to ulcers and gangrene
- neuropathy

- peripheral nerve damage—diabetic neuropathy (microvascular)
- predisposition to infections.

## Macrovascular disease

Compared with non-affected people of the same age and sex, individuals with diabetes suffer from an increased severity of atherosclerosis, probably due to the increased plasma levels of cholesterol and triglycerides.

The main clinical sequelae of this are seen in:

- heart → ischaemic heart disease
- brain → cerebral ischaemia
- legs and feet → gangrene—ischaemia of toes and areas on the heel is a characteristic feature of diabetic gangrene
- kidney → chronic nephron ischaemia, an important component of the multiple renal lesions in diabetes.

## Diabetic nephropathy

Diabetes is now one of the most common causes of end-stage renal failure. Associated renal disease can be divided into three forms:

- Complications of diabetic vascular disease—macrovascular atherosclerosis affecting aorta and renal arteries → ischaemia; microvascular glomerular capillary basement membrane thickening (hyaline arteriolosclerosis) → ischaemic glomerular damage. Microalbuminuria is a reliable marker of the progression of diabetic nephropathy.
- Diabetic glomerulosclerosis (diffuse and nodular types)—↑ leakage of plasma proteins through capillary wall into glomerular filtrate → proteinuria and progressive glomerular hyalinization with eventual chronic renal failure.
- Increased susceptibility to infections → papillary necrosis. Acute pyelonephritis is a common complication of diabetes mellitus and occurs as a result of the relative immunosuppression of diabetes together with reduced neutrophil function.

## Eye disease

Diabetes is the most common cause of acquired blindness in the Western world. It can affect the eyes in five main ways:

1. Background retinopathy—small vessel abnormalities in the retina leading to hard exudates, haemorrhages and microaneurysms. Does not usually affect acuity.
2. Proliferative retinopathy—extensive proliferation of new capillaries in the retina. Sudden deterioration in vision may result from vitreous haemorrhage as a consequence of proliferating new vessels or from the development of retinal detachment.
3. Maculopathy—caused by oedema, hard exudates or retinal ischaemia and results in a marked reduction of acuity.
4. Cataract formation—greatly increased incidence in individuals with diabetes.
5. Glaucoma—increased incidence in those with diabetes due to neovascularization of the iris (rubeosis iridis).

## Predisposition to infections

Patients with diabetes have an increased tendency to develop infections, usually of a bacterial or fungal nature. The main target organs are:

- skin—folliculitis, erysipelas, cellulitis and superficial fungal infections
- oral and genital mucosae—especially with *Candida*
- urinary tract—increased predisposition to acute pyelonephritis, often associated with recurrent lower urinary tract infections.

Persistent glycosuria in individuals with poorly controlled diabetes predisposes to urinary and genital infection.

## Diabetic neuropathy

Clinically, most cases of diabetic neuropathy affect the peripheral nervous system, although central nervous system pathology does occur. The main effects are:

- microvascular thickening of basement membrane and microthrombi formation in small vessels supplying peripheral nerves
- axonal degeneration with patchy, segmental demyelination
- thickening of Schwann cell basal lamina.

The presentation may be of polyneuropathy (classically 'glove and stocking' sensory impairment), mononeuropathy (e.g. carpal tunnel syndrome) or autonomic neuropathy (symptoms include postural hypotension, nausea, vomiting, impotence and gustatory sweating).

### Clinical Note

Blood glucose control in diabetes lowers the incidence and progression of vascular complications. This can be achieved by:
- diet alone—in type II patients
- diet and oral hypoglycaemic drugs (e.g. sulphonylureas, biguanides, thiazolidinediones)—in type II patients who fail on diet alone
- diet and insulin—all type I patients and some type II.

Pancreatic transplantation is curative in type I diabetes but is limited by organ availability. Islet cell transplants are a potential future therapy.

# Islet cell tumours

These tumours are rare compared with those of the exocrine pancreas. They occur most commonly in individuals aged 30–50 years.

## Insulinomas

The most common tumour of the islet cells. Insulinomas are derived from pancreatic β-cells:

- Produce hypoglycaemia through hypersecretion of insulin
- May produce attacks of confusion, stupor and loss of consciousness
- C-peptide is characteristically increased (commercial insulin preparations removes C-peptide).

## Zollinger–Ellison syndrome

This syndrome of gastric hypersecretion, multiple peptic ulcers and diarrhoea is caused by the gastrin-secreting tumour (gastrinoma) of the pancreatic G cells. Tumours are multiple in 50% of cases and are often malignant, with 10–20% occurring in other sites, e.g the duodenum.

It may also be part of the MEN I syndrome, with adenomas also present in other endocrine glands (see below).

## Other islet cell tumours

For a summary of islet cell tumours see Figure 10.22.

## VIPomas

These produce vasoactive intestinal polypeptide (VIP), resulting in a syndrome of watery diarrhoea, hypokalaemia and achlorhydria (WDHA).

### Glucagonomas

These glucagon-secreting tumours are derived from pancreatic α-cells and cause secondary diabetes mellitus (usually mild), necrolytic migratory erythema (skin rash) and uraemia.

### Somatostatinomas

These somatostatin-producing tumours derived from pancreatic δ-cells are associated with diabetes mellitus, cholelithiasis and steatorrhoea.

## MULTIPLE ENDOCRINE NEOPLASIA SYNDROMES

These are syndromes in which patients develop tumours in a number of different endocrine organs. Patients are younger than those who develop single sporadic tumours and usually have a strong family history of multiple endocrine tumours with autosomal dominant inheritance.

There are three main types of MEN syndrome:

1. MEN I (Wermer's) syndrome
2. MEN IIa (Sipple's) syndrome
3. MEN IIb (sometimes called MEN III) syndrome.

## MEN I (Wermer's) syndrome

Patients usually show a combination of hyperparathyroidism (chief cell hyperplasia and adenomas), pituitary adenomas (usually prolactinomas) and pancreatic tumours (gastrin and insulin producing). Rarely, there may also be thyroid tumours and adrenal cortical adenomas. MEN I syndrome is caused by a germ-line mutation in the MEN-1 tumour suppressor gene.

**Fig. 10.22** Summary of islet cell tumours

| Islet cell tumour | Occurrence | Clinical features |
| --- | --- | --- |
| Insulinoma | 70–75% | Hypoglycaemia |
| Gastrinoma | 20–25% | Zollinger–Ellison syndrome: gastric hypersecretion, multiple peptic ulcers and diarrhoea |
| VIPoma | Rare | Water diarrhoea, hypokalaemia and achlorhydria |
| Glucagonoma | Rare | Secondary diabetes mellitus, necrolytic migratory erythema and uraemia |
| Somatostatinoma | Rare | Diabetes mellitus, cholelithiasis and steatorrhoea |

## MEN IIa (Sipple's) syndrome

Patients have a combination of phaeochromocytoma (50% bilateral) and medullary carcinoma of the thyroid and hyperparathyroidism due to parathyroid hyperplasia. MEN IIa and IIb syndromes have been linked to mutations in the *RET* oncogene, with near 100% disease penetrance.

## MEN IIb (MEN III) syndrome

In contrast to MEN IIa it does not induce hyperparathyroidism, and has the additional features of mucocutaneous neuromas and ganglioneuromas.

Genetic screening of at-risk family members in MEN II families now allows prophylactic thyroidectomy in those with RET mutations to avoid the near certainty of medullary carcinoma.

# Pathology of the reproductive system 11

## Objectives

In this chapter, you will learn to:
- Describe infection and neoplasia of the vulva, vagina and cervix, particularly cervical cancer.
- Understand inflammatory and neoplastic disease of the uterus and endometrium.
- Recall disorders of the ovary and fallopian tubes, with the focus on ovarian cancer.
- Describe ectopic pregnancies, spontaneous abortion and other disorders of the placenta and pregnancy.
- Understand the common forms of breast disease, particularly breast carcinoma.
- Briefly describe disorders of the penis.
- Recall testicular cancer and other disorders of the testis and epididymis.
- Describe benign prostatic hyperplasia and prostatic carcinoma.

# DISORDERS OF THE VULVA, VAGINA AND CERVIX

## Infections of the lower genital tract

### Bartholin's cyst

This common, benign, mucus-secreting cyst on the vulva is derived from Bartholin's glands (mucus secreting glands in the posterior part of the labia majora). Frequently there is superimposed infection—Bartholin's abscess.

## Viral infection

Viral infections of the vulval skin are typically due to either herpes simplex virus (HSV) or human papillomavirus (HPV).

### Herpes simplex virus

HSV type 2 infection of the vulva (herpes vulvitis) produces initially painless blisters, which subsequently break down to form a painful, sore, eroded area. HSV-2 infection is now a major sexually transmitted disease and is becoming more common in young women.

### Human papillomavirus

This sexually transmitted disease may present with a thickening of the vulval skin and mucosa (flat condyloma) in the labia minora, or as multiple protuberant warts (condylomata acuminata) that can be either sessile or pedunculated. There is a strong link between HPV infections of the vulva and intraepithelial neoplastic change in both the vulva (see below) and cervix.

## Bacterial and protozoal infections

### Gardnerella vaginalis

This Gram-negative coccobacillus is often associated with other sexually spread infections. The patient complains of a foul-smelling discharge, which is thin, greyish and sometimes shows bubbles. Examination confirms both the discharge and the odour.

### Chlamydia trachomatis

One of the most common sexually transmitted diseases in the UK; 80% of women are asymptomatic, increasing the likelihood of silent spread amongst the population. Ascending infection into the upper genital tract (pelvic inflammatory disease) is increasingly common; this is an important cause of tubal infertility.

Genital infection with *Chlamydia trachomatis* may produce painful superficial groin nodes (lymphogranuloma venereum), which develop over weeks from initially painless vulval papules. Later, chronic lymphatic obstruction may lead to non-pitting oedema of the external genitalia.

### Trichomonas vaginalis

This sexually transmitted flagellated protozoan is typically asymptomatic in men, but in women it often produces an intensely irritating vaginal discharge with inflammation of the vulva, vagina and cervix. The discharge is often frothy and offensive.

### Treponema pallidum

Now rarely sexually transmitted, this spirochaetal bacterium is responsible for syphilis. This granulomatous disease typically involves three stages (primary, secondary and tertiary). It affects the penis in the primary stage:

- Primary—small indurated lesions (chancres) develop at the site of entry but then spontaneously heal.
- Secondary—occurs several weeks later and is characterized by multiple, moist, warty, vulvovaginal lesions (condylomata lata), with skin rashes and generalized illness (fever, malaise).
- Tertiary—develops in untreated individuals and often involves the CNS (see Chapter 5).

## Fungal and yeast infection

Fungal infections are usually caused by either superficial dermatophytes or *Candida albicans*. There is usually associated fungal vaginitis, presenting with a copious vaginal discharge and vulval reddening and soreness.

### *Candida albicans*

This is a normal commensal of the vagina but its proliferation is usually suppressed by commensal vaginal flora.

Conditions that predispose to candidal overgrowth are:

- pregnancy/oestrogen contraceptives—high concentration of oestrogens in the blood
- immunosuppressive therapy, e.g. cytotoxic drugs and corticosteroids
- glycosuria, e.g. diabetes, pregnancy (due to lowering of the renal threshold for sugar)
- antibiotic therapy—destruction of normal commensal bacteria
- chronic anaemia—iron stores are needed to maintain an adequate immune reaction.

Macroscopically, white plaques of fungal hyphae develop on inflamed vaginal mucosa. Vaginal discharge is associated with severe vulval irritation. Infections are often severe in people with diabetes.

### Dermatophytes

Infection of vulval skin with dermatophytic fungi produces a similar superficial inflammation and soreness.

### *Treatment*

Both candidal infections and dermatophytes can be treated with antifungal pessaries or systemic therapy.

Figure 11.1 shows the organisms that cause infections of the lower genital tract.

## Dysplastic and neoplastic disorders of the vulva and vagina

### Tumours of the vulva

#### Squamous cell carcinoma

This is the most common malignant tumour of the vulva, typically occurring in elderly women and often showing extensive local invasion and metastases to

| Fig. 11.1 Organisms that cause infections of the lower genital tract | |
|---|---|
| Infection | Organism |
| Viruses | HPV<br>HSV |
| Bacteria | *Gardnerella vaginalis*<br>*Chlamydia trachomatis*<br>(lymphogranuloma venereum)<br>*Treponema pallidum* (syphilis) |
| Protozoa | *Trichomonas vaginalis* |
| Fungi and yeast | Dermatophytes, *Candida albicans* |

the inguinal lymph nodes. The majority of cases appear to arise *de novo*, but some form from dysplastic epithelium amounting to carcinoma in situ, known as vulval intraepithelial neoplasia.

It is also thought that squamous cell carcinoma may develop from areas of lichen sclerosus (atrophic lesions that are most common after the menopause).

### Vulval intraepithelial neoplasia

This is generally seen in patients younger than those with invasive tumours. In 90% of cases there is coexistent evidence of incorporated HPV DNA (especially serotypes 16 and 18), usually with visible warty change in the affected and adjacent epithelium. Although invasive carcinoma and vulval intraepithelial neoplasia (VIN) do occasionally coexist in elderly women, it is thought that progression of VIN to invasive carcinoma is not common.

## Tumours of the vagina

### Dysplastic

Vaginal intraepithelial neoplasia (VAIN) is rare compared with cervical intraepithelial neoplasia (CIN). Most cases are found in women previously treated for CIN or invasive cervical cancer.

### Neoplastic

Primary malignant tumours of the vagina are extremely rare, but include squamous cell carcinomas and adenocarcinomas.

Secondary tumours are more common, particularly from malignant tumours of the cervix, endometrium and ovary. Vaginal bleeding after hysterectomy for uterine or ovarian malignancy should always be investigated and biopsied because of the frequency of metastatic tumour in the residual vaginal vault.

# Inflammation of the cervix

## Acute and chronic cervicitis

Acute and chronic inflammation of the cervix is particularly common in the presence of an intrauterine contraceptive device.

### Acute cervicitis

There is acute inflammation of the cervix with erosion. It is occasionally seen in herpes simplex infection, typically with herpetic disease of the vulva and vagina.

### Chronic cervicitis

This chronic inflammation of the cervix is typically caused by the same organisms responsible for infective vaginitis: *Trichomonas, Candida* and *Gardnerella* species and the gonococci. It is characterized by a heavy plasma cell and lymphocytic infiltrate.

## Endocervical polyps

These common abnormalities derived from the endocervix affect up to 5% of women. Large polyps may protrude from the cervix through the external os and can cause intermenstrual bleeding from erosion and ulceration.

Macroscopically, these are smooth, rounded or pear-shaped polyps about 1–2 cm in diameter.

Microscopically, they are composed of endocervical stroma and glands. The surface of the polyp may show ulceration and inflammation, often accompanied by squamous metaplasia.

# Neoplasia of the cervix

## Cervical intraepithelial neoplasia

Cervical intraepithelial neoplasia (CIN) is the pre-neoplastic (dysplastic) proliferation of epithelium of the transformation zone of the cervix.

*Aetiology*—there is a strong association with HPV infection, particularly serotypes 16 and 18.

Risk factors are:

- sexual intercourse—very low incidence in virgins, with increased risk in those who have had multiple sexual partners and first intercourse at an early age.
- human papillomavirus—DNA from HPV types 16, 18, 31 or 33 has been identified in over 90% of cervical carcinomas. Proteins produced by HPV are thought to inactivate products of tumour suppressor genes thereby facilitating tumour development. For example, the viral protein E6 of HPV subtype 16 can bind and inactivate the function of the *p53* tumour suppressor protein (see Chapter 3). It is likely that new HPV vaccines targeted against

serotypes 16 and 18 will reduce HPV infection and CIN development

- combined oral contraceptive pill—prolonged use is associated with an increased risk in those who carry HPV infection (may be linked to increased sexual risk-taking when on contraceptive pill)
- smoking—associated with increased risk
- immunosuppression—predisposes to carcinoma of the cervix, e.g. HIV patients.

### Classification

Three grades of severity are recognized. Grading depends on the proportion of the cervical epithelium wall that is replaced by atypical cells:

1. CIN I (mild dysplasia)—upper two-thirds of the epithelium normal, basal third atypical cells
2. CIN II (moderate dysplasia)—upper third of the epithelium normal, atypical cells occupy the lower two-thirds
3. CIN III (severe dysplasia)—corresponds to carcinoma in situ. Atypical cells extend throughout the full thickness of the epithelium with minimal differentiation and maturation on the surface.

### Progression

CIN is associated with a risk of progression to an invasive carcinoma, the risk for CIN I being lowest and for CIN III being the highest.

The natural history of CIN is important as it determines how often screening is required to detect progression of the disease.

### Clinical Note

Cervical screening aims to detect preinvasive atypical cells by cytological examination of surface epithelial cells. Smears repeated every 3 years are considered adequate for population screening (from 20 to 65 years old). In the UK it is estimated that regular attendance at screening prevents up to 90% of cervical cancer. Management of CIN is by the local destruction of abnormal epithelium using cryotherapy, laser therapy or cone biopsy following histological confirmation of its nature.

## Squamous cell carcinoma

The vast majority of cervical carcinomas are squamous cell carcinomas arising from the transformation zone or ectocervix.

There are around 3000 cases of cervical cancer in the UK each year, with 1300 deaths. This equates to a lifetime risk of around 1% (similar across the developed world), compared to 5% in parts of the developing world where screening programmes do not exist. This type of carcinoma occurs in all ages from late teens onwards, but the average age is 45 years.

The carcinoma is preceded by the preinvasive phase of CIN (see above and Fig. 11.2). Risk factors are as for CIN.

Macroscopically, tumours demonstrate the following features (Fig. 11.1):

- Early—areas of granular irregularity of the cervical epithelium, with progressive invasion of the stroma causing abnormal hardness of the cervix
- Late—fungating ulcerated areas, which destroy the cervix.

Microscopically, lesions may be keratinizing or non-keratinizing.

The common presenting symptom is vaginal bleeding in the early stages. Advanced neglected tumours may cause urinary obstruction due to bladder involvement.

Invasive carcinomas are managed according to the degree of local invasion and survival is related to the stage of the disease (Fig. 11.3).

Early invasive carcinoma is usually managed by radical hysterectomy and/or radiotherapy, whereas advanced disease is usually only amenable to radiotherapy and/or chemotherapy. Involvement of the para-aortic lymph nodes is associated with a very poor prognosis.

# DISORDERS OF THE UTERUS AND ENDOMETRIUM

## Inflammatory disorders

### Chronic endometritis

An inflammation of the endometrium, chronic endometritis is typically associated with menstrual irregularities and is often found in women who are being investigated for infertility.

Microscopically there is lymphoid and plasma cell infiltration of the endometrium.

*Risk factors*—the majority of cases are associated with a definite clinical risk factor for developing inflammation:

- recent pregnancy; miscarriage or instrumentation (50% of cases)
- chronic pelvic inflammatory disease, e.g. following chlamydial infection (25% of cases)
- use of an intrauterine contraceptive device (about 20% of cases)
- tuberculosis in developing countries (5% of cases).

**A. Cervical intra-epithelial neoplasia**

grade I    grade II    grade III

basement membrane

**B. Early stromal invasion 1A**

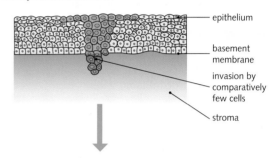

epithelium

basement membrane

invasion by comparatively few cells

stroma

**C. Microinvasive carcinoma stage 1A**

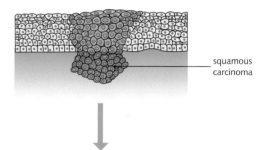

squamous carcinoma

**D. Occult invasive carcinoma stage 1B**

**Fig. 11.2** Cervical intraepithelial neoplasia (CIN) and invasive squamous carcinoma. (A) Increasing dysplasia of CIN grades I–III. (B) Early stromal invasion of < 1 mm. (C) Micro-invasive carcinoma with invasion of < 3 mm. (D) Occult invasive carcinoma with invasion > 500 mm³. There is some risk of spread to the lymph nodes but the tumour is still clinically undetectable. (Adapted from Underwood, 2000.)

| Fig. 11.3 Stages and prognosis for carcinomas of the cervix | | |
|---|---|---|
| **Stage** | **5-year survival (%)** | **Degree of local invasion** |
| I | 85–90 | Confined to cervix |
| II | 60 | Invasion of upper part of vagina or adjacent parametrial tissues |
| III | 40 | Spread to pelvic side wall, lower vagina or ureters |
| IV | 15 | Invasion of rectum, bladder wall or outside pelvis |

## Disorders of the endometrium

### Adenomyosis

This is a condition in which the endometrium grows down to develop deep within the myometrium, occurring in 20% of women. This may cause enlargement of the uterus and is sometimes associated with menstrual abnormalities and dysmenorrhoea.

Macroscopically, there are small, irregular, endometrial lesions—some of which are cystic—that can be seen within the affected myometrium. Involvement of the myometrium may be diffuse (more common) or focal with deep nodules of endometrium (nodular adenomyosis).

Microscopically, irregular nests of endometrial stroma are found deep within muscle but in continuity with surface endometrium.

### Endometriosis

This is defined as endometrial glands or stroma occurring outside the uterus, and still capable of responding to cyclical hormonal stimulation. Phases of proliferation and breakdown are associated with the development of the fibrous adhesions and accumulation of haemosiderin pigment. This affects 1 in 15 women of reproductive age. There are numerous sites:

- Common—ovaries, fallopian tubes, round ligaments, pelvic peritoneum
- Less common—intestinal wall, bladder, umbilicus, laparotomy scars.

#### Theories of origin

The aetiopathogenesis of endometriosis remains unclear but three main theories operate to various degrees:

1. Retrograde menstruation—fragments of endometrium migrate along the fallopian tubes during menstruation
2. Metaplasia of peritoneal epithelium—differentiation of peritoneal epithelium into endometrium

3. Metastatic spread of endometrium, via the blood or lymphatic vessels.

Macroscopically, the foci of endometriosis appear as cystic and solid masses, which are characteristically dark brown because of accumulated iron pigment from repeated bleeding.

Microscopically, solid masses of endometriosis are composed of endometrial glands and stroma, fibrosis and macrophages containing iron pigments.

Endometriosis may present with cyclical pelvic pain, dysmenorrhoea and infertility.

The complications are:

- infertility (about 30% of cases)—often due to adhesions and blockages affecting ovulatory pathways
- bowel obstruction—due to fibrous adhesions between adjacent organs
- chocolate cysts—the whole of the fallopian tube and ovary may be converted into a cystic mass containing brown, semi-liquid material.

Endometriosis is dependent on oestrogen for continued growth and proliferation, with the disease becoming inactive after oophorectomy or onset of the menopause. Thus, induction of the hypo-oestrogenic state by suppression of ovulation is effective in many cases (e.g. continuous progesterone therapy).

### Functional endometrial disorders

#### Anovulatory cycle

An anovulatory cycle is one that is not associated with the development and release of the ovum from the ovary. This is normal and common at both the start and end of reproductive life. Several follicles may start to develop and for a time produce hormones. However, the attempt ends in atresia and the atretic follicle is absorbed.

It is associated with irregular menstruation, although the effects of excessive oestrogen stimulation are manifest in the endometrium as the proliferation of glands.

Other causes of anovulation are listed in Figure 11.4.

**Fig. 11.4** Non-physiological causes of anovulation

| Type | Cause | Clinical feature |
|---|---|---|
| Primary ovarian dysfunction | Genetic | e.g. Turner's syndrome, autoimmune |
| Secondary ovarian dysfunction | Disorders of gonadotrophin regulation | Hyperprolactinaemia |
| | Gonadotrophin deficiency | Pituitary tumour Pituitary infarction Pituitary ablation |
| | Functional | Weight loss Exercise |
| | Polycystic ovary syndrome | Associated with obesity and insulin resistance |

**Fig. 11.5** Types of endometrial hyperplasia

| Degree of hyperplasia | Morphological features | Progression to adenocarcinoma (%) | Time taken (years) to develop into adenocarcinoma |
|---|---|---|---|
| Mild (most common) | Cystic glandular hyperplasia with characteristic appearance of 'Swiss cheese'. (Previously known as metropathia haemorrhagica.) Cells show no cytological atypia | 1 | 10 |
| Moderate | Crowding of glands in a back-to-back fashion. Epithelium is stratified and mitoses are relatively frequent. Cells show no cytological atypia | 5 | 7 |
| Severe | Cellular atypia is prominent, glands are distorted by intraglandular polypoid formations, and mitoses are frequent | 30 | 4 |

### Inadequate luteal phase

The irregular ripening of a follicle is associated with infertility. This may be caused by failure of the production of progesterone by the corpus luteum or by defective receptors for progesterone within the endometrium. Examination of the endometrium in the second half of the menstrual cycle shows inadequate or absent development of secretory changes.

### Endometrial hyperplasia

Hyperplasia of the endometrium typically occurs in the third and fourth decades of life, in response to oestrogenic stimulation. It presents with haemorrhage but the severity or frequency is not related to the degree of pathological change. Certain types of endometrial hyperplasia are associated with a degree of risk for malignant change (severe/atypical hyperplasia).

Figure 11.5 shows the different types of endometrial hyperplasia.

**HINTS AND TIPS**

The importance of endometrial hyperplasia is that it is associated with an increased risk of the development of endometrial adenocarcinoma, i.e. it is thought to be preneoplastic.

# Neoplastic disorders

## Benign

### Endometrial polyps

These localized overgrowths of endometrial glands and stroma are very common and are typically seen in the perimenopausal age range. They are caused by inappropriate proliferation of glands in response to oestrogenic stimuli.

Macroscopically, they are found in the uterine fundus projecting into the endometrial cavity; their size is variable but they are usually 1–3 cm in diameter. They have a firm, smooth, nodular appearance within the endometrial cavity but occasionally prolapse through the cervical os. They may ulcerate or undergo torsion.

Microscopically, they are cystically dilated endometrial glands in a vascular stroma.

Clinical features are associated with menstrual abnormalities and dysmenorrhoea.

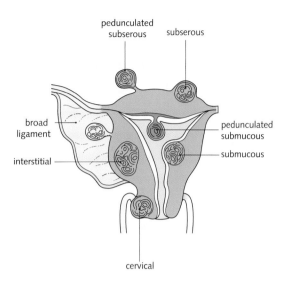

**Fig. 11.6**  Fibroids within the uterus.

### Fibroids (leiomyomas)

These benign, smooth muscle tumours arise in the muscle wall of the uterus (myometrium). They are the most common of all pelvic tumours, affecting over half of all women over the age of 30, usually becoming symptomatic in the decade before the menopause. Their cause is unknown but risk factors include:

- age—rare under 30 years
- race—more common in Afro-Caribbean populations
- parity—more common in nulliparous and women with low fertility
- genetic—often a family history.

Leiomyomas have the following features:

- oestrogen sensitive
- fast growing in pregnancy
- shrink at menopause or with antigonadotrophic hormone therapy.

Sites within the uterus (Fig. 11.6) are:

- subserous—just beneath the peritoneum on the outer uterine surface
- interstitial (most common)—surrounded by smooth muscle
- submucous—lying immediately below the endometrium.

Macroscopically, they are:

- rounded, rubbery, pale nodules with whorled appearance on cut surface
- well circumscribed with pseudocapsule that may become pedunculated forming polyps
- variable in size. Most common are 2–4 cm but they range from < 1 cm to 20–30 cm in diameter
- typically multiple.

Microscopically they are seen as:

- islands of smooth muscle cells with intervening collagenous stroma
- lacking cellular atypia and with very few mitoses (compared to malignant leiomyosarcomas). Malignant change in leiomyomas is considered extremely rare.

*Clinical features*—leiomyomas may present with abnormal menstrual bleeding, dysmenorrhoea and infertility.

Complications occur following ischaemic degeneration, pregnancy and compression.

Investigations are by ultrasound and laparoscopy. Management is:

- surgical—women who no longer wish to conceive usually undergo hysterectomy
- medical—uterine leiomyomas may be shrunk by gonadotrophin-releasing hormone (GnRH) agonists, which induce hypo-oestrogenism. This allows easier surgical removal by myomectomy.

> **HINTS AND TIPS**
>
> Remember that fibroids are not fibromas. Fibroids are benign tumours of smooth muscle (leiomyomas).

## Malignant

### Endometrial carcinoma

Adenocarcinomas of the endometrium are the second most common gynaecological malignancy. The mean age of presentation is 56 years and 80% of women are postmenopausal.

**Fig. 11.7** Clinical staging of endometrial cancer

| Stage | Proportion of cases (%) | Degree of invasion | 5-year survival (%) |
|---|---|---|---|
| I | 75 | Corpus of uterus only | 85 |
| II | 10 | Corpus and cervix | 65 |
| III | 10 | Invasion confined to pelvis | 40 |
| IV | 5 | Invasion outside pelvis or involves bladder or rectal mucosa | 10 |

Endometrial carcinoma is associated with:

- hyperoestrogenic state—obesity, diabetes, late menopause, prolonged use of unopposed oestrogens, oestrogen-secreting tumours
- previous pelvic irradiation
- lower parity.

There are two main groups: hyperoestrogenic and non-hyperoestrogenic tumours.

*Hyperoestrogenic tumours (type 1 disease)*—these are associated with a generally good prognosis. They occur in patients close to the menopause, associated with an abnormal oestrogenic stimulation of the endometrium and endometrial hyperplasia. Most tumours are adenocarcinomas (60%) and are graded (I-III) according to the amount of glandular and solid pattern within the tumour. High-grade tumour is associated with a worse prognosis.

*Non-hyperoestrogenic tumours (type 2 disease)*—these are more often associated with a poor prognosis, occur in older postmenopausal women and are not associated with oestrogenic stimulation or endometrial hyperplasia.

Macroscopically, there are:

- small tumours—diffuse, solid areas or polypoid lesions in the endometrium
- larger tumours—fill and distend the endometrial cavity with soft, white, friable tissue.

Microscopically, they are seen as:

- hyperoestrogenic tumours—typically well-differentiated adenocarcinomas composed of hyperplastic endometrial glandular tissue with only superficial myometrial invasion at diagnosis
- non-hyperoestrogenic tumours—typically poorly differentiated with deep myometrial invasion.

The condition classically presents as postmenopausal bleeding.

The main route of spread is by local invasion to the fallopian tubes, ovaries, bladder or rectum.

If venous and lymphatic invasion occurs, there may be involvement of the vagina and para-aortic nodes.

Widespread haematogenous metastasis is uncommon except with papillary serous carcinomas and clear cell carcinomas.

The amount of direct invasion into the myometrium is closely correlated with prognosis.

The prognosis of uterine carcinoma is related to stage (Fig. 11.7).

## DISORDERS OF THE OVARY AND FALLOPIAN TUBE

## Inflammatory disorders and infections

### Salpingitis

Inflammation of the fallopian tube(s).

#### Suppurative salpingitis
*Aetiology*—it is almost always caused by ascending infection from the uterine cavity.

Predisposing factors are:

- following pregnancy and endometritis
- following insertion of an IUD
- sexually transmitted disease (*Mycoplasma, Chlamydia* and gonococci).

Macroscopically, tubes are swollen and congested, and the serosal surface appears red and granular due to vascular dilatation.

Microscopically, tubal epithelium shows neutrophil infiltration and the lumen may contain pus.

Chronic inflammation may supervene, with sequelae of fibrosis and occlusion of the tubal lumen on resolution.

Complications are:

- infertility—fibrosis causes distortion of mucosal plicae and occlusion of tubal lumen
- pyosalpinx—massive distension of tubal lumen by pus

- hydrosalpinx—dilatation of a fallopian tube by clear watery fluid (product of the proteolysis of pus on resolution of an infection).

## Pelvic inflammatory disease

Pelvic inflammatory disease (PID) is a combined infection of the fallopian tubes, ovaries and peritoneum. It is typically a result of ascending infection or, less commonly, postoperative infection. Predisposing factors are as for suppurative salpingitis (see above).

*Neisseria gonorrhoeae* and *Chlamydia trachomatis* are the most common responsible organisms, although anaerobic organisms are often found in pelvic abscesses.

Inflammation is initially acute and, without prompt treatment, may progress to chronic PID, which often results in tubal infertility.

Clinical features are:

- symptoms—gradual onset of pelvic pain, irregular bleeding, vaginal discharge, fever
- signs—abdominal tenderness and guarding; extreme tenderness of the adnexa.

Treatment is by the removal of an IUD (if present) and the use of broad-spectrum antibiotics.

## Cysts

### Ovarian cysts

Ovarian cystic lesions are extremely common. They can be either neoplastic or non-neoplastic. The majority of non-neoplastic cysts arise from developing Graafian follicles; a minority is derived from surface epithelium.

### Follicular cysts

These unruptured, enlarged Graafian follicles are lined by granulosa cells, with an outer coat of thecal cells. Normal ovaries commonly contain one or more small cysts ($< 5$ cm in diameter), which typically disappear by the resorption of fluid. However, multiple follicular cysts are found in:

- mild endometrial (cystic) hyperplasia—also termed metropathia haemorrhagica
- polycystic ovary syndrome (see below).

Most cysts are clinically insignificant though some may be a cause of hyperoestrogenism.

### Polycystic ovary syndrome

This is a complex adrenal-ovarian disorder in which multiple small follicular cysts develop beneath a thickened, white ovarian capsule as a result of increased androgenic activity. This is thought to be secondary to a decrease in peripheral insulin sensitivity (promoted by obesity) causing hyperinsulinaemia.

*Clinical features*—patients have a persistent anovulatory state, high levels of luteinizing hormone (LH) and oestrogen, low levels of follicle-stimulating hormone (FSH) and high levels of circulating androgen.

Common presenting symptoms are:

- menstrual irregularity
- infertility
- hirsutism
- acne
- occasional galactorrhoea.

*Complications*—high oestrogen levels may cause endometrial hyperplasia and increase the risk of the development of endometrial carcinoma. Cardiovascular disease, diabetes mellitus and breast cancer are also increased in this group.

## Neoplastic disorders of the ovary

Ovarian cancer is responsible for more deaths than any other gynaecological malignancy (5000 cases per year in the UK, with 3700 deaths), largely because it often presents at an advanced stage. The ovarian tumour marker CA125 is used routinely to monitor for relapse in patients who have undergone treatment. CA125, along with other markers, may be used in future screening programmes for ovarian cancer.

Primary ovarian cancers account for 6% of all malignancies in women, but only 5–10% have a direct hereditary component. In these women, mutations are usually found on either the *BRCA1* or *BRCA2* tumour suppressor genes (see Chapter 3). Ninety-five per cent of ovarian cancer cases are sporadic and show complex genetic abnormalities including a high incidence of *p53* mutation (50% of cases) and amplification of the *erbB-2 (HER-2/neu)* oncogene (30% of cases). There are several different tumour types.

> **Clinical Note**
>
> A logical way of classifying ovarian tumours is according to the normal tissue constituents from which they are derived:
> - surface epithelial tumours (70% of all cases)
> - germ cell tumours (20% of all cases)
> - sex cord and stromal tumours (10% of all cases).

### Surface epithelial stromal tumours

Epithelial tumours of the ovary comprise about 70% of all ovarian tumours and about 90% of malignant tumours. They are typically found in adult life.

As with all ovarian tumours, it appears that there is a decreased risk associated with pregnancy and the oral contraceptive pill. This is part of the 'incessant ovulation' hypothesis, whereby continuous monthly re-pair of the ovarian epithelium has been suggested as one factor in the development of ovarian cancer.

*Types*—epithelial tumours are derived from surface epithelium, which in turn is derived from embryonal coelomic epithelium. Tumours with this origin can differentiate along different pathways into different types of tumours: tubal differentiation (serous tumours), endometrial differentiation (endometrial and clear cell tumours), endocervical differentiation (mucinous tumours) and transitional differentiation (Brenner tumours).

Microscopically, these tumours are classified into benign, malignant and borderline (abnormal tissue architecture with atypical cells but no evidence of invasion). The majority of borderline tumours behave in a benign fashion but some appear capable of low-grade malignancy.

### Serous tumours of the ovary

These ovarian cystic tumours of tubal differentiation contain a watery fluid; the majority (70%) are benign:

- Benign (serous cystadenoma)—thin-walled, uni-locular cystic tumour lined by cuboidal regular epithelium.
- Malignant (serous cystadenocarcinoma)—characterized by pleomorphic cells and mitoses with invasion of the ovarian stroma. Over half of cases occur bilaterally. A frequent histological finding is concentrically laminated calcified concretions called psammoma bodies.
- Borderline serous tumours—presence of cellular atypia but with no invasion.

### Mucinous tumours of the ovary

These multilocular cystic ovarian tumours of endo-cervical differentiation contain gelatinous material:

- Benign (mucinous cystadenoma)—no atypical features or mitoses.
- Malignant (mucinous cystadenocarcinoma)—invasion of the ovarian stroma. Less than 10% of mucinous tumours are malignant.
- Borderline mucinous tumours—presence of cellular atypia but with no invasion.

### Endometrioid tumours

These ovarian tumours show endometrial differentiation. The vast majority are malignant (endometrioid carcinomas), accounting for 20% of all ovarian carcinomas.

The clear cell carcinoma is a variant of endometrioid carcinoma, characterized by the presence of cells with clear cytoplasm and containing abundant glycogen.

### Brenner tumours of the ovary (transitional cell)

Tumours are composed of nests of epithelium resembling the transitional cell epithelium of the urinary tract; they are associated with a spindle-cell stroma. The epithelial component may be benign, borderline or malignant. The majority are unilateral and benign.

Germ cell and sex-cord stromal tumours are illustrated in Figure 11.8.

## Metastatic

The ovary is a common site of tumour metastasis. This may be of Müllerian origin (e.g. uterus, fallopian tubes) or from extra-Müllerian sites (typically the breast and gastrointestinal tract).

### Krukenberg's tumour

This describes bilaterally enlarged ovaries containing metastatic signet ring-cell adenocarcinoma (typically of gastric origin).

## DISORDERS OF THE PLACENTA AND PREGNANCY

## Ectopic pregnancies

This describes any fertilized ovum that is implanted outside the uterine cavity. Ectopics occur in about 1 in 300 pregnancies. The fallopian tube (especially in the ampulla) is by far the most common site for this; other sites of abnormal implantation are very rare but include the peritoneal cavity, the ovary and the cervix.

The aetiology is uncertain but ectopic pregnancies are possibly the result of some structural abnormality of the fallopian tube, e.g. scarring or adhesions resulting from previous episodes of salpingitis or endometriosis, or previous tubal surgery for contraceptive purposes, i.e. sterilization. However, half of ectopic pregnancies occur without such predisposing factors.

*Pathogenesis*—following implantation, the proliferation of trophoblasts erodes the submucosal blood vessels, precipitating severe bleeding into the tubal lumen (haematosalpinx). The muscular wall of the fallopian tube is unable to undergo hypertrophy or distension, and so tubal pregnancy almost always results in the rupture of the fallopian tube and death of the fertilized ovum. This typically occurs in the early stages of pregnancy and often before the patient is even aware of being pregnant.

The types of rupture are:

- into the lumen of the fallopian tube—common in ampullary pregnancy. Conceptus is extruded towards the fimbriated end of the tube. Mild

**Fig. 11.8** Germ cell and sex-cord stromal ovarian tumours

| Tumour | Features |
| --- | --- |
| **Germ cell tumours** | |
| **Teratoma** | |
| Benign cystic teratomas (dermoid cyst) | Cysts may be lined by structures such as the skin, hair, teeth, bone, or respiratory tract tissue |
| Solid teratomas | Composed of a variety of tissues, including cartilage, smooth muscle, or epithelium |
| **Dysgerminoma** | |
| | Similar to seminoma of the testis |
| **Yolk-sac tumours** | |
| | Cystic, solid, and haemorrhagic; secrete α-fetoprotein |
| **Sex-cord stromal tumours** | |
| Granulosa cell tumours | Composed of granulosa cells derived from follicles |
| Sertoli–Leydig cell tumours | Mixture of cell types usually seen in the testis |
| Gonadoblastomas | Primitive germ cells and sex-cord stromal derivatives are present |
| Steroid cell tumours | Composed of cortical adrenal like cells containing abundant lipid |

haemorrhage into the peritoneal cavity occurs, which may collect as a clot in the pouch of Douglas
- into the peritoneal cavity—occurs most commonly from the isthmus of the tube, either spontaneously or as a result of pressure (e.g. straining at the stool, coitus or pelvic examination). Haemorrhage is likely to be severe. Retroperitoneal (rare)—rupture occurs into the potential space between the leaves of the broad ligament. Haemorrhage into the site is more likely to be controlled.

# Spontaneous abortion

Many fertilized ova fail to implant successfully. It has been estimated that around 40% of all conceptions fail to convert into recognizable pregnancies. Of those that survive this far, 15% terminate in a clinically recognized spontaneous abortion.

*Aetiology*—causes of spontaneous abortion differ according to the stage of pregnancy, as shown in Figure 11.9.

**Clinical Note**

Clinical features of an ectopic rupture are:
- severe lower abdominal pain—usually localized to the side of the ectopic pregnancy
- vaginal bleeding—occurs after fetal death, and is an effect of oestrogen withdrawal
- signs of anaemia—due to internal blood loss
- shock may occur if haemorrhage is severe and rapid, e.g. due to large vessel erosion. This is the most dangerous and dramatic consequence of tubal pregnancy.

**HINTS AND TIPS**

To remember the causes of abortion at different stages of pregnancy, learn the following rules of thumb:
- First trimester causes—majority are associated with abnormal fetuses.
- Second trimester causes—mainly due to uterine abnormalities.
- Third trimester causes—mainly the result of maternal abnormalities.

**Fig. 11.9** Causes of spontaneous abortion

| Time | Cause |
| --- | --- |
| First trimester | Abnormal chromosomal karyotypes, particularly Turner's syndrome<br>Structural developmental abnormalities, e.g. neural tube defects<br>Maternal SLE<br>Transplacental infection, e.g. *Brucella*, *Listeria*, rubella, *Toxoplasma*, cytomegalovirus and herpes |
| Second trimester | Chorioamnionitis<br>Rupture of membranes<br>Placental haemorrhages<br>Structural abnormalities of the uterus, e.g. congenital uterine malformations<br>Large submucosal leiomyomas<br>Incompetence of the cervix<br>Abnormal placentation (but more common in third trimester) |
| Third trimester | Uncontrolled hypertension<br>Eclampsia<br>Placental abnormalities, e.g. placental haemorrhage, abruption and infarction |
| At any time | Endocrine abnormalities: diabetes, hypothyroidism, deficiency of progesterone or luteinizing hormone<br>Trauma: surgical operation, blow to abdomen, or hypotensive shock |

Note: SLE, systemic lupus erythematosus.

# Pre-eclampsia and eclampsia

## Pre-eclampsia

This is high blood pressure (> 140/90 mmHg), peripheral oedema and proteinuria, developing during pregnancy in a woman whose blood pressure was previously normal. An increase in blood pressure alone is termed gestational hypertension. Hypertensive disorders occur in about 10% of all pregnant women. The aetiology is unknown.

Risk factors are:

- first pregnancy (primigravidae)—increased risk
- multiple pregnancies (e.g. twins)
- medical comorbidities—diabetes, pre-existing hypertension, systemic lupus erythaematosus (SLE)
- extremes of maternal age—older or younger women
- family history.

The pathogenesis is unclear but probably relates to inadequate placental invasion by spiral arteries, leading to placental ischaemia. This is thought to release a chemical factor that triggers vasoconstriction and endothelial damage to promote hypertension.

Endothelial cells of kidney arterioles become swollen and fibrin deposition occurs in glomeruli leading to proteinuria (Fig. 11.10).

Pre-eclampsia may be mild or severe according to the level of blood pressure derangement. Severe proteinuria leads to peripheral oedema.

### Effects of pre-eclampsia

Reduced placental blood flow causes an increased risk of fetal hypoxia in late pregnancy, particularly during labour, with resultant perinatal mortality. The fetus may also suffer intrauterine growth retardation and have a low birth weight.

Maternal problems are less common, being largely confined to severe pre-eclampsia, which may progress into full-blown eclampsia (see below).

The disease resolves immediately after delivery.

## Eclampsia

This is the occurrence of one or more convulsions not caused by other conditions such as epilepsy or cerebral haemorrhage in a woman with pre-eclampsia.

Incidence is rare; only a small proportion of patients with severe pre-eclampsia develop eclampsia.

Clinical features are severe systemic disturbance, i.e. frontal headaches, visual disturbance, rapid and sustained rise in blood pressure, severe epigastric pain,

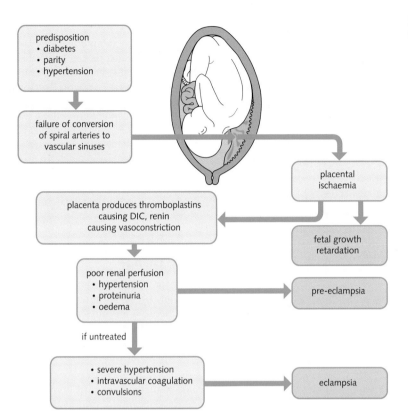

**Fig. 11.10** Pathogenesis of pre-eclampsia.

shock, anuria and fits. A main cause of death is intracerebral haemorrhage.

There is disseminated intravascular coagulation with widespread occlusion of blood vessels, fibrinoid necrosis of vessel walls and, in fatal cases, widespread microinfarcts in the brain, liver, kidneys and other organs.

Eclampsia is associated with a maternal mortality of 2% and a neonatal mortality of 3.5%. However, fatal eclampsia is now rare because of screening and treatment for the pre-eclamptic syndrome.

## Neoplastic disorders of trophoblastic origin

### Hydatidiform mole

This is the abnormal development of a gestational trophoblast leading to the formation of a benign mass of cystic vesicles derived from chorionic villi. It occurs in 1 in 2000 pregnancies in the UK and USA, but it is seen more frequently amongst some racial groups such as the Japanese population.

The disease is the result of an error in embryogenesis. There are two types:

1. Partial—a partial mole is triploid with most containing one maternal and two paternal haploid sets of chromosomes. Cystic vesicles are found in only a part of the placenta. Fetal parts and some normal placental villi are present along with the abnormal trophoblastic tissue. There is a low risk of subsequent development of a malignant tumour of the trophoblast (choriocarcinoma).

2. Complete—a complete mole is entirely of paternal origin (no maternal genetic contribution) and usually forms a bulky mass that may fill the uterine cavity. No fetal parts or normal placental villi are present. The risk of subsequent choriocarcinoma is greater than in a partial mole, occurring in about 3% of cases.

The aetiopathogenesis is unknown.
Clinical features are:

- amenorrhoea and other symptoms of pregnancy, followed by continuous or intermittent vaginal bleeding. Many molar pregnancies spontaneously miscarry
- enlarged soft uterus (often larger than dates would suggest).

Diagnosis is by elevated human chorionic gonadotrophin (hCG) excretion in urine (typically much greater than in normal pregnancies) and by ultrasound for the absence of the fetus. Very high hCG levels may cause extreme morning sickness (hyperemesis gravidarum) and promote pre-eclampsia.

Treatment is by evacuation of the uterus, with a second aspiration or curettage 2–4 weeks later to ensure complete removal of the mole.

Follow-up is by regular estimations of hCG for at least a year. Detection of hCG after 1 month may suggest incomplete removal and the persistence of trophoblastic disease. Untreated, this carries a risk of subsequent choriocarcinoma.

## Invasive mole (chorioadenoma destruens)

This is a hydatidiform mole that invades through the decidua into the myometrium and associated blood vessels. Perforation of the uterus may occur, resulting in invasion of the parametrium. True malignant transformation is rare.

## Choriocarcinoma

These malignant tumours of trophoblastic tissue have a propensity for invading vessel walls and blood-borne metastases occur early to many sites, particularly the lung and brain.

They are rare in the UK and USA (at 1 per 50 000 pregnancies) but more common in Asia, South America and Africa.

*Aetiology*—about 50% develop from a hydatidiform mole and about 20% arise after a normal pregnancy with a variable time lag (a few months to many years).

The prognosis is excellent as the tumours respond well to cytotoxic chemotherapy (particularly if post-treatment monitoring of hCG levels is carried out).

## Placental site trophoblastic tumour

This is a rare tumour in which the bulk of the tissue consists of chorionic epithelium but with very few villi. Typically benign, it may undergo malignant change.

## DISORDERS OF THE BREAST

## Inflammatory disorders and infections

### Acute mastitis and breast abscess

These are uncommon and are usually complications of lactation. The most frequent organism is *Staphylococcus aureus,* which gains access through cracks and fissures of the nipple and areola. An abscess may form if drainage is inadequate.

## Mammary duct ectasia

There is an abnormal progressive dilatation of the large breast ducts, which accumulate inspissated (thickened) secretions. The aetiology is unknown and it affects older women (perimenopausal age range). Patients develop a firm breast lump, but this does not mimic a carcinoma. There may also be a clear or green-coloured discharge.

## Fat necrosis

This is usually caused by trauma. Histology shows necrosis with multinucleated giant cells and later fibrosis. It may cause a discrete lump mimicking a carcinoma.

## Fibrocystic changes

### Simple fibrocystic change

This is a generic term for a number of benign lesions that may occur together, producing lumpiness in the breast tissue. Peak incidence is around the menopause. It is thought that fibrocystic change is caused by hormonal imbalance.

The histological changes that may be present include:

- cysts—ranging in size from microscopic to palpable lesions 1–2 cm in diameter. Diagnosis is confirmed by needle aspiration of clear fluid (blood-stained aspirate requires further investigation)
- apocrine metaplasia—epithelial lining of hyperplastic ducts undergoes metaplasia to that of normal apocrine glands
- fibrosis—replacement of breast tissue by dense fibrous tissue, which can be due to cyst rupture
- sclerosing adenosis—marked proliferation of specialized hormone-responsive stromal tissue and myoepithelial cells, i.e. the number of acini per lobule increases. This forms localized areas of irregular stellate, collagenous sclerosis in which epithelial elements are also present. Occasionally difficult to distinguish from some patterns of invasive carcinoma.

There is no increased risk of a carcinoma unless there is accompanying epithelial hyperplasia (see below).

### Epithelial hyperplasia

This describes the proliferation of epithelial cells within ducts or lobules (ductal hyperplasia and lobular hyperplasia respectively). There are two types:

1. Hyperplasia of the usual type—normal cytology and tissue architecture with no signs of malignancy
2. Hyperplasia of atypical type—biological spectrum between some abnormalities of cytology/architecture and carcinoma in situ.

The risk of subsequent invasive breast carcinoma is increased in individuals with florid usual hyperplasia, further increased in subjects with atypical hyperplasia and much higher in those specifically with lobular carcinoma in situ.

Epithelial hyperplasia can only be diagnosed histologically.

---

**Clinical Note**

Breast lumps are relatively common presentations. The following benign pathologies may cause discrete breast lumps or nipple discharge that mimic carcinomas:
- Fat necrosis
- Intraduct papilloma
- Fibroadenoma.
  The best form of management is so-called 'triple assessment.' This consists of:
- history and examination (both the lump and regional nodes)
- imaging (mammography or ultrasound)
- tissue sampling if required (fine-needle aspiration or core biopsy).

---

## Neoplasms of the breast

### Fibroadenoma

This is the most common benign tumour of the female breast. There is proliferation of both stroma and epithelium, usually in young women (most frequently the 25–35 age group). It produces discrete but mobile breast lumps typically 1–4 cm in size, often multiple and bilateral.

### Phyllodes tumour

This is a tumour composed of both stroma and epithelium, but the stroma is more cellular than in fibroadenomas. It is less common than fibroadenoma and occurs in the older age group (peak incidence being 45 years of age). Clinically, the tumour presents as a breast lump.

Macroscopically, there are rubbery white lesions consisting of a whorled pattern of slit-like spaces and solid areas.

Microscopically, there is a variable appearance, classified into benign (90% of cases), or of borderline malignant potential or definitely malignant.

There is the potential for local recurrence with increasing aggressiveness, and the tumour may eventually metastasize. Phyllodes tumours are therefore excised with a wide margin or, if necessary, are treated by mastectomy.

### Intraductal papilloma

Epithelial proliferation within ducts produces papillary structures. These occur in older women and may produce a blood-stained nipple discharge. Papillomas are usually solitary with no increased risk of a carcinoma. However, a rare condition of multiple intraduct papillomas is premalignant.

## Carcinoma

*Incidence*—this comprises 30% of all cancers in women and is the most common cause of death in 35- to 55-year-old women, increasing with age steeply to 45 years and continuing to increase less steeply thereafter. There are around 40 000 cases each year in the UK; 5-year survival is 80%.

There is a 200-fold female preponderance, with the highest rates in America, Western Europe and the Antipodes, and the lowest rates in Africa and Southeast Asia.

### Predisposing factors
These include:

- atypical epithelial proliferation—4- to 5-fold increased risk in severe atypia
- mutations of *BRCA1* (chromosome 17) and *BRCA2* genes (chromosome 13)—5% of cases
- first-degree relative with breast cancer—increased risk independent of *BRCA* mutations
- long interval between menarche and menopause, i.e. early menarche and/or late menopause
- older age at first pregnancy
- ionizing radiation, as seen in those receiving intensive radiotherapy for Hodgkin's disease (up to 30% risk of breast cancer within 30 years of treatment)
- obesity and dietary factors—postmenopausal obesity risk linked to higher oestrogen levels. Role of dietary fat is controversial.

### Carcinoma in situ
All breast carcinomas are adenocarcinomas derived from epithelial cells of the terminal ductal lobules. Carcinoma in situ refers to neoplastic cells confined to the ducts and lobules, with no evidence of invasion through the basement membrane. Ductal carcinoma in situ (DCIS) is the more common form, presenting as microcalcifications on mammography. Lobular carcinoma in situ (LCIS) is more common in younger women and is more likely to affect both breasts. LCIS is not associated with calcifications on mammography or a mass, and is therefore often an incidental finding on biopsy.

DCIS may progress to invasive carcinoma, but is highly treatable at the in situ stage. LCIS may progress to invasive carcinoma, but is predominantly thought to be a strong risk marker for carcinoma in either breast.

### Invasive carcinoma
Invasive carcinomas are tumours that have eroded through the basement membrane of their tissue of origin to invade surrounding structures. The most common presentation is a painless palpable mass,

excluding those detected early by mammographic screening (see below). Large masses may cause skin dimpling or interfere with lymphatic drainage to produce classic skin changes (e.g. *peau d'orange*). Nipple retraction can also occur. Axillary lymph nodes may be palpable, reflecting metastasis from the primary site.

Investigation is by ultrasound, mammography, core biopsy or fine-needle aspiration cytology. Invasive carcinomas are categorized histologically:

- Invasive ductal (most common at 75%)
- Invasive lobular
- Mucinous
- Tubular
- Medullary
- Papillary.

The classification of breast cancer is summarized in Figure 11.11.

*Macroscopic features*—a discrete lump with tethering to the skin or surrounding connective tissue. The macroscopic appearance of the tumour depends on the amount and type of stroma within the carcinoma.

Spread is as follows (Fig. 11.12):

- Direct—skin and muscles of the chest wall
- Lymphatic—axillary lymph nodes, internal mammary lymph nodes
- Blood—lungs, bone, liver, and brain
- Transcoelomic—pleural cavities and pericardium.

### Management and prognosis

The mainstay of treatment is surgical excision, often with axillary node clearance. Radiotherapy and chemotherapy are often used after surgery to reduce the risk of relapse.

*Prognosis*—related to tumour grade and type (tubular has the best prognosis), size of the tumour, lymph node status and oestrogen receptor status (usually responds to tamoxifen if positive). *C-erbB-2 (HER-2)* is a proto-oncogene that is found in 15–20% of breast cancers. It is associated with poorer prognosis but this

**Fig. 11.11** Types of breast carcinoma

| Character | Neoplasm |
|---|---|
| Non-invasive | Ductal carcinoma *in situ* <br> Lobular carcinoma *in situ* |
| Invasive | Invasive ductal carcinoma (85%) <br> Invasive lobular carcinoma (10%) <br> Mucinous <br> Tubular <br> Medullary <br> Papillary |

**Fig. 11.12** Spread of breast carcinoma

| Spread | Area |
|---|---|
| Direct | Skin |
| Lymphatic | Axillary lymph nodes <br> Internal mammary lymph nodes <br> Supraclavicular lymph nodes |
| Haematogenous | Liver <br> Lung <br> Opposite breast <br> Bone <br> Brain |

may be improved by novel monoclonal antibody therapy (Herceptin).

Figure 11.13 shows the TNM staging used for breast carcinoma.

## Screening for breast carcinoma

There is no direct screening method equivalent to the cytology of the uterine cervix. The primary screening modality is mammography which is more effective in older women with less radiodense breast tissue. Abnormalities seen on mammograms include calcification and soft tissue deformity. In the UK there is a National Health Service Breast Screening Programme with 3-yearly mammography for all women over the age of 50 (until 70 years). Long-term studies suggest that such screening successfully reduces the mortality from breast carcinoma; it is possible that the age range screened may be extended in the future.

## The male breast

### Gynaecomastia

This is the benign enlargement of breast tissue.

*Aetiology*—hormonal influences including increased oestrogen production or receptor sensitivity. It is associated with liver cirrhosis, stilboestrol therapy for prostate carcinoma and drugs such as chlorpromazine.

### Carcinoma

Less than 1% of breast carcinomas occur in men. The condition is associated with Klinefelter's syndrome and is usually of the ductal type; the lobular type is extremely rare.

**Fig. 11.13** Tumour, node, metastases (TNM) staging of breast carcinoma

| Tumour | Nodes | Metastases |
|---|---|---|
| T1 tumour 20 mm or less; no fixation or nipple retraction | N0 node negative | M0 no distant metastases |
| T2 tumour 20–50 mm, or less than 20 mm with fixation | N1 axillary nodes mobile | M1 distant metastases present |
| T3 tumour 50–100 mm, or less than 50 mm with fixation | N2 axillary nodes fixed | |
| T4 greater than 100 mm, or chest wall invasion | N3 supraclavicular nodes positive or arm oedema | |

## DISORDERS OF THE PENIS

## Inflammation and infection

### Viral infection

Common viral infections of the penis include genital herpes and genital warts (condyloma acuminatum).

#### Genital herpes

This is an acute infection of the penile mucosa by the herpes simplex virus with the formation of typical herpetic vesicles on the glans penis. The vesicles soon burst to produce shallow painful ulcers.

The virus may remain latent for many years. Recurrent herpes infections are caused by reactivation of the virus, which may be precipitated by a febrile illness, immune suppression, emotional stress or UV light.

#### Condyloma acuminatum (genital warts)

These cauliflower-like warts are seen on the penis and around the perineum. They are caused by the human papillomavirus subtypes HPV6 and HPV11, which are sexually transmitted.

### Bacterial infection

Inflammation of the glans (balanitis) and prepuce (posthitis) can be caused by a variety of bacterial organisms, the most common of which are staphylococci, coliforms, gonococci and *Chlamydia*.

The appearance is that of marked congestion and oedema with exudate on the surface of the glans. Ulceration with chronic scarring may occur if untreated; this is a common cause of phimosis.

### Fungi

Infection with *Candida albicans* is common in men with diabetes mellitus.

## Neoplastic disorders

## Malignant

### Carcinoma in situ

Penile carcinoma in situ is seen in two forms: Bowen disease (opaque plaques with shallow ulceration) affecting the shaft and scrotum, and erythroplasia of Queyrat, which is restricted to the glans, presenting with flat, red, glistening plaques. There is a spectrum of changes from dysplasia to carcinoma in situ grouped together as penile intraepithelial neoplasia. Many cases are associated with HPV infection (most commonly serotype 16).

Penile carcinoma in situ is a precancerous condition and may lead to invasive cancer unless treated vigorously with local irradiation or 5-fluorouracil cream.

### Squamous cell carcinoma

This is a well-differentiated, keratinising, invasive tumour usually seen in elderly men. It occurs most commonly in uncircumcised men and is thought to be associated with a previous infection with human papillomavirus.

It presents as a warty, cauliflower-like growth that bleeds easily. It is typically slow growing but it is often neglected because of patient embarrassment.

## DISORDERS OF THE TESTIS AND EPIDIDYMIS

## Congenital abnormalities and regression

### Cryptorchidism (undescended testis)

This is a condition caused by maldescent of the testes, affecting about 5% at birth, and 1% by the first birthday.

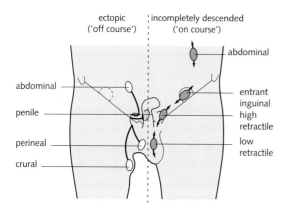

ectopic ('off course') | incompletely descended ('on course')

abdominal

abdominal

penile

perineal

crural

entrant inguinal

high retractile

low retractile

**Fig. 11.14** Maldescended testes showing common sites of arrest. (Adapted with permission from Lecture Notes on Urology, 5th edn, by J Blandy, Blackwell Science, 1998.)

In the embryo, the testes develop from the genital ridge high on the posterior wall.

At about 7 months' gestation, the testes migrate down the posterior abdominal wall. They are guided by a cord (the gubernaculum) through the inguinal ring into the scrotum.

Occasionally, migration fails to occur and one (75% of cases) or both (25% of cases) testes become arrested somewhere along the route (Fig. 11.14). There are three conditions:

1. Abdominal testicle—usually found just inside the internal ring
2. Inguinal testicle—in the inguinal canal, particularly exposed to trauma
3. Retractile testicles (most common)—either high or low, depending on ability to be manoeuvered into correct position. Usually settles at puberty and does not need an operation.

The complications are:

- infertility—temperature of aberrant locations is higher than in the scrotum and prevents normal germ cell development. The testis remains small and incapable of producing effective spermatozoa
- malignancy—more common in an undescended testis; about 1 in 10 of all testicular tumours arise in association with cryptorchidism
- inguinal hernia—there is nearly always a patent tunica vaginalis that predisposes to the development of an inguinal hernia
- torsion of the testicle (see below).

Management is by detection and correction of testicular maldescent. This is important because of the increased risk of testicular carcinoma. Some restoration of function may be achieved by 'orchidopexy' at an early stage (the testis is surgically pulled down and fixed to the scrotum).

## Abnormalities of the tunica vaginalis

The tunica vaginalis and tunica albuginea (membrane sheaths surrounding the testes) are invested with mesothelial cells and may be the site of fluid accumulation, inflammation or (uncommonly) tumour formation.

### Hydrocele

Fluid accumulates in the cavity bounded by the tunica vaginalis. This is the most common cause of swelling within the scrotum.

This is often idiopathic, but the aetiology may involve:

- congenital patency of the processus vaginalis, often with continuity into the peritoneal cavity
- secondary to tumours, epididymitis, mumps or acute orchitis.

### Haematocele

Blood accumulates in the cavity bounded by the tunica vaginalis, usually due to trauma or torsion and rarely due to tumour spread.

### Chylocele

Accumulation of lymph secondary to obstructed drainage.

### Hernias

Indirect inguinal hernias (described in Chapter 8) typically occur as a result of patent processus vaginalis.

## Trauma and vascular disturbances

### Torsion

There is twisting of a testicle on its pedicle with obstruction of venous return such that blood continues to enter the testis but cannot leave. The testis is engorged and painful, eventually becoming infarcted (venous infarction). In advanced torsion, the testis is almost black as a result of vascular congestion.

Early detection and surgical relief are required to save testicular viability. Surgical removal is necessary for advanced disease.

### Varicocele

This describes variceal dilatation of the veins of the pampiniform plexus of the spermatic cord.

## Neoplastic disorders

Tumours of the testis, although relatively uncommon, are important because many occur in young men; they are the most common tumour among 15- to 35-year-olds.

The exact aetiology is unknown but there are links with testicular maldescent and/or dysgenesis, possibly with some genetic susceptibility.

Clinical presentations are:

- painless unilateral enlargement of testis (majority)
- secondary hydrocele
- symptoms of metastases—especially in malignant teratoma, e.g. haemoptysis from lung deposits
- endocrine effects—gynaecomastia, precocious puberty (typically from Leydig or Sertoli cell tumours).

There are two main groups of testicular tumour:

1. Germ cell tumours (97% of cases)—derived from multipotential germ cells of the testis arising mainly as teratomas and seminomas
2. Non-germ cell tumours (3% of cases)—derived from specialized and non-specialized support cells of the testis.

## Germ cell tumours

### Seminoma
The most common malignant testicular tumour, accounting for about 50% of all malignant germ cell tumours, with a peak age of onset between 30 and 40 years. The tumour shows spermatogenic differentiation.

Histological types of seminoma are:

- classic seminoma (most common subtype)—characteristic feature is the presence of fibrous septa with lymphocytic infiltrate
- spermatocytic seminoma—larger tumour cells with some small cells resembling spermatocytes
- anaplastic seminoma—cells show marked pleomorphism and increased mitotic activity.

### Teratoma
This tumour of germ cell origin is composed of several types of tissue representing endoderm, ectoderm and mesoderm. The tumours retain their totipotentiality for differentiation and are more aggressive than seminomas. The peak age of onset is 20–30 years.

Teratomas are classified according to their histological pattern; two systems exist (Fig. 11.15), with the British classifications described below:

- Differentiated teratoma—a rare type of teratoma of mature and well-differentiated tissue, producing a wide range of organoid structures (e.g. skin, hair, cartilage and bone). Lesions are usually seen in young children. They behave in a benign fashion.
- Malignant teratoma intermediate—partly solid and partly cystic tumour, with less maturity and areas of malignancy with cellular pleomorphism and necrosis.
- Malignant teratoma undifferentiated—completely undifferentiated tumour with marked nuclear pleomorphism and a high mitotic rate.
- Malignant teratoma trophoblastic—identical to choriocarcinoma in the placenta (see page 215), this highly malignant tumour contains areas of syncytiotrophoblast and cytotrophoblast cells. hCG and α-fetoprotein (AFP) are useful markers.
- Yolk sac tumour (orchioblastoma)—the pure form is seen in children up to 3 years old and has a good prognosis. The adult (mixed) form is more aggressive. AFP is a useful marker.

### Combined germ cell tumour
Between 10 and 15% of germ cell tumours consist of a mixture of seminomatous and teratomatous elements.

### Prognosis of germ cell tumours
The prognosis of testicular teratomas has improved greatly with the use of cytotoxic chemotherapy, and it is related to histological type, as well as to tumour stage. Seminomas are more likely to respond to radiotherapy. In general, germ-cell tumours containing trophoblastic, yolk sac and undifferentiated elements have the worst prognosis.

**Fig. 11.15** Comparison of the British and WHO classifications of teratomas

| Type of differentiation | British | WHO |
|---|---|---|
| Somatic | Differentiated teratoma | Mature teratoma |
| | Malignant teratoma intermediate | Immature teratoma or mixed teratoma and embryonal carcinoma |
| None | Malignant teratoma undifferentiated | Embryonal carcinoma |
| Extra-embryonic | Yolk sac tumour | Yolk sac tumour |
| | Malignant teratoma trophoblastic | Choriocarcinoma |
| WHO, World Health organization | | |

## Non-germ cell tumours

### Interstitial (Leydig) cell tumour

This rare tumour arises from the interstitial or Leydig cells of the testis. It may produce androgens, oestrogens or both, causing precocious development of secondary sexual characteristics in childhood or loss of libido/gynaecomastia in adults. Ninety per cent are benign.

### Sertoli cell tumour (androblastoma)

This well-circumscribed tumour is composed of cells resembling normal Sertoli cells of the tubules. Most lesions are benign.

### Malignant lymphomas

The non-Hodgkin's-type lymphoma is usually a poorly differentiated B cell lymphoma with a diffuse pattern. These comprise about 5% of testicular tumours with a peak incidence between 60 and 80 years of age.

### Metastatic tumours

The spread of other tumours to the testis may occasionally occur, particularly in acute leukaemia.

Figure 11.16 provides a summary of testicular tumours.

Many testicular tumours have useful cell markers:
• Trophoblastic germ cell tumours—↑ hCG
• Yolk sac tumours—↑ α-fetoprotein
• 90% of patients with malignant teratoma undifferentiated—↑ α-fetoprotein, ↑ hCG or both
• 50% of patients with malignant teratoma intermediate—↑ α-fetoprotein, ↑ hCG or both.

## DISORDERS OF THE PROSTATE

### Benign prostatic hyperplasia

Non-neoplastic enlargement of the prostate is the most common disorder of the prostate, affecting almost all men over the age of 70. However, it is found with increasing frequency and severity from about 45 years.

The aetiopathogenesis is uncertain but believed to be a result of androgen-oestrogen imbalance. Central (periurethral) prostatic glands are hormone sensitive and they undergo hyperplasia. Their continuing enlargement compresses peripheral prostatic glands leading to their collapse, leaving only fibrous supporting stroma (Fig. 11.17).

Affected lobes are:

• two lateral lobes (majority of cases)
• posterior lobe (uncommon), causing an obstruction of the urinary outflow tract at the internal urinary meatus at the bladder neck.

| **Fig. 11.16** Summary of testicular tumours | |
|---|---|
| **Germ cell tumours (97% of cases)** | |
| Seminomas | Classic seminoma<br>Spermatocytic seminoma<br>Anaplastic seminoma<br>Seminomas with trophoblastic giant cells |
| Teratomas | Differentiated teratoma<br>Malignant teratoma intermediate<br>Malignant teratoma undifferentiated<br>Malignant teratoma trophoblastic<br>Yolk sac tumour |
| Combined | Mixture of seminomatous and teratomatous elements |
| **Non-germ cell tumours (3% of cases)** | |
| Sex-cord and stromal tumours | Interstitial (Leydig) cell tumour<br>Sertoli cell tumour |
| Others | Malignant lymphomas<br>Metastatic tumours |

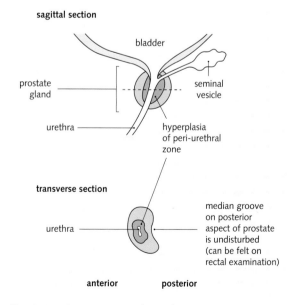

**Fig. 11.17** Benign prostatic hyperplasia.

**Fig. 11.18** Complications of benign prostatic hyperplasia

| | |
|---|---|
| Bladder wall | Hypertrophy of smooth muscle<br>Trabeculation: due to prominent bands of thickened smooth muscle<br>Diverticula: protrude between trabeculae |
| Bladder size | Dilation: due to failure of bladder wall compensatory mechanisms |
| Ureteric changes | Dilation of ureters |
| Urinary infection (cystitis) | Bladder fails to empty completely after micturition, and residual urine is liable to infection |
| Kidney disease | Pyelonephritis: from ascending infection<br>Impaired renal failure<br>Hydronephrosis<br>Calculi |

Histologically:

- Nodular pattern of hyperplastic glandular acini lined with tall columnar epithelial cells and separated by fibrous stroma
- Some nodules are cystically dilated and contain a milky fluid
- Other nodules contain numerous calcific concretions (corpora amylacea).

Infarction causes necrotic areas with a haemorrhagic margin. There is often muscular hypertrophy particularly in the region of the bladder neck.

*Clinical presentation*—compression of the prostatic urethra by the enlarged prostate causes difficulties with micturition, mainly hesitation, poor stream and terminal dribbling.

*Complications*—prolonged prostatic obstruction can lead to several complications, which are outlined in Figure 11.18.

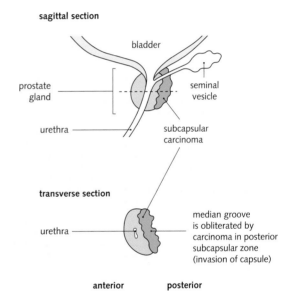

**Fig. 11.19** Prostatic carcinoma.

## Neoplastic disorders

### Prostatic carcinoma

This is an adenocarcinoma of the prostate and it is shown in Figure 11.19. It is the second most common cause of cancer death in males and its detected incidence is increasing (30 000 per year in the UK). It is rare before 55 years of age with a peak incidence between 60 and 85 years; 5-year survival is 65%.

Its aetiology is uncertain but there is probably hormonal involvement (reduced androgens).

Unlike benign hyperplasia, carcinoma usually arises in the peripheral zone of the prostate and it is, therefore, often well established before the development of urinary symptoms. Indeed, some tumours may remain silent even in the presence of widespread metastases.

Types are divided into three groups on the basis of their behaviour:

1. Latent—small foci of well-differentiated carcinoma, frequently an incidental finding in prostatic glands of elderly men. Remain confined to the prostate for a long period
2. Invasive—invade locally and metastasize
3. Occult—not clinically apparent in primary site (small tumour) but present as widespread symptomatic metastatic disease.

Macroscopically, there are diffuse areas of firm, white tissue merging into fibromuscular prostatic stromal tissues. Distortion and extension outside the prostatic capsule is common, producing a firm, craggy mass that can be palpated on rectal examination.

Microscopically, the majority has a well-differentiated glandular pattern (good prognosis); a minority has poorly differentiated sheets of cells with no acinar pattern (poor prognosis).

Spread is:

- direct—to the base of the bladder and adjacent tissues. May cause obstruction of the urethra (difficulty in micturition) and may block the ureters, causing hydronephrosis
- lymphatic—to pelvic and para-aortic nodes
- haematogenous—most commonly to bone, but also to the lungs and liver. Bone metastases are typically sclerotic with bone production (dense on radiograph) rather than lytic with bone destruction.

Diagnosis is by:

- Imaging—ultrasound, X-ray, isotope bone scan (for bony metastases).
- Needle biopsy—histological examination together with immunohistochemical detection of prostate-specific antigen (PSA) and prostate-specific acid phosphatase (PSAP) in biopsy material.
- Serology—PSA and PSAP may also be used as serum markers for disease, levels being particularly raised when there is metastatic disease. However, raised PSA alone is relatively non-specific for prostate carcinoma, meaning that screening programs are likely to have a high false-positive rate.

### Clinical Note

The clinical features of prostatic carcinoma:
- Urinary symptoms (hesitancy, poor stream, terminal dribbling)
- Hard, craggy prostate on rectal examination
- Bone metastases: pain (especially back pain), fracture, anaemia.

*Treatment*—if tumour is confined to prostate, radical prostatectomy or radiotherapy may be curative. If spread has occurred, androgen suppressing drugs (e.g. luteinizing hormone releasing hormone analogues) suppress testosterone and improve survival from this slow-growing tumour. Orchidectomy is occasionally performed for the same effect.

# Pathology of the musculoskeletal system

## Objectives

In this chapter, you will learn to:
- Describe common disorders of bone structure, particularly osteoporosis and Paget's disease.
- Recall the infectious causes of bone disease and their manifestations.
- Describe fractures and bone healing, including the complications that may occur.
- Briefly describe the tumours of bone.
- Understand the causes of disruption to the neuromuscular junction.
- Describe inherited and acquired myopathies.
- Describe in detail osteoarthritis, rheumatoid arthritis and the wider effects of rheumatoid disease.
- Understand ankylosing spondylitis and arthritis associated with systemic disease.
- Recall the pathologies of the crystal arthropathies.
- Understand the causes and effects of septic arthritis.

## DISORDERS OF BONE STRUCTURE

## Achondroplasia

This hereditary disorder of endochondral ossification is the most common cause of true dwarfism, occurring in approximately 1 per 50 000 births.

*Aetiology*—autosomal dominant with a high incidence of spontaneous mutation accounting for the 80% of cases in which an achondroplastic child is born to unaffected parents (increased incidence with paternal age). The affected gene is for fibroblast growth factor receptor (chromosome 4).

*Pathogenesis*—the mutation suppresses cartilage proliferation in the growth plate, resulting in diminished lengthening of cartilage bones (e.g. long bones, base of the skull and pelvis). Periosteal bone formation is normal. Cartilage bones are, therefore, shortened but thick and strong. Membranous bone (such as the vault of the skull) is not affected.

## Disorders of the bone matrix

### Osteogenesis imperfecta (brittle bone disease)

This heterogeneous group of rare congenital disorders is characterized by abnormal collagen formation with unusually brittle and fragile bones.

*Aetiology*—mutation of genes coding for type I collagen results in abnormal collagen formation in the osteoid. The pattern of inheritance can be either dominant or recessive, and it involves mutation at sites on chromosomes 7 and 17.

*Appearance*—there is a marked variation in severity but widespread weakness of bone results in multiple fractures frequently leading to severe deformity. Lax joint ligaments, blue sclera and hearing loss are also often seen, once more reflecting decreased collagen synthesis.

## Osteoporosis

This slowly progressive disorder is characterized by reduced bone mass as a result of a relative increase in bone erosion. The bone structure remains qualitatively normal, but there is less of it.

*Incidence*—the most common metabolic bone disease. Peak bone mass is achieved in early adulthood, with bone density decreasing with age from the third or fourth decade of life. A high peak bone mass protects against future osteoporosis.

Osteoporosis is widespread in the elderly, where it is an important cause of morbidity and even mortality, as weakened bone predisposes to minimal trauma fractures. Bone loss in women is accelerated by oestrogen deficiency, making postmenopausal women a high-risk group for osteoporosis. Hormone replacement therapy is partly protective (see Chapter 11). The risk factors for osteoporosis are illustrated in Figure 12.1.

*Macroscopically*—bones are lighter in weight, less dense on radiography (Fig. 12.2) and show thinning of the cortex. Lumbar vertebral bodies are more biconcave than normal, such that the intervertebral disc space appears more spherical ('fish vertebrae').

*Microscopically*—bone trabeculae are thinner and reduced in number, and there is a decrease in the number of osteoblasts. Mineralization is not affected.

Complications are:

- bone pain—especially in the back because of compression of vertebral bodies. This may reduce overall height and cause an anteroposterior bending of the spine (kyphosis)

- pathological fractures—following minimal trauma, especially of the femur (hip fracture), neck and at the wrist.

Osteoporosis may also develop in a localized area of bone secondary to disuse, surrounding inflammation or in conditions such as myeloma (see Chapter 13).

Diagnosis is by bone densitometry scanning at the hip and spine to show the degree of bone loss. Osteopenia describes reduced bone density that has not yet reached osteoporotic levels.

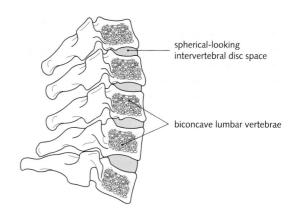

spherical-looking intervertebral disc space

biconcave lumbar vertebrae

**Fig. 12.2** Radiographic appearance of lumbar vertebrae in osteoporosis.

**Fig. 12.1** Type and associated risk factors for osteoporosis

| Type | Risk factors |
|---|---|
| Idiopathic | Female<br>Early menopause<br>Small stature<br>Thin physique<br>Family history<br>Advanced age<br>Nulliparity |
| Secondary: generalized | **M**etabolic: low calcium intake, impaired supply of protein (e.g. nephritic syndrome or cirrhosis of liver), scurvy<br>**A**ssorted endocrine disorders: thyrotoxicosis, panhypopituitarism and Cushing's syndrome<br>**S**teroid therapy<br>**C**igarette smoking<br>**A**lcohol abuse<br>**R**educed physical activities<br>**A**luminium antacids |
| Secondary: localized | Disuse atrophy: especially in neurological limb paralysis or post fracture |

*The mnemonic 'MASCARA' can be used to help remember the causes of secondary generalized osteoporosis.*

*Management*—emphasis is on prevention rather than treatment, namely avoidance of risk factors, with encouragement of physical exercise and adequate calcium intake. Bisphosphonates are highly effective drugs for reducing the rate of decline in osteoporosis.

## Osteomalacia and rickets

Osteomalacia is a disease of defective bone mineralization that is most commonly seen in the developing world. It is usually due to a lack of vitamin D or disturbances in its metabolism (e.g. conversion to active vitamin D via the liver and kidney).

Bone is incompletely calcified, with the development of wide 'seams' of osteoid. The bone is weak and prone to fracture.

Rickets—the same disorder—occurs in the growing bones of children, leading to characteristic skeletal changes, e.g. bowing of long bones.

Both disorders are potentially reversible with early dietary supplementation to correct deficiencies or treatment of underlying disorders of vitamin D metabolism.

## Disorders of osteoclast function

### Osteopetrosis (marble bone disease; Albers–Schönberg disease)

This rare inherited disorder is characterized by increased density of all cartilaginous bones, especially the vertebrae, pelvic bones and ribs.

*Pathogenesis*—defective resorption of bone by osteoclasts produces diffuse symmetrical skeletal sclerosis.

*Appearance*—there is no discernible differentiation of cartilaginous bones into cortex and medulla: the cortical compact bone extends into the medulla, which is thus devoid of cancellous bone.

*Effect*—bones are excessively dense, yet extremely brittle and prone to fracture. There is a lack of bone marrow function predisposing to infection and increased risk of cranial nerve compression within the base of the skull.

### Paget's disease of the bone (osteitis deformans)

This chronic disease of excessive uncontrolled resorption and deposition of bone particularly affects the skull, backbone, pelvis and long bones. It is rare before 40 years of age, but increases in incidence with age thereafter. It is relatively common in the UK, affecting 3% of those over 40, but rare in Asia, Africa and the Middle East.

*Aetiology*—unknown, but recent evidence suggests a paramyxovirus infection of the osteoclasts. Electron microscope studies have demonstrated probable viral inclusions in the nuclei of osteoclasts.

*Pathogenesis*—large, abnormal, multinucleated osteoclasts cause excessive bone erosion with destruction of trabecular and cortical bone. Each wave of bone destruction is followed by a vigorous but uncoordinated osteoblastic response, producing new osteoid to fill the defects left by the osteoclasts. However, both osteoclastic erosion and osteoblastic deposition are random, haphazard and unrelated to functional stresses on the bone, resulting in greatly distorted bone architecture.

*Morphology*—bone shows a characteristic woven, non-lamellar pattern indicative of rapid reparative deposition. Well-marked 'cement lines' are often visible, producing the characteristic 'mosaic' or 'crazy-paving' appearance. The bone becomes increasingly sclerotic and brittle, thereby prone to fracture.

Disruption of bone architecture is followed by progressive increased vascularity in the spaces between the thickened bone trabeculae.

The effects of Paget's disease can be widespread (affecting many bones) or localized (15% of cases confined to one area in a single-bone—monostotic—Paget's disease).

Most patients present with one or both of the following features:

- Bone pain—usually localized to site of most active disease
- Bone deformity—following extensive disease, most commonly enlargement of skull, kyphosis or bowing of tibia.

*Complications*—some patients occasionally present with the complications of Paget's disease:

- Nerve compression symptoms—usually seen in association with Paget's disease of the skull, in which enlargement of the pagetic bone can lead to cranial nerve palsies (e.g. CN VIII compression results in deafness). Spinal stenosis may compress spinal nerve roots
- Pathological fracture—bone is increased in bulk but is weaker than normal and more likely to fracture with trivial trauma
- Cardiac hypertrophy—due to increased vascularity of bones
- Malignant tumour (1% of cases)—usually osteosarcoma, which may develop in areas of long-standing active Paget's disease. This is the most common cause of osteosarcoma in the elderly and has a poor prognosis.

---

**Clinical Note**

Investigations in Paget's disease are:
- serology—normal calcium and phosphate, increased alkaline phosphatase
- urine—increased urinary excretion of hydroxyproline
- abnormal isotope bone scans

- X-ray—localized bone enlargement, altered trabecular pattern and alternating areas of rarefaction and increased density.

  Management is by analgesia for bone pain, and calcitonin or bisphosphonates for severe bone pain not controlled by analgesics. The latter inhibit bone resorption.

# INFECTIONS AND TRAUMA

## Osteomyelitis

This infection of bone typically affects the cortex, medulla and periosteum, and it is most commonly encountered in children under the age of 12 years. Adult onset is usually due to compromised host resistance (e.g. severe debilitation, immunosuppression). The most common causative organisms are *Staphylococcus aureus* (over 80% of identified cases), *Mycobacterium tuberculosis*, *Escherichia coli* (particularly in infants and the elderly) and *Salmonella* species (particularly in patients with sickle-cell disease).

Infective organisms gain access to the medullary cavity of the bone by two main routes:

1. Direct access through an open wound, particularly when open fractures are involved. This route is also important in postoperative orthopaedic patients (particularly those with prosthetic joint replacements).
2. Blood-borne spread: following bacteraemia from a focus of sepsis elsewhere.

*Clinical features*—abrupt onset of severe pain at the site of bone infection accompanied by fever and malaise.

Complications and sequelae:

- Resolution—with appropriate antibiotic therapy, ideally based on blood cultures or aspiration material
- Pathological fracture—purulent acute inflammatory exudate formed in closed compartment of marrow cavity causes compression of vessels with necrosis of medullary bone trabeculae, resulting in increased predisposition to fractures
- Adjacent sepsis—destruction of cortical bone may lead to discharge of pus into extraosseous connective tissue, and infection may track through to the skin surface producing a chronic discharging sinus. Spread may also occur to other bones (malignant osteomyelitis) or neighbouring joints (septic arthritis – see later)
- Chronicity—in chronic osteomyelitis, the organisms may remain viable within the marrow cavity for many years. Chronicity results in extensive bone destruction, marrow fibrosis and recurrent focal suppuration (Brodie's abscess). There is also reactive new bone formation, particularly around inflamed periosteum, leading to a thickened and abnormally

shaped bone. Given that osteomyelitis is most common in children, growth disturbance may occur if the physis is damaged.

Diagnosis is by blood culture and isotope scan.

Management is by analgesia, antibiotic therapy and potential surgical drainage of abscesses.

# Fractures

A fracture is a break in the structural continuity of bone. Note that any break, even of only one cortex, constitutes a fracture. Fractures are the most common abnormality of bone and they are caused by physical trauma.

## Types of fracture

Fractures can be classified into two main types according to their relation to surrounding tissues:

1. Simple (closed)—without contact with external environment, i.e. skin or mucous membrane overlying bone is intact. Simple fractures are less likely to become infected.
2. Compound (open)—with direct contact between the fracture and external environment, e.g. a fracture of the tibia with laceration of overlying skin. Compound factures are more likely to become infected.

Other descriptive terms for fractures are:

- comminuted—more than two fragments present
- complicated—involvement of a nerve, artery or viscus
- pathological—fracture occurring in abnormal bone, e.g. in osteoporosis or due to a bone tumour
- stress—slowly developing fracture resulting from repeated application of minor force
- greenstick—usually seen in children, this is where only one side of a bone is fractured, leaving it bent but intact.

## Processes of healing

Bone fractures heal by granulation tissue formation with fibrous repair, followed by new bone formation in the fibrous granulation tissue (see Chapter 2 for wound healing of the skin).

The sequence of events in healing of a simple undisplaced fracture is illustrated in Figure 12.3.

**Fig. 12.3** Healing of a simple fracture. (A) Haematoma formation, due to tearing of medullary blood vessels. (B) Organization: migration of neutrophils and macrophages into fracture with organization of haematoma within about 24 hours. Capillaries and fibroblasts proliferate forming fibrovascular granulation tissue. New osteoprogenitor cells (derived from mesenchymal precursor cells) mature into osteoblasts, and they migrate into granulation tissue. (C) Callus formation: osteoblasts deposit large quantities of osteoid collagen in a haphazard way producing a woven bone pattern. Fracture is bridged on outside by external callus (may contain cartilage) and it is bridged in medullary cavity by internal callus (rarely contains cartilage). However, direct ossification may occur between fractured ends if they are closely apposed. (D) Remodelling: about 3 weeks post fracture, callus is well established and undergoes remodelling. Osteoclastic resorption and osteoblastic osteoid synthesis removes surplus calcified callus, replacing bulky, woven bone with compact, organized, lamellar bone. Process takes several months.
(E) Completion: formation of new lamellar trabecular bone is complete. Bone is orientated in a direction determined by stresses to which it is exposed with mobilization. However, even after remodelling, cortical irregularities and minor marrow space fibrosis persist at site of fracture.

## Complications of healing

Bones show great capacity for healing, but certain complications can occur:

- Malunion—poor anatomical alignment of fractures results in deformity, angulation or displacement.
- Delayed union—this is common, and it is said to have occurred when a fracture has not united in a reasonable time (defined as 25% longer than the average time).
- Non-union—if union has not occurred within 1 year then the terminology is changed from one of 'delayed union' to one of 'non-union'. The defect is typically filled with fibrous tissue/fibrous ankylosis.

### Causes of complications

Efficient healing of fractures requires optimal conditions. Factors that prevent efficient healing are:

- poor apposition of fractured bone ends—a fracture is 'reduced' to achieve the best alignment possible
- inadequate immobilization—immobilization should be achieved by splinting
- interposition of foreign bodies or soft tissues
- infection
- corticosteroid therapy
- poor general nutritional status
- poor blood supply.

## TUMOURS OF THE BONES

## Metastatic disease of the skeleton

Most common tumours in bone are blood-borne metastases from other primary sites or are tumours of the haemopoietic cells located within the marrow spaces of bones, particularly myeloma.

## Carcinomas

There are five common carcinomas that have a predilection for metastasizing to bone:

1. Adenocarcinoma of the breast
2. Carcinoma of bronchus (particularly small cell, undifferentiated carcinoma)
3. Adenocarcinoma of the kidney
4. Adenocarcinoma of the thyroid
5. Adenocarcinoma of the prostate.

Metastases are typically multifocal, occurring most commonly in parts of the skeleton that contain vascular marrow, especially vertebral bodies, ribs, the pelvis, and upper ends of the femur and humerus.

### Osteolytic versus osteosclerotic metastases

Most metastatic tumour cells within bone marrow spaces lead to erosion of bone (osteolytic metastases), through the release of substances that promote osteo-clastic resorption (e.g. prostaglandins, parathyroid-hormone-related peptide; PRHRP). However, prostatic carcinoma (and very rarely breast carcinoma) produces metastatic deposits in which there is osteoblastic stimulation of new bone formation (osteosclerotic metastases) particularly in the lumbosacral vertebrae.

Clinical features:

- Bone pain—usually localized to site of deposits.
- Pathological fractures—erosion of trabecular bone either directly, or through osteoclast-stimulated bone erosion (osteolytic metastases) → bone weakness → fracture.

Complications are:

- leucoerythroblastic anaemia—a result of extensive replacement of bone marrow
- symptoms of hypercalcaemia—caused by the release of calcium from bone by osteolytic process
- nerve and spinal cord compression—particularly in vertebral metastases.

## Haematopoietic malignancies

Haematopoietic malignancies found in bone (e.g. myelomas, lymphomas, leukaemias) are discussed in Chapter 13.

### HINTS AND TIPS

Secondary tumours of bone are more common in adults than children, whereas primary tumours of bone are generally more common in children than adults.

## Bone-forming tumours

These are rare primary bone tumours, derived from cells involved in bone formation and modelling.

## Osteoma

Benign, smooth, rounded bone tumour is seen on the surface of long bones or skull bone. Apart from visible or palpable swelling, there are usually no symptoms. Such tumours are slow-growing and do not undergo malignant transformation. Patients with Gardner's syndrome have multiple osteomas and intestinal polyps.

## Osteoid osteoma and osteoblastoma

### Osteoid osteoma

Rarely causing severe bone pain, this typically arises between the ages of 10 and 30 years. It is more common in males. Most frequently it affects long bones of the lower leg but it may occur in any bone except the skull.

Tumours are composed of active osteoblasts, which deposit large, irregular masses of osteoid collagen in a haphazard manner.

Osteoid osteomas are painful; pain is usually relieved by aspirin but not by rest. Radiographs characteristically show a central dense area surrounded by a halo of translucency. Excision is usually curative and lesions do not recur.

### Osteoblastoma (giant osteoid osteoma)

This large tumour with identical histological features to osteoid osteoma mainly affects the bones of the hands, feet and vertebrae. Tumours are typically more locally aggressive, generating a dull achy pain that is unresponsive to aspirin.

## Osteosarcoma

This malignant tumour of osteoblasts occurs most often in adolescent children, with a second peak in the fifth decade of life linked to highly active Paget's disease. Some cases are associated with familial cancer syndromes of retinoblastoma syndrome (defect in *RB1*) and the Li–Fraumeni syndrome (defect in *p53*). The majority arise around the knee (lower femur or upper tibia) and a minority in other long bones such as the upper end of humerus or femur.

Symptoms are bone pain increasing gradually with tumour growth, but the tumour is often well-advanced at the time of diagnosis. A progressively enlarging bony lump may be palpable.

*Spread*—the tumour grows rapidly within the medullary cavity, eventually eroding through the cortical plate into soft tissue. Metastasis occurs early via the bloodstream, usually to the lung.

Prognosis has improved with the adoption of earlier surgical treatment combined with chemotherapy. However, 5-year survival is still only 50%.

## Cartilage-forming tumours

### Osteochondroma

This is the most common tumour of bone. It is benign, growing as an exophytic nodule from metaphyses of long bones. It is also known as a 'cartilage-capped exostosis' as it is composed of protuberant bone covered with a cap of cartilage and an outer layer of perichondrium.

Lesions are found most commonly in the humerus, femur and the upper end of the tibia. They may be solitary or multiple (typically autosomal dominant condition, hereditary multiple exostoses). Solitary lesions usually first develop in adolescence. Chondrosarcomatous change is rare in solitary lesions but more common in hereditary multiple exostoses.

## Chondroma

This is a benign tumour of hyaline cartilage, composed of well-circumscribed nodules of cytologically benign chondrocytes embedded in a cartilaginous matrix.

Tumours are thought to originate from residual nests of cartilage cells left behind in metaphysis as bone growth proceeds. They are found most commonly in small bones of hands and feet.

They may be single (solitary enchondroma) or multiple (enchondromatosis or Ollier's disease). The term 'enchondroma' is used to indicate that the tumour arises and grows within the medullary cavity of bone (compared to osteochondroma, which grows as a nodular exophytic lesion). A solitary chondroma rarely undergoes malignant change, but occasionally it occurs in multiple enchondromatosis.

## Chondrosarcoma

This slow-growing malignant tumour often reaches a large size, eventually breaking through the periosteum into surrounding soft tissue, but usually maintaining a clearly defined border.

Macroscopically, there is a glistening white appearance, similar to that of normal cartilage.

Microscopically:

- The majority are low-grade, well-differentiated tumours that metastasize very late, and are histologically similar to benign cartilaginous tumours. Radical local surgery may be curative.
- The minority are high-grade, poorly differentiated tumours with marked pleomorphism, high mitotic activity and grow rapidly with early blood-borne metastases.

## Other tumours

### Ewing's sarcoma

A highly malignant bone tumour probably derived from primitive neuroendocrine cells, this affects children between the ages of 5 and 15 years. It has a characteristic chromosomal translocation—t(11;22) (q24; q12)—that results in the fusion of the *FLT-1* gene from chromosome 11 with the *EWS* gene on chromosome 22. The sarcoma usually arises in the diaphyses of long bones, particularly the femur.

Areas of osteolytic bone destruction surrounded by layers of new periosteal bone give the tumour a characteristic 'onion skin' appearance on X-ray. Pain, swelling and tenderness may be associated with fever and leucocytosis (thus tumours are sometimes mistaken for osteomyelitis). Effective chemotherapy, radiotherapy and surgical excision (often amputation) has increased 5-year survival to 75%.

**Fig. 12.4** Summary of bone tumours

| Type | Tumour | Clinical features |
|---|---|---|
| Metastatic (secondary) | Carcinoma of bronchus (especially small cell) Adenocarcinomas of the breast, kidney and thyroid Prostate | Metastases occur most commonly to vertebral bodies, ribs, pelvis and upper ends of femur and humerus |
| Primary | Bone-forming tumours | Osteoma Osteoid osteoma Osteoblastoma Osteosarcoma |
| | Cartilage-forming tumours | Osteochondroma Chondroma Chondroblastoma (Codman's tumour) Chondrosarcoma Chondromyxoid fibroma |
| | Fibrous and fibro-osseous tumour | Fibroma Fibrous dysplasia Fibrosarcoma Malignant fibrous histiocytoma |
| | Others | Ewing's sarcoma Giant cell tumour (osteoclastoma) |

## Giant cell tumour (osteoclastoma)

Osteolytic lesions arise in the epiphyses of long bones, typically in young and middle-aged adults. It only occurs in bones where the epiphyses have fused.

The tumour is composed of a mass of large multinucleated giant cells resembling large osteoclasts embedded in a supporting spindle-celled stroma. There is a gradual expansion of lesions into the metaphysis and the erosion of cortical bone; penetration of the periosteum or articular cartilage may occur.

Osteoclastoma is generally classed as benign, although a significant number become locally invasive and tend to recur after removal. About 10% of cases are truly malignant and metastasize to the lung via the bloodstream.

Figure 12.4 provides a summary of bone tumours.

## DISORDERS OF THE NEUROMUSCULAR JUNCTION

### Overview

Several diseases of muscle have been shown to result from disorders affecting transmission at the neuromuscular junction (NMJ).

Clinical presentation of NMJ dysfunction:

- Fatigability—primarily affecting proximal limb muscles, extraocular muscles (causing ptosis or diplopia) and muscles of mastication, speech and facial expression
- Periodic paralysis—sudden reversible attacks of paralysis and flaccidity.

Disorders can be classified into two types, pre- and postsynaptic abnormalities, depending on which of the synaptic membranes is affected.

## Presynaptic abnormalities

### Botulism

This rare form of food poisoning is caused by ingestion of a toxin produced by the bacterium *Clostridium botulinum*, found in imperfectly treated tinned food or preserved fish contaminated with the microbe.

*Pathogenesis*—the toxin binds irreversibly to those presynaptic nerve terminals of axons whose impulse transmission is acetylcholine (ACh) mediated. These include the NMJ, autonomic ganglia and parasympathetic nerve terminals. Binding of the toxin prevents fusion of ACh vesicles with the neuronal membrane, thereby preventing ACh release.

Clinical symptoms are chiefly vomiting and paresis of skeletal, ocular, pharyngeal and respiratory muscles. Antitoxin is available, but it has no effect once the toxin is bound. Recovery of transmission is achieved by terminal axonal sprouting and the formation of new synaptic contacts. Mortality can be high.

## Lambert–Eaton myasthenic syndrome

This autoimmune disorder is characterized by abnormal fatigability and is often found in patients with lung cancer (when it is considered a paraneoplastic syndrome). Autoantibodies are thought to bind to presynaptic voltage-dependent calcium channels at motor nerve terminals to cause functional loss. This in turn causes the reduced release of ACh in response to nerve stimulation. Small cell lung carcinoma cells express calcium channels, suggesting that cross-reactive autoantibody production is triggered by these tumour antigens.

## Postsynaptic abnormalities

### Myasthenia gravis

This autoimmune disease is characterized by a progressive failure to sustain a maintained or repeated contraction of striated muscle. Prevalence is about 1 in 30 000. The disease usually appears between the ages of 15 and 50 years, and females are more often affected than males.

*Aetiology*—autoantibodies against the post-synaptic acetylcholine receptor are produced by B lymphocytes that are defectively controlled by T lymphocytes as a result of a disorder of the thymus gland. As a result of this interaction, receptors are degraded via a complement reaction, or blocked to activation by acetylcholine. This severely hampers neurotransmission. About 15% of cases have a thymoma (see Chapter 13) and 65% of patients have thymic gland hyperplasia.

There is a strong link to other autoimmune diseases, including thyrotoxicosis (Graves' disease), diabetes mellitus, rheumatoid arthritis (RA), and systemic lupus erythaematosus (SLE). There is linkage with various human leucocyte antigens (HLA), such as A1, B7 and DRw3.

*Presentation*:

* Early symptoms—intermittent ptosis or diplopia, weakness of chewing, swallowing, speaking or of moving the limbs. Movement is initially strong, but it rapidly weakens by the end of the day or after exercise
* Later symptoms—respiratory muscles may be involved and respiratory failure is not an uncommon cause of death. Asphyxia occurs readily as the cough may be too weak to clear foreign bodies from the airways. Muscle atrophy may occur in long-standing cases.

The disease runs a remitting/relapsing course, and relapses may be precipitated by emotional disturbances, infections, pregnancy or severe muscular effort.

The prognosis is variable. If the disorder is confined to eye muscles, then the prognosis for life is normal and disability slight. A prognosis of myasthenia associated with thymoma is markedly worse.

**Clinical Note**

Investigations in myasthenia gravis:
* Tensilon test—short-acting, anticholinesterase drug trial increases acetylcholine (ACh) concentrations in the synaptic cleft and transiently relieves symptoms
* Autoantibody screen—elevated ACh receptor antibody in 80% of cases
* Electromyography (EMG)—characteristic decremental response
* CT thorax scan—identify thymomas
* Autoimmune screening—especially for thyroid diseases.
  Management:
* Medical—anticholinesterase drugs (prevent ACh breakdown); immunological treatment: plasma exchange (removes autoantibody), intravenous immunoglobulin, immunosuppressant treatment
* Surgical—thymectomy.

## MYOPATHIES

### Definition

Myopathy is any condition that primarily affects muscle physiology, structure or biochemistry.

### Inherited myopathies

#### X-linked muscular dystrophy

Muscular dystrophy is the term used to describe inherited degenerative muscle diseases.

X-linked muscular dystrophy is characterized by the progressive degeneration of single muscle cells over a prolonged period of time. It results in muscle fibre destruction with the development of fibrosis.

#### Duchenne muscular dystrophy

The pattern of inheritance is X-linked recessive (p21 region); hence the disorder is almost exclusively seen in males. This is the most common form of muscular dystrophy in childhood, affecting 1 in 3500 male births.

The disorder is due to a mutation of the gene coding for dystrophin, a protein that normally anchors the actin cytoskeleton of muscle fibres to the basement membrane via a membrane glycoprotein complex (Fig. 12.5). Dystrophin helps to transmit the forces of

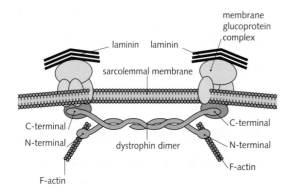

Fig. 12.5   Anchorage role of dystrophin. Dystrophin molecule is a long, rod-shaped protein, one end binding to membrane glycoprotein, the other to actin, with middle rod region.

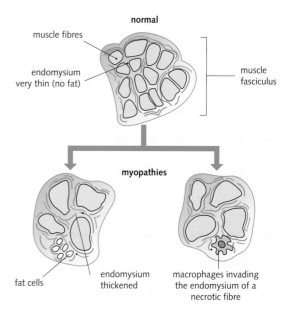

Fig. 12.6   Changes in muscle associated with Duchenne muscular dystrophy.

contraction, meaning that muscle fibres in Duchenne patients are liable to tearing with repeated contraction.

Different degrees of severity of Duchenne dystrophy result from different mutations within the dystrophin gene:

- Severe Duchenne dystrophy—complete failure to produce dystrophin as a result of mutations causing gene frameshifts
- Moderate to severe forms of Duchenne dystrophy—dystrophin is produced but anchorage is inefficient because of mutations in binding sites for either membrane glycoprotein complex or actin cytoskeleton
- Mild form of Duchenne dystrophy (Becker's dystrophy)—mutation in the middle rod region produces an abnormally weighted dystrophin protein which is still capable of anchoring muscle to basement membrane. Becker's dystrophy has a later onset than Duchenne.

*Morphological features*—muscle changes associated with Duchenne are illustrated in Figure 12.6.

*Clinical features*—childhood onset of muscle weakness is associated with a high serum creatine phosphokinase level (caused by muscle necrosis) and calf hypertrophy due to fatty replacement of muscle (pseudo-hypertrophy; Fig. 12.4). Cardiac muscle is also affected leading to cardiomyopathy (see Chapter 6).

The prognosis depends on the degree of severity. For severe Duchenne it is very poor; most affected individuals are wheelchair dependent in their early teens and dead by their early twenties.

## Myotonic disorders

Myotonic disorders are diseases in which there is a continuing contraction of muscle after voluntary contraction has ceased.

### Myotonic muscular dystrophy

This autosomal dominant disorder is characterized by muscle weakness, myotonia (inability to relax muscles) and several non-muscle features including cataracts, frontal baldness in males, gonadal atrophy, cardiomyopathy and (in some cases) dementia.

This is the most common inherited muscle disease of adults, affecting 1 in 8000.

The genetic abnormality is an unstable CTG repeat sequence in a cAMP-dependent protein kinase located on chromosome 19. The disease shows anticipation, meaning that it appears at a younger age in each succeeding generation. The mechanism by which this mutation causes myotonia is unknown.

Microscopically, affected muscles show abnormalities of fibre size with fibre necrosis, abundant internal nuclei and replacement by fibrofatty tissue.

The disorder usually becomes apparent in adolescence or early adulthood with facial weakness and disturbed gait.

*Prognosis*—death is commonly due to involvement of respiratory muscles in middle-age.

## Acquired myopathies

### Idiopathic inflammatory myopathies

There is primary inflammation of muscle with resulting fibre necrosis. The inflammatory infiltrate is mainly composed of T lymphocytes and monocytes as part of an abnormal autoimmune response. There are three main types of inflammatory myopathies, any of which may occur as part of an immune-mediated systemic disease such as systemic sclerosis.

## Polymyositis

This inflammatory muscle disorder is characterized by weakness, pain and swelling of proximal limb muscles and facial muscles, often with ptosis and dysphagia. It is the most common inflammatory muscle disorder, though still relatively rare. It occurs most frequently in adults, with females affected more than males by 3:1.

*Aetiology*—cytotoxic T cells and other lymphoid cells are found within the endomysium suggesting autoimmune injury of myocytes, but the mechanism of sensitization is unknown.

Associations:

- Increased predisposition in people with HLA-B8/DR3
- Connective tissue diseases such as SLE, RA or scleroderma
- Dermatomyositis—see below
- Malignancy—particularly in association with non-Hodgkin's lymphoma, lung and bladder cancer.

Microscopically, there is a lymphocytic infiltration of muscle with fibre necrosis.

*Clinical features*—an insidious onset in the third to fifth decade of life, with symmetrical proximal muscle weakness initially affecting the lower limbs. Progression is typically slow but it may eventually involve pharyngeal, laryngeal and respiratory muscles leading to dysphagia, dysphonia and respiratory failures.

*Investigations*—blood: increased muscle enzymes (e.g. creatine kinase); tests for rheumatoid factor and antinuclear factor are often positive. Electromyography: useful for demonstrating myopathy without neuropathy. Muscle biopsy: muscle necrosis and regeneration in association with inflammatory cell infiltrate. Magnetic resonance imaging: non-invasive detection of active myositis.

*Treatment*—it may respond to immunosuppressive treatment such as corticosteroids and azathioprine.

## Dermatomyositis

This has the muscle components of polymyositis accompanied by periorbital oedema and a characteristic purple 'heliotrope' rash on the upper eyelids. Often, there is also an erythaematous, scaling rash on the face, shoulders, upper arms and chest with red patches over the knuckles, elbows and knees. Arthralgia, weight loss and fever sometimes occur.

Dermatomyositis has an even stronger association with malignancy than polymyositis, especially affecting the ovary, pancreas, colon, lung and stomach.

## Inclusion body myositis

This slowly progressive inflammatory muscle disorder is similar to polymyositis, but typically affects distal muscles in an asymmetric pattern. It also occurs mainly in the elderly. By light microscopy, histological features also appear similar to polymyositis, but with electron microscopy vacuoles containing filamentous inclusion bodies can be seen within fibres.

## Endocrine myopathies

There is a weakness and wasting of muscle associated with endocrine disease. The main causes are:

- corticosteroid-induced myopathy—either therapeutic or in Cushing's disease.Corticosteroids are associated with type 2 muscle fibre atrophy
- myopathies of thyroid dysfunction—associated with both hyperthyroidism and hypothyroidism
- myopathy of osteomalacia—painful myopathy often without much wasting or weakness.

Changes are usually reversible with appropriate therapy.

## ARTHROPATHIES

## Osteoarthritis

Osteoarthritis (OA) is a degenerative disease of articular cartilage. It is associated with secondary changes in underlying bone resulting in pain and impaired function of the affected joint. Although the name suggests that primary OA is an inflammatory process, its main effects on the erosion of cartilage are independent of acute or chronic inflammation, even though inflammatory cells may be present in the affected joint.

It is extremely common—80% of the elderly population show radiographic evidence of OA, although only around 25% of these are symptomatic.

Females are affected more than males, except at the hip where both genders are equally prone to OA. It is increasingly common above 60 years of age, but it may also occur in younger age groups following any form of mechanical derangement.

OA affects joints that are constantly exposed to wear and tear, typically large weight-bearing joints (e.g. those of the hip and knee), but also small joints in the hands, particularly the base of the thumb. The aetiology is as follows:

- Primary—no obvious causes or predisposing factors (majority of cases)
- Secondary—arising as a complication of other joint disorders, mainly inflammatory joint disease, congenital joint deformities, trauma to joints, avascular necrosis of bone.

Secondary OA is also an important component of occupational joint disease, e.g. OA of the fingers in typists and of the knee in professional footballers.

Risk factors for the development of OA are:

- fixed—ageing, genetic predisposition, female gender (except hip OA), abnormal joint structure
- modifiable—abnormal load on joints, repetitive loading, trauma.

## Pathological changes

Pathological changes involve cartilage, bone, synovium and joint capsule with secondary effects on muscle (Fig. 12.7).

Early stage:

- Erosion and destruction of articular cartilage— degenerate superficial cartilage splits along lines of fibres to produce fronds (fibrillation). Narrowing of the joint space can be seen on radiography

**Fig. 12.7** Pathological changes in osteoarthritis (OA). (A) Normal joint. (B) Early stages of OA. (C) Later stages of OA.

- Inflammation and thickening of the joint capsule and synovium.

Later stages:

- Sclerosis of subarticular bone—caused by constant friction of naked bone surfaces which now articulate in the absence of cartilage (bone eburnation).
- Osteophytes form around the periphery of the joint by irregular outgrowth of bone. Some may break off to form loose bodies within the joint. In distal interphalangeal joints of the fingers, osteophytes appear as small nodules (Heberden's nodes); in proximal interphalangeal joints, they are called Bouchard's nodes.
- Small cysts may develop in areas where the bone is not thickened as a result of synovial fluid accumulation in underlying bone.
- Reactive thickening of synovium and joint capsule due to inflammation caused by bone and cartilage debris.
- Disuse atrophy of muscle due to immobility of the diseased joint.

OA can be classified according to the main presenting features as follows:

- Primary generalized OA—usually associated with development of Heberden's nodes on fingers. It is most common in postmenopausal women
- Erosive inflammatory OA—form of OA in which there is severe inflammation and erosion of cartilage, with rapid progression
- Hypertrophic OA—florid osteophyte formation and bone sclerosis, but with slow progression and a relatively good prognosis.

## Clinical features

The main symptoms of OA are pain and limitation in the movement of the affected joint, which often leads to functional impairment (e.g. difficulty walking in hip OA). Sometimes OA is associated with visible swelling around the joint margins (usually as an effect of osteophytes).

In OA of the cervical vertebrae (cervical spondylosis), osteophytes compressing emerging spinal nerves are responsible for much of the symptomatology.

### Clinical Note

OA diagnosis is largely clinical, although there are four classic X-ray signs (of which one or more may be seen):
1. Narrowed joint space
2. Osteophytes (at bone margins)
3. Cysts
4. Sclerosis.

Treatment:
- Lifestyle—reduce pressure across joint (e.g. weight loss, walking stick) and encourage strengthening exercises
- Medical—analgesics and NSAIDs for pain relief; intra-articular or periarticular corticosteroid injections if severe pain (especially knee OA)
- Surgical—joint replacement for advanced hip or knee disease.

## Rheumatoid arthritis

Rheumatoid arthritis (RA) is a chronic inflammatory joint disease caused by a multisystem connective tissue autoimmune disorder, rheumatoid disease (see below). It affects about 1% of the UK population, females more than males by about 3:1. Onset is typically between 35 and 45 years of age, but it follows a normal distribution curve and no age group is exempt.

RA mainly affects peripheral synovial joints such as the fingers and wrists, but it can also affect the knees and more proximal joints. The most common presentations are symmetrical.

The aetiology is autoimmune and there is an association with HLA-DR4 haplotype in most ethnic groups. The condition is characterized by autoimmune-mediated activation of CD4+ T cells within affected joints. The antigen for this reaction is unknown, but once it has been triggered, the release of proinflammatory cytokines drives the destruction of the joint.

Many RA patients have a circulating autoantibody directed against the Fc portion of native immunoglobulins (rheumatoid factor). The presence of rheumatoid factor (seropositive arthritis) helps to distinguish RA from several other inflammatory joint diseases (seronegative arthritis), but not all RA patients are rheumatoid factor positive. The exact role and underlying stimulus of rheumatoid factor is uncertain. However, immunological techniques have demonstrated it in plasma cells located in the synovium of affected joints. There is increasing evidence to suggest that RA is a disease of both cellular and humoral immune mechanisms.

## Pathological changes

There are three main pathological changes (Fig. 12.8):

1. Rheumatoid synovitis
2. Articular cartilage destruction
3. Focal destruction of bone.

### Rheumatoid synovitis

The synovium becomes swollen and shows a villous pattern. Chronic inflammatory cells (mainly lymphocytes and plasma cells) increase in number within the synovial

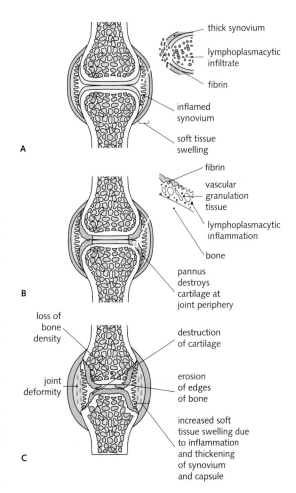

**Fig. 12.8** Pathological changes in rheumatoid arthritis (RA). (A) Rheumatoid synovitis. (B) Articular cartilage destruction. (C) Focal destruction of bone.

stroma, often forming an exudate that effuses into the joint space. Fibrin is deposited on the surface of the synovium, which undergoes hypertrophy. Soft tissue swelling from synovial inflammation may be marked.

### Articular cartilage destruction

Inflammatory granulation tissue grows across the surface of the cartilage (pannus) from the edges of the joint. The articular surface shows the loss of cartilage beneath the extending pannus, most marked at joint margins.

### Focal destruction of bone

Osteolytic destruction of bone occurs at the edges of the joint. Bone 'erosions' can be seen on radiography and are associated with joint deformity. There is also increased soft tissue swelling due to inflammation and thickening of the synovium and capsule.

# Clinical features

## Symmetrical polyarthritis

The insidious onset of arthritis first attacks finger joints (mainly metacarpophalangeal and proximal interphalangeal joints) followed by metatarsophalangeal joints and joints of the ankles, wrists, knees, shoulders, elbows and hips (in decreasing order of frequency). RA can also affect synovial joints of the spine (particularly cervical). Affected joints become swollen, painful and warm, often with redness of overlying skin. Stiffness tends to be worse in the mornings or following inactivity.

> **HINTS AND TIPS**
>
> In the hands, rheumatoid arthritis tends to affect metacarpophalangeal (MCP) and proximal interphalangeal (PIP) joints whereas OA tends to affect PIP and distal interphalangeal (DIP) joints.

## Joint deformities

As the disease progresses, muscle atrophy and joint destruction result in limitation of joint motion, joint instability, subluxation and deformities. Subluxation is the partial dislocation of a joint such that the bone ends still make contact, but are misaligned. There are also flexion contractures of small joints of the hands and feet, knees, hips and elbows.

Of the hands:

- Anterior subluxation of the metacarpophalangeal (MCP) joints with ulnar deviation of the fingers
- 'Swan neck' deformity—hyperextension of proximal interphalangeal (PIP) joint with fixed flexion at distal interphalangeal (DIP) joints
- Boutonnière (buttonhole) deformity—fixed flexion of proximal interphalangeal joint and extension of the terminal interphalangeal joint
- Z deformity of the thumbs—fixed flexion at metacarpophalangeal joint and hyperextension at interphalangeal joint.

In the wrists there is often a fixed flexion deformity with a prominent, tender ulnar styloid process and pain on pronation/supination.

In the knees, Baker's cyst (cystic swelling in the popliteal fossa) is seen.

In the cervical spine, there is atlantoaxial subluxation.

Deformities are initially correctable but permanent contractures eventually develop such that joints become completely disorganized.

## Rheumatoid nodules

Joint changes are often associated with development of subcutaneous rheumatoid nodules, usually located over the extensor aspect of the forearm but occasionally found overlying other bony prominences. Nodules are composed of extensive areas of fibrinoid material surrounded by a giant cell granulomatous reaction. They occur elsewhere in the body as part of the rheumatoid disease (see below).

# Complications

- Secondary OA as a result of loss of articular surface, particularly in weight-bearing joints such as the knee
- Septic arthritis—infection of the joint secondary to invasion from an ulcerated nodule or infected skin lesion
- Amyloidosis—found in 25–30% of RA patients at autopsy
- Carpal tunnel syndrome
- Ruptured extensor tendons of the hand.

# Investigations and diagnosis

## Investigations

- Radiography—periarticular osteopenia, loss of articular cartilage (joint space), erosions, subluxation and ankylosis
- Serology—rheumatoid factors (IgG- or IgM-type immunoglobulins that react with the Fc portion of IgG). This is present in 60–80% of those with RA and in 10% of people without RA
- Measuring acute phase response—usually present in widespread RA as measured by, e.g. erythrocyte sedimentation rate (ESR), C-reactive protein (CRP).

## Diagnosis

Diagnosis of RA can be made with four or more of the following criteria (which have been taken from the American Rheumatism Association, 1988 revision):

- Morning stiffness (> 1 hour), of at least 6 weeks' duration
- Arthritis of three or more joint areas, of at least 6 weeks' duration
- Arthritis of hand joints, of at least 6 weeks' duration
- Symmetrical arthritis, of at least 6 weeks' duration
- Rheumatoid nodules
- Rheumatoid factor
- Radiological changes.

> **Clinical Note**
>
> RA treatment involves:
> - symptom management—analgesics, NSAIDs, intra-articular steroid injections
> - disease-modifying anti-rheumatic drugs (DMARDs)—improve symptoms and reduce radiological progression, e.g. sulfasalazine, methotrexate. Newer anti-TNFa monoclonal antibody agents are used in refractory disease
> - surgery—for advanced painful joint disease.

RA is associated with increased mortality, reducing lifespan by an average of 8–15 years. Worse prognosis is associated with being female, being positive for rheumatoid factor and having MTP joint or systemic involvement.

## Extra-articular features (rheumatoid disease)

### Lungs
Pulmonary involvement causes interstitial pneumonitis and fibrosing alveolitis, which eventually leads to a pattern of interstitial pulmonary fibrosis. Also, patients may develop lesions similar to the subcutaneous rheumatoid nodule, both within the lungs and on the pleural surfaces. These rheumatoid granulomas are particularly common in patients who already have industrial lung disease caused by inhaling various types of silica; the association of coal-worker's lung with rheumatoid granulomas in seropositive miners is called Caplan's syndrome. Pleural effusions, bronchitis and bronchiectasis are all more common in rheumatoid patients.

### Blood vessels
There may be development of vasculitis which is either:

- acute neutrophilic vasculitis, presenting with purpura and occasional foci of ulceration

  Or

- lymphocytic vasculitis, producing a more low-key erythaematous patchy rash.

### Eyes
Dry eye syndrome (keratoconjunctivitis sicca) is caused by lymphocytic inflammation of both lacrimal and mucous glands (secondary Sjögren's syndrome, present in 15% of all RA patients). Lack of tears leads to secondary inflammation of the cornea. In addition, sight-threatening scleritis may occur because of degeneration of collagenous tissue in the eye.

### Haemopoietic and lymphoreticular systems
Anaemia of chronic disease is common in rheumatoid patients and a minority develops hypersplenism or lymphadenopathy. The risk of lymphoma is also increased in longstanding rheumatoid disease. Felty's syndrome describes splenomegaly, lymphadenopathy, anaemia and leucopenia with RA. Sepsis is an important and common cause of death in these patients.

### Neurological system
Hypertrophied synovium and joint deformities increase the likelihood of peripheral compression neuropathies. Bilateral carpal tunnel syndrome is a relatively common early manifestation of RA. Spinal nerve compression also occurs; severe and potentially fatal cord compression may follow atlantoaxial subluxation.

### Heart
About one-third of RA patients develop asymptomatic pericarditis, which occasionally becomes complicated by a pericardial effusion. Rheumatoid nodules may cause heart block, cardiomyopathy and ischaemia (by coronary artery compression).

A summary of the effects of rheumatoid disease is provided in Figure 12.9.

## Juvenile rheumatoid arthritis

This accounts for approximately 15% of cases of juvenile chronic arthritis. By definition, it begins before 16 years of age. Clinical features are similar to those of adults but smaller joints tend to be spared, rheumatoid nodules are usually absent and rheumatoid factor is often negative. Systemic manifestations are more common and prognosis is considered worse than for adults.

## Ankylosing spondylitis

This is an example of a seronegative arthritis (rheumatoid factor negative). It is an inflammatory arthritic disorder characterized by a rigid spine due to ossification of the spinal joints and ligaments. The condition begins in the lumbar vertebral spine and sacroiliac joints, extending upwards to involve thoracic and cervical vertebrae over a period of months or years. There may also be involvement of peripheral joints, mainly the hips and knees.

It affects 0.5% of the population in the UK, typically presenting in late adolescence and young adults (age 15–30 years of age), and in males more than females by 3:1.

The aetiology is unknown but more than 90% of individuals with ankylosing spondylitis have the HLA-B27 antigen (less than 10% of the normal population have this antigen), which suggests an autoimmune disorder. HLA-B27 positivity is a common feature of the seronegative arthritides.

*Morphological changes*—chronic inflammation of vertebral ligaments slowly heals by dense fibrosis and ossification ('bony ankylosis') to form a rigid shell that links the periphery of the vertebral bodies. Eventually the vertebral column becomes fused, inflexible and rigid ('bamboo spine').

There is typically an insidious onset of recurring episodes of low back pain and stiffness, sometimes radiating to the buttocks or thighs. Symptoms are characteristically worse in early morning and after inactivity.

Systemic manifestations include aortic valve incompetence (as a result of rheumatoid aortitis), anterior uveitis and amyloidosis.

**Fig. 12.9** Clinical features of rheumatoid disease.

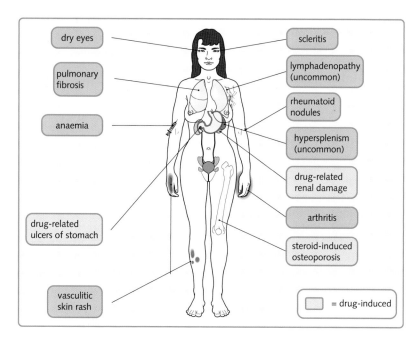

On investigation, ESR and CRP are usually raised but may be normal, serology is negative for rheumatoid factor and X-rays may show sacroiliitis and bridging syndesmophytes between vertebrae.

The disease progresses slowly but unremittingly. Management is by:

- lifestyle—regular physiotherapy and exercise (e.g. non-weight-bearing sports like swimming) to maintain as full mobility as possible and prevent deformity
- medical—mainly NSAIDs for symptomatic relief
- surgery for associated hip disease, including hip replacement.

Seventy-five per cent of individuals with ankylosing spondylitis maintain a good quality of life with minimal disability.

A comparison of joint diseases is provided in infection (Fig. 12.10).

## Arthritis in association with other systemic disease

### Reiter's syndrome

This inflammatory syndrome is characterized by the triad of arthritis, urethritis and conjunctivitis. It complicates 0.8% of urethral infection in males and 0.2% of cases of dysentery. It occurs in males more than females by 15:1 and the usual age of onset is 20–40 years of age. More than 80% of patients are HLA-B27 positive.

Classification is on the basis of aetiology:

- Genital type—usually follows non-specific (non-gonococcal) urethritis or, less commonly, cystitis or prostatitis
- Intestinal or postdysenteric type—in some parts of the world it may follow dysentery or occasionally non-specific diarrhoea, occurring 10–30 days after intestinal manifestations.

The underlying pathological mechanism is unknown but is probably autoimmune, triggered by the prior infection.

Clinical features are:

- arthritis, usually affecting knee or ankle, and developing within weeks of the infectious episode. Clinically and histologically, arthritis resembles rheumatoid arthritis with chronic inflammatory synovitis
- dysuria and penile (or vaginal) discharge
- conjunctivitis (in 30% of cases).

*Prognosis*—the first attack typically resolves spontaneously within 6 months. However, 50% of patients relapse and some have continued relapsing chronic arthritis, causing disability but seldom deformity. In a minority of cases, there is development of severe spondylitis and features very similar to ankylosing spondylitis.

### Psoriatic arthritis

About 5% of psoriasis patients develop arthropathy, which characteristically involves the distal interphalangeal joints (see Chapter 14).

**Fig. 12.10** Comparison of joint diseases

|  | Osteoarthritis | Rheumatoid disease | Ankylosing spondylitis |
|---|---|---|---|
| Affected age group | Elderly | Any age | Onset usually before 30 years |
| Rheumatoid factor | Negative | Positive | Usually negative |
| Sex | Females > males | Females > males | Males > females |
| HLA association | None known | HLA-DR4 | HLA-B27 |
| Hands | Heberden's nodes (DIP) Bouchard's nodes (PIP) | Ulnar deviation of MCP joints Swan neck deformity Boutonnière deformity Z deformity of thumbs Prominent ulnar styloid process | — |
| Affected joints | Mainly hip, knees and spine. Usually asymmetrical. | Any Usually symmetrical | Mainly spine |
| Joint pathology | Erosion of cartilage Osteophytes | Destruction of joints | Bony ankylosis |
| Synovial pathology | Slight synovial hyperplasia | Florid synovial hyperplasia; pannus | — |
| Associated diseases | — | Rheumatoid disease Sjögren's syndrome Interstitial lung fibrosis | Aortic valve incompetence Uveitis Amyloidosis |

*Note: DIP, distal interphalangeal; MCP, metacarpophalangeal; PIP, proximal interphalangeal*

## Arthritis associated with gastrointestinal disease

### Bacterial gastroenteritis
Like Reiter's syndrome, this is a reactive arthritis, occurring after infection with *Salmonella*, *Yersinia* or *Campylobacter* species. HLA-B27 antigen is again present in 80% of affected patients.

### Inflammatory bowel disease
Enteropathic arthritis is seen at some stage in up to 20% of patients with ulcerative colitis and Crohn's disease. Typically it involves knee joints, but occasionally also ankles, elbows and small digital joints. Sacroiliitis and ankylosing spondylitis are also much more frequent in patients with inflammatory bowel disease.

## Others

### Neuropathic (Charcot's) joint disease
This joint disease occurs secondary to the loss of pain and position sense within the joint, which is swollen and deformed but not painful. Possible causes of loss of joint sensation include diabetic neuropathy, tabes dorsalis, syringomyelia, leprosy and cauda equina lesions (e.g. myelomeningocele).

### Sarcoid arthritis
Arthritis occurs in 10% of patients with sarcoidosis, with onset typically in the first year of the disease. It may be of two types:

1. Early acute transient type—polyarticular symmetrical arthritis typically affecting knees and ankles, and usually associated with erythema nodosum. Arthritis is typically self-limiting
2. Chronic persistent type—polyarticular associated with chronic sarcoidosis.

## Crystal arthropathies

These diseases are characterized by deposition of crystals in joints and soft tissues. Affected patients usually present with an episode of acute arthritis, inflammation being caused by the deposition of the crystals, sometimes called a 'chemical arthritis'. With time, inflammatory changes lead to the development of chronic arthritis with features of OA (secondary OA).

**Fig. 12.11** Comparison of true gout and pseudogout

|  | True gout | Pseudogout |
| --- | --- | --- |
| Crystal type | Urate | Calcium pyrophosphate |
| Underlying process | Hyperuricaemia | Chondrocalcinosis |
| Joints affected | Small | Large |
| Pain | Severe | Moderate |

## Nomenclature

The term 'gout' is used as a clinical description of joints affected by crystal deposition. This term is then refined by demonstrating the type of crystal involved. There are two main types of crystal arthropathies: urate gout ('true gout' or simply 'gout') and calcium pyrophosphate gout ('pseudogout'). A comparison of the two types is shown in Figure 12.11.

## Gout

This acute inflammatory crystal arthropathy is caused by the deposition of urate crystal in joints and soft tissues as a result of hyperuricaemia. Prevalence is about 1% of the UK population and it is largely confined to men (90%), although some women develop the condition postmenopausally, It can present at any time above the age of 20.

*Aetiology*—uric acid is normally derived from the breakdown of purines and is excreted in the urine. Increased concentrations of serum uric acid (hyperuricaemia) can result in gout.

There are two main causes of hyperuricaemia:

1. Underexcretion of uric acid (most common)—of uncertain origin but clinically associated with hyperlipidaemia, renal failure, lactic acidosis (alcohol, exercise, starvation, vomiting) and thiazide diuretics
2. Overproduction of uric acid (least common)—a result of either high cell turnover (e.g. leukaemia, chemotherapy, severe psoriasis) or rare congenital enzyme defects of purine metabolism.

However, it should be noted that the majority of patients who have a raised blood uric acid level will never develop gout or any of its complications. The condition has a familial tendency, and it is believed to be polygenically inherited.

### Pathogenesis

Gout affects the joints, soft tissues and kidney, as discussed below.

*Joints*—supersaturation of urate in synovial fluid results in the precipitation of urate crystals in certain joints, forming white powdery deposits on the surface of articular cartilage, beneath which degenerative changes can be seen. Crystal release into the synovial fluid stimulates an acute inflammatory reaction leading to the excruciating pain, oedema and the redness seen in acutely inflamed joints. Microscopically, neutrophil polymorphs can be seen to phagocytose urate crystal in the joint fluid. Repeated acute attacks eventually produce chronic arthritis and large urate crystal aggregations (tophi).

*Soft tissues*—uric acid crystals are also deposited in the soft tissues around joints, where their presence excites a foreign body, giant cell reaction. These soft tissue masses may also enlarge to produce tophi, especially around the pinna of the ear.

*Kidney*—in 10% of patients, urate crystals deposited in the kidney may lead to an interstitial nephritis and to renal calculi composed of uric acid. Crystals may also cause urinary obstruction, increasing the likelihood of complications such as pyelonephritis.

### Clinical features

Characteristics of gout are:

* intermittent attacks of excruciating pain, oedema and redness (acute gouty arthritis)
* monoarthropathy (90%); polyarthropathy (two or more affected joints) 10%
* metatarsophalangeal joint of the big toe is most commonly affected (podagra, 75% of cases), but gout occasionally affects the ankle and, less commonly, the knee and hip.

Recurrent attacks affecting the same joint eventually lead to articular cartilage destruction, chronic synovial thickening and secondary OA-chronic gouty arthritis.

Diagnosis:

* Clinical features (as above)
* Raised serum urate level
* Presence of crystals of sodium urate in aspirated synovial fluid from joint (detected with polarizing light).

*Management*—analgesia for acute attacks: NSAIDs (e.g. indometacin) and colchicine. Preventative measures in recurrent disease:

- Allopurinol—suppresses uric acid synthesis by inhibiting xanthine oxidase
- Uricosuric agents—e.g. probenecid
- Diet—excessive purine intake and overindulgence in alcohol should be avoided.

*Prognosis*—some patients have only a single attack or suffer another only after an interval of many years. More often there is a tendency towards recurrent attacks that increase in frequency and duration so that, eventually, attacks merge and the patient remains in a prolonged state of subacute gout.

## Pseudogout

This acute inflammatory crystal arthropathy is caused by deposition of calcium pyrophosphate crystals in articular cartilage of joints (chondrocalcinosis). It is most common in the elderly and affects males more than females.

The aetiology can be sporadic, metabolic or familial:

- Sporadic—in the vast majority of cases, the cause of pyrophosphate deposition is unknown but it is probably an age-related phenomenon
- Metabolic—in patients under the age of 60 years, the disease is often associated with hyperparathyroidism, haemochromatosis or other less common metabolic or endocrine disorders
- Familial—in a minority of patients, the disease is inherited as an autosomal dominant disorder.

### Pathogenesis

Chondrocalcinosis is often asymptomatic. However, if crystals are shed into the joint space, patients develop an acute arthritis similar to that seen in urate gout. This shedding of crystals may be precipitated by trauma or intercurrent illness, or it may be spontaneous.

With time, damage to cartilage leads to the development of secondary OA.

*Clinical features*—as with gout, the affected joint becomes suddenly painful, warm, swollen and tender. However, the most commonly affected joint is the knee (> 50% of cases), followed by the wrist, shoulder and ankle. The duration of the attack can vary from days to weeks and recurrent attacks are uncommon.

Diagnosis is by X-ray – cartilaginous calcification is usually obvious on X-ray – and by the presence of calcium pyrophosphate dihydrate crystals in aspirated synovial fluid from the joint (detected with polarizing light).

Intra-articular aspiration and corticosteroids are the most effective treatment for acute pseudogout (anti-inflammatory drugs and colchicine also work but are often avoided in the elderly).

## Infective (septic) arthritis

This inflammation of a joint is caused by infection—typically bacterial. This may affect any age group but children and young adults are the most commonly affected. It is a medical emergency, with a mortality rate of 10%. In older adults, most cases are associated with penetrating injury. Males are affected more often than females by 2:1. The knee and hip are the most common sites.

*Aetiology*—a wide range of bacteria may be responsible, but *Staphylococcus aureus*, streptococci and *Haemophilus* species are the most important. Patients who have developed septic arthritis always have bacteraemia.

Risk factors are diabetes, RA, joint puncture, surgery and immunosuppressive treatment.

Bacteria gain access to a joint via:

- local trauma—well-recognized complication of penetrating injury such as open fractures, insertion of surgical prosthesis and non-sterile, intra-articular injection of steroids for established autoimmune arthritis
- spread from adjacent infective foci—especially in neonates with epiphyseal osteomyelitis
- haematogenous spread—most common route, usually from the skin or upper respiratory tract. Intravenous drug users are particularly likely to develop septic arthritis associated with Gram-negative bacteraemia.

*Clinical features*—there is an abrupt onset of severe pain, tenderness, swelling and erythema. The majority of cases affect a single joint only but some cases of gonococcal arthritis and arthritis in intravenous drug abusers may affect more joints.

*Complications*—untreated, it proceeds rapidly to joint destruction often with osteomyelitis, sinus formation, ankylosis and dislocation of the hip.

### Clinical Note

Septic arthritis is one of a group of conditions that may cause gait abnormalities in children (the limping child'). Trauma and septic arthritis occur throughout childhood, but other disorders are relatively age-specific:

- 1–5 years—developmental dysplasia of the hip (DDH): unstable hip joints more common in girls
- 5–10 years—Perthes' disease: avascular necrosis of the femoral head
- 10–15 years—slipped upper femoral epiphysis (SUFE): displaced femoral head, most commonly in pubertal boys.

*Diagnosis*—radiographs are normal at first but useful to exclude fractures or other bony injury. Later in the course of the disease, features of periarticular osteoporosis, joint space narrowing, periostitis and articular erosions may become apparent. Examination and culture of aspirated joint space fluid is essential for identification of the causative organism.

Treatment is by antibiotic therapy (intravenous or intramuscular).

The prognosis for recovery without joint damage is directly related to the speed with which antibiotic therapy is instituted.

In this chapter, you will learn to:
- Describe the patterns of common autoimmune diseases.
- Discuss the causes of primary and secondary immunodeficiency.
- Understand amyloidosis and its widespread effects.
- Recall the causes of increased and decreased numbers of white blood cells.
- Discuss neoplasms of white blood cells, focusing on lymphomas, leukaemias and myelomas.
- Describe disorders of the spleen and thymus.
- Logically describe the causes for the common clinical presentation of anaemia.
- Recall the mechanisms that produce polycythaemia.
- Discuss common disorders of haemostasis affecting blood vessel walls, platelets and clotting factors.

## AUTOIMMUNE DISEASE

Autoimmune diseases that cause damage in many tissues and organs, involving a number of systems, are termed 'multisystem' or 'systemic' autoimmune diseases (Fig. 13.1).

### Systemic lupus erythematosus

This inflammatory disorder of connective tissues is associated with autoantibodies to a variety of autoantigens. Many tissues are affected but synovial joints, skin, kidneys and the brain are the major target organs (Fig. 13.2).

Systemic lupus erythematosus (SLE) affects 30 per 100 000 of the UK population, and it presents most commonly in the young and middle-aged with a peak incidence between 20 and 30 years of age. Females are more affected than males by about 8:1.

The aetiology is unknown but there is a strong familial tendency. Drugs (hydralazine, phenytoin, procainamide), chemicals and unidentified viral infections have all been postulated as the sensitizing stimulus to autoantibody production.

*Pathogenesis*—SLE appears to be a disorder of immune system self-tolerance, as patients develop autoantibodies to a wide array of self-antigens. Antibodies are produced against components of both nucleic acids and cytoplasmic phospholipids:

- Anti-dsDNA—antibody against double-stranded DNA (most frequently detected)
- Anti-DNA histone—drug induced SLE

- Antibodies to other nuclear components—anti-Ro, anti-La and anti-Sm
- Antiphospholipid (cardiolipin)—causes thrombotic tendency, recurrent abortions and false-positive test for syphilis
- Rheumatoid factors—antibodies directed against self-IgG antibodies.

None of these antibodies is specific for SLE and most have been detected in other connective tissue disorders or in diseases with an immunological basis.

Microscopically, fibrinoid necrosis is typically seen in vessels of affected organs, especially small arteries, arterioles and capillaries. In chronic SLE, fibrous thickening of vessels may lead to luminal narrowing.

The disease commonly presents with malaise, weight loss, fever, marked musculoskeletal symptoms and a rash. However, the range of features that may occur is vast as demonstrated in the list below.

### The American Rheumatism Association's list of diagnostic criteria for SLE

The criteria are listed in order of specificity:

- Discoid skin rash—round ('discoid'), red, scaly, telangiectatic plaques, usually on the face and scalp and less commonly on the hands.
- Neurological disorder—most common feature is non-organic psychiatric disorder, thought to be due to vasculitides in the brain. Vessel occlusion due to the prothrombotic action of antiphospholipid antibody on platelets can cause infarction and neuronal loss; this may present with symptoms such as seizure or psychosis.

**Fig. 13.1** Summary of systemic autoimmune diseases

| Disorder | Sex ratio | Type of autoimmunity | Clinical features |
|---|---|---|---|
| SLE | 8F : 1M | Antibodies directed against components of nucleic acids and cytoplasmic phospholipids | Skin rashes, neurological disorders, glomerulonephritis, haematological disorders, etc |
| Rheumatoid disease | 3F : 1M | Rheumatoid factors: autoantibodies directed against native IgG | Chronic polyarthritis, subcutaneous nodules, vasculitis, interstitial pulmonary fibrosis, splenomegaly, etc. |
| Polymyositis and dermatositis | 3F : 1M | Cell-mediated autoimmunity | Weakness, pain and swelling of proximal limb muscles and facial muscles Ptosis and dysphagia Dermatomyositis (= additional features of erythematous, scaling rash) |

**Fig. 13.2** Multisystem manifestations of systemic lupus erythematosus (SLE).

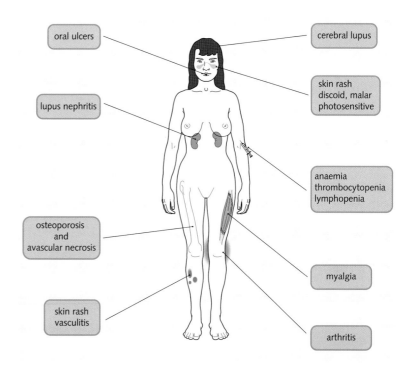

- Malar skin rash—symmetrical erythematous rash on the cheeks and the bridge of the nose (butterfly rash).
- Skin photosensitivity—malar or discoid rash on sun-exposed areas. Caused by immune complex deposits on the dermal side of the basement membrane.
- Oral ulceration—red erosions closely resembling oral lichen planus.

- Renal abnormality (lupus nephritis)—variable pattern from asymptomatic proteinuria to severe glomerular disease leading to renal failure (see Chapter 9).
- Evidence of immunological disorder—presence of autoantibodies, particularly of the antinuclear type.
- Haematological disorders—normocytic hypochromic anaemia, autoimmune haemolytic anaemia,

leucopenia (usually due to lymphopenia), thrombocytopenia (sometimes associated with anti-platelet antibodies), predisposition to thrombosis (especially if antiphospholipid antibody positive).

- Serosal inflammation—pleurisy, pericarditis.
- Arthritis, bone disease and/or myalgia—often mis-diagnosed as rheumatoid arthritis, SLE arthritis is non-erosive and involves two or more peripheral joints. Myalgia in the form of skeletal muscle pain is common and it is thought to be caused by a lymphocytic vasculitis.

## Clinical features

Diagnosis is based on a combination of clinical features and the result of laboratory investigation, primarily the identification of autoantibodies, especially those directed against nuclear DNA. The condition is frequently underdiagnosed.

Treatment is by systemic corticosteroid therapy for acute and life-threatening manifestations of SLE. Immunosuppressive drugs are often used to aid maintenance with less exposure to severe steroid side effects. Lifelong warfarin is needed in antiphospholipid syndrome to reduce the risk of thrombosis.

The disorder follows a protracted course of relapses and remissions. Renal, CNS and cardiac lesions are the most important prognostically. With treatment, in excess of 90% of patients can be anticipated to survive for 10 years.

## Rheumatoid disease

Rheumatoid disease is a common and important autoimmune presentation with widespread effects on the musculoskeletal, cardiovascular, respiratory, haematological, ocular and neurological systems. It is covered in detail in Chapter 12.

## Organ-specific or cell-type specific disease

Autoimmune diseases involving a single organ or cell-type are known as organ-specific or cell-type specific autoimmune diseases. Figure 13.3 is an overview of these conditions, providing page references to the detailed discussions of each condition elsewhere.

**HINTS AND TIPS**

Although organ-specific autoimmune diseases specifically affect one organ, they frequently occur together, e.g. Addison's disease is often associated with autoimmune gastritis.

### Hashimoto's thyroiditis

This causes hypothyroidism as a result of antibody-mediated destruction of the thyroid gland.

**Fig. 13.3** Organ-specific autoimmune diseases.

| Disease | Associated autoantibody | Comment | Full discussion |
|---|---|---|---|
| Graves' disease | Anti-TSH receptor antibody (TRAb) | Hyperthyroidism | p. 211 |
| Hashimoto's disease | Anti-thyroid hormones | Hypothyroidism | p. 213 |
| Type I diabetes mellitus | Anti-islet β-cell antibody | Insulin-responsive hyperglycaemia | p. 223 |
| Addison's disease | Antiadrenal antibodies | Hypoadrenocorticalism | p. 222 |
| Autoimmune gastritis | Antiparietal cell and/or anti-intrinsic factor antibodies | Pernicious anaemia | p. 135 |
| Vitiligo | — | Hypopigmentation | p. 332 |
| Myasthenia gravis | Anti-acetylcholine receptor antibody | Muscle fatigue | p. 262 |

Note: *TSH, thyroid-stimulating hormone.*

## Graves' disease

Thyrotoxicosis is due to overstimulation of thyroid-stimulating hormone (TSH) receptors by autoantibodies. This condition is discussed in more detail in Chapter 10.

## Type I diabetes mellitus

Type I (insulin-dependent) diabetes mellitus is characterized by hyperglycaemia, which is responsive to insulin. The disorder is caused by antibody-mediated destruction of the insulin-secreting β-cell population of the pancreas.

As well as being an organ-specific disease (of the pancreas), the resultant hyperglycaemia has effects on many other systems. Consequently, diabetes mellitus is also classified as a multisystem disease.

## Addison's disease

This rare condition of chronic adrenal insufficiency is most commonly caused by the autoimmune-mediated destruction of the adrenal cortex. It is often associated with other autoimmune endocrine disease, e.g. of the thyroid.

## Autoimmune gastritis

Chronic inflammation of the gastric mucosa is caused by the autoimmune destruction of gastric parietal cells, with or without intrinsic factor autoantibodies (cause pernicious anaemia).

## Vitiligo

The autoimmune destruction of melanocytes causes patchy loss of pigmentation.

## Myasthenia gravis

The autoimmune destruction of acetylcholine receptors occurs at the neuromuscular junction.

## Diseases of immunodeficiency

Immunodeficiency can be defined as the occurrence of, or increased susceptibility to, severe and prolonged infection caused by a specific defect in the immune system. Primary immunodeficiencies are a rare group of diseases, which usually result from genetic defects in one or more of the effector components of the immune system. Symptoms commonly develop in infancy, after the initial protection of maternal antibodies has ended (Fig. 13.4). More than 95 inherited immunodeficiency disorders have now been identified. Secondary immunodeficiencies are acquired disorders that result from extrinsic or environmental causes. There are many origins of secondary immunodeficiencies.

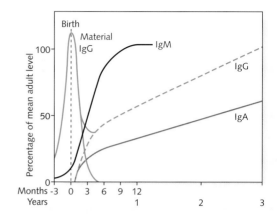

**Fig. 13.4** Serum immunoglobulin levels in the neonate. (Adapted with permission from Lecture Notes in Paediatrics 8th Ed., by S Newell, Blackwell Publishing, London, 2008).

**HINTS AND TIPS**

The type of infection associated with diseases of immune deficiency depends on the category of immune disorder:
- B cell deficiencies (defective antibody response)—increased susceptibility to opportunistic infections caused by extracellular organisms
- T cell deficiencies (defective cell-mediated immunity)—increased susceptibility to opportunistic infections caused by intracellular organisms
- Mixed B and T cell deficiencies (defective antibody response and cell-mediated immunity)—increased susceptibility to most infections.

## Primary immunodeficiencies

### Transient physiological agammaglobulinaemia of the neonate

This natural transient trough in antibody levels usually occurs between 3 and 6 months of age. It is caused by falling levels of maternally derived IgG prior to the appearance of the infant's own antibody (IgM followed by IgG and IgA; see Fig. 13.4). It can be more prolonged and more severe in premature infants.

### X-linked agammaglobulinaemia of Bruton

In this X-linked recessive disorder, affected males present with recurrent infections from between 4 months and 2 years of age (maternal IgG protects against earlier infection). Pre-B cells are unable to differentiate into mature B cells because of a lack of an enzyme called

Bruton's tyrosine kinase (located on chromosome Xq22). This kinase normally transduces maturation signals from the antigen receptor of a pre-B cell. The disease is characterized by:

- deficiency of B cells and plasma cells
- negligible levels of immunoglobulins
- small lymph nodes and absent tonsils.

T cell numbers and functions are normal and infections are, therefore, primarily bacterial. Recurrent bacterial infections of the upper respiratory tract (e.g. by *Streptococcus pneumoniae*) are a common first presentation.

Treatment is with long-term prophylactic immunoglobulin-replacement therapy and the rigorous use of antibacterial agents.

## Common variable immunodeficiency

This is a heterogeneous group of conditions, many of which are inherited, although sporadic cases do occur. The common feature is agammaglobulinaemia, characterized by an increased susceptibility to bacterial infections, and presenting in late childhood or adolescence. Both sexes are affected equally.

The marrow contains normal numbers of immature B cells but there is a failure of differentiation of B cells into plasma cells. This may be due to a defect in T cell signalling.

The disease is more common and more variable than the X-linked form (hence the name); however, the pattern of infection is similar, chiefly affecting the lungs, sinuses and gastrointestinal (GI) tract. The risk of autoimmune disease is also increased in these patients.

Treatment is as for X-linked deficiency.

## Isolated IgA deficiency

The commonest form of immunodeficiency, this affects 1 in 700 Caucasians. Circulating B cells bearing surface IgA are immature and fail to differentiate into IgA-secreting plasma cells.

Patients are prone to sinopulmonary infections and bowel colonization with *Giardia*, *Salmonella* and other enteric pathogens.

## DiGeorge syndrome (thymic hypoplasia)

This rare, congenital disorder is caused by the arrested development of the third and fourth branchial arches, resulting in an almost complete absence of the thymus and parathyroid gland. The genetic defect has been mapped to chromosome 22q11.

Immunoglobulin levels are normal, but affected individuals have decreased circulating levels of T lymphocytes, resulting in impaired cell-mediated immunity.

Patients typically develop a triad of infections: candidiasis, pneumocystis pneumonia and persistent diarrhoea.

The syndrome is also characterized by tetany from hypocalcaemia (due to hypoparathyroidism) and is associated with abnormalities of the great vessels (e.g. transposition or Fallot's tetralogy).

Treatment requires transplantation of thymic tissue.

## Severe combined immunodeficiency

This inherited deficiency of lymphocytic stem cells is characterized by:

- deficiency of both T and B cells
- negligible circulating immunoglobulins
- greatly reduced cell-mediated immunity
- hypoplastic thymus.

The condition can be X-linked (gamma chain of interleukin-2 receptor at Xq13–21.1) or an autosomal recessive disorder. It presents during the first few months of life with a failure to thrive and persistent infections. In addition infants are at risk from graft-versus-host disease. One example of this occurs when maternal T cells cross the placenta; another involves T cells in non-irradiated blood products.

Death usually occurs within the first 2 years of life from multiple infections, although a bone marrow transplant can be an effective cure in some cases. X-linked SCID has become the first human disease to be successfully corrected by gene therapy, although work is continuing on a possible increased risk of leukaemia following such procedures.

## Secondary immunodeficiencies

Secondary immunodeficiencies are those that result from extrinsic or environmental causes, as listed in Figure 13.7. The pathologies of most of these diseases are covered in other chapters.

## Acquired immunodeficiency syndrome

Acquired immunodeficiency syndrome (AIDS) is caused by infection with the human immunodeficiency virus (HIV). It is characterized by a profound defect in cell-mediated immunity with lymphopenia and diminished T lymphocyte responses.

The usual cause is HIV-1 (Fig. 13.5). Routes of transmission are threefold: sexual contact, blood-borne (transfusions or contaminated needles) and maternal (placental or via breast milk).

### Pathogenesis

HIV is an enveloped RNA retrovirus that binds to CD4 receptors present on T helper cells and various cells of the monocyte/macrophage system via its cell surface heterodimer of glycoproteins, gp120/gp41:

- Following cell entry, the virus loses its coat and utilizes its enzyme, reverse transcriptase, to make

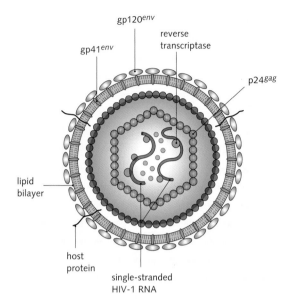

**Fig. 13.5** Structure of the human immunodeficiency virus (HIV)-1.

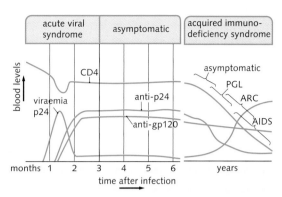

**Fig. 13.6** CD4 count, viral antigen (p24) and antibody levels following HIV infection. (AIDS, acquired immunodeficiency syndrome; ARC, AIDS-related complex; p24, nucleocapsid protein; PGL, persistent generalized lymphadenopathy.)

viral DNA, which is inserted into the host chromosome.

- Viral replication is initially repressed by intracellular factors and by cell-mediated immunity mediated by CD8+ cytotoxic T cells, and so the virus can remain latent (i.e. dormant) for months or even years.
- Activation of latently infected T cells triggers viral replication, and infectious virus particles are - released, resulting in the infection of more CD4+ cells.

Eventually, there is depletion of T helper cells, which results in a severely impaired cell-mediated immunity, with a high risk of multiple opportunistic infections.

There is a correlation between the fall in the CD4 cell count and increasing viral antigen levels (Fig. 13.6).

### Clinical features

The clinical outcome of HIV infection has been classified into four stages (Figure 13.8).

The duration of each stage is highly variable – some patients pass directly through stages II and III to AIDS-related conditions or even to fully developed ('full blown') AIDS, whereas others remain in the earlier stages for months or years. Opportunistic infections tend to develop when the CD4 count drops below 200 cells/mm³. A small proportion of HIV-infected patients do not develop clinical AIDS.

The reasons for these variations in the course of the disease are poorly understood and the factors that determine progression from one stage into the next remain unclear.

### Prognosis and treatment

The prognosis for HIV patients with access to combination anti-retroviral therapy (cART) is dramatically improved. Combination means administering two or more anti-HIV drugs, so as to minimize the development of drug resistance. These include a reverse transcriptase and a protease inhibitor, as well as newer drugs targeting other parts of the virus replication cycle. In addition, antimicrobial therapy is given with the aim of preventing or treating infection (prophylactic antibiotics or antifungals). The intention is to attain a near-normal life expectancy – similar to treatment of insulin-dependent diabetes mellitus.

In the initial stages of HIV infection, viral load and CD4 cell counts are monitored only; cART treatment is generally delayed unless the patient is critically ill, has developed an opportunistic disease, or their CD4 count has dropped below a critical level (currently 350 cells/cu mm³). Unfortunately, many AIDS patients in developing countries have a very poor prognosis because these expensive therapies are unavailable.

cART is not risk-free, there being many toxicities, which dominate the management of HIV-infected patients in rich countries. These include liver fibrosis and steatosis, kidney damage and deranged lipid metabolism. Also, as the patient's cellular immune status improves on cART, there is a risk of immunological over-reaction to infection antigens, with severe imflammatory reactions and organ damage: this is termed 'IRIS' – the immune reconstitution inflammatory syndrome. It is most commonly seen with tuberculosis co-infection.

Figure 13.7 provides a summary of immune deficiencies.

**Fig. 13.7** Summary of immune deficiencies

| Category | Deficiency | Example |
|---|---|---|
| Primary | B cell (antibody deficiency) | Transient hypogammaglobulinaemia of infancy<br>X-linked agammaglobulinaemia<br>Acquired common variable hypogammaglobulinaemia<br>Selective IgA or IgG subclass deficiencies |
| | T cell | Thymic hypoplasia (DiGeorge syndrome) |
| | Mixed B and T cell | Severe combined immune deficiency |
| Secondary | B cell (antibody deficiency) | Myeloma<br>Protein deficiency |
| | T cell | AIDS<br>Hodgkin's disease<br>Non-Hodgkin's lymphoma<br>Drugs, e.g. steroids, ciclosporin, azathioprine |
| | Mixed B and T cell | Chronic lymphocytic leukaemia<br>Post-bone marrow transplantation<br>Post-chemotherapy/radiotherapy<br>Chronic renal failure<br>Splenectomy |

**Fig. 13.8** Classification of HIV infection

| Stage I | Initial infection; can be either:<br>• Symptomatic seroconversion: mononucleosis-like syndrome, mild meningoencephalitis<br>• Asymptomatic seroconversion |
|---|---|
| Stage II | Chronic asymptomatic infection: laboratory tests typically normal but may have anaemia, neutropenia, thrombocytopenia, low CD4 lymphocytes, lymphopenia and hypergammaglobulinaemia |
| Stage III | Persistent generalized lymphadenopathy:<br>with or without laboratory test abnormalities<br>as in stage II |
| Stage IV | AIDS-related complex: generalized lymphadenopathy with persistent fever, weight loss, unexplained diarrhoea, CNS manifestations and haematological abnormalities including thrombocytopenia, leucopenia and anaemia<br>Fully developed AIDS:<br>• Wide spectrum of opportunistic infections including *Pneumocystis carinii*, toxoplasmosis, *Cryptococcus*, cryptosporidiosis, atypical mycobacteria, herpes simplex or zoster, oral hairy leucoplakia, histoplasmosis, candidiasis, cytomegalovirus, *Salmonella*<br>• Secondary cancers, e.g. Kaposi's sarcoma, non-Hodgkin's lymphoma, squamous carcinoma of the mouth or rectum |

## AMYLOIDOSIS

## Definition and chemical nature of amyloid

Amyloidosis is the pathological deposition of abnormal extracellular fibrillar protein, amyloid, in different tissues. Amyloid is composed of a meshwork of rigid, straight fibrils formed from precursor peptides (immunoglobulin light chains, serum amyloid protein A, peptide hormones) lined up in a cross-β-pleated sheet structure. The β-pleated sheet structure is important because enzymes in the body are incapable of digesting such large molecules in this form. It is detected histologically as a bright pink hyaline material that readily takes up Congo red stain, which is used in diagnosis.

### HINTS AND TIPS

It is important to note that it is the physical arrangement of the constituent amino acids that make a protein an amyloid rather than any specific amino acid sequence.

There are many different types of amyloid, each being formed from different precursor amino acids with the precursors themselves often being fragments of larger proteins.

## Amyloid formation

Fifteen distinct forms of amyloid have been described, but three predominate:

1. AA (amyloid associated)—synthesized in liver (non-immunoglobulin)
2. AL (amyloid light chain)—immunoglobulin light chains derived from plasma cells
3. Aβ amyloid—forms the cerebral lesion of Alzheimer's disease.

Amyloid formation occurs because of the production of either:

- abnormal amounts of normal precursor peptide (common), e.g. immunoglobulin light chains in multiple myeloma or serum amyloid A protein in acute-phase response. It may be a result of overproduction, reduced degradation or reduced excretion of protein

or

- normal amounts of abnormal (amyloidogenic) peptide (rare), e.g. due to transthyretin polymorphisms, which make these proteins more prone to misfolding and aggregation.

Normally, misfolded proteins would be degraded by proteosomes within a cell or by macrophages extracellularly. In amyloidosis, however, the macrophage control mechanisms appear to fail and the misfolded proteins aggregate extracellularly.

## Classification of amyloidosis

Clinically, amyloidosis presents with organ involvement that is either:

- systemic—may involve many tissues as it is particularly deposited in the blood vessel walls and basement membranes. Usually fatal, death generally occurring from renal or cardiac disease

or

- localized—affects only one organ or tissue. Rarely, it may be found without any obvious predisposing cause. The skin, lungs and urinary tract are the most frequent sites.

In both cases, the progressive accumulation of amyloid leads to cellular dysfunction by preventing the normal processes of diffusion through extracellular tissues and by physical compression of functioning parenchymal cells.

## Systemic amyloidosis

### Reactive systemic amyloidosis

This amyloid is composed of protein A and is termed the AA type. It is derived from serum amyloid A (SAA) protein, which is an acute-phase reactant synthesized in the liver. SAA increases are seen in response to a variety of diseases, invariably featuring chronic inflammation:

- Rheumatoid arthritis (most common cause): in up to 3% of rheumatoid patients
- Chronic infections (e.g. tuberculosis)
- Hodgkin's disease
- Inflammatory bowel disease
- Bronchiectasis.

Such reactive disease in response to chronic inflammatory disorders tends to produce more severe systemic involvement when compared to other forms of amyloidosis. AA-type amyloid is deposited in many organs, but it has a predilection for the liver, spleen and kidney. It results in hepatosplenomegaly with or without renal vein thrombosis and nephrotic syndrome.

### AL amyloidosis

This amyloid is composed of immunoglobulin light chains (and/or parts of their variable regions) and is termed AL type. Immunoglobulin light chains are formed by proliferating plasma cells usually in association with:

- multiple myeloma—occurs in up to 15% of patients with this condition
- Waldenström's macroglobulinaemia
- heavy-chain disease
- primary amyloidosis.

Primary amyloidosis is a myeloma-associated amyloidosis that occurs in the absence of any clinically obvious myeloma. It is caused by a clinically occult plasma cell tumour, which is revealed only by serum electrophoresis showing the presence of a monoclonal immunoglobulin band. It is also known as benign monoclonal gammopathy.

AL-type amyloid is deposited in many organs, including the tongue, skin, heart, nerves, kidneys, liver and spleen. It has a predilection for connective tissue within these organs.

A common presentation of advanced AL amyloidosis is nephrotic syndrome and biventricular cardiac failure. Macroglossia (enlarged tongue), peripheral neuropathy, carpal tunnel syndrome and overt renal failure are also seen.

### Hereditary amyloidosis

Hereditary forms of amyloidosis are rare, and they include familial Mediterranean fever (AA type) and familial neuropathic forms (pre-albumin, AF type).

## Localized amyloidosis

### Alzheimer's disease

The most common example of amyloid deposition occurs in the nervous system, in both Alzheimer's disease (see Chapter 5) and in normal ageing (cerebral angiopathy). The amyloid (Aβ) is composed of peptide fragments termed β-protein or A4 protein, both of which are derived from a normal, neuronal membrane protein—amyloid precursor protein (APP).

### Senile amyloidosis

Minute deposits of amyloid usually derived from serum transthyretin (pre-albumin) are found in the heart and in the walls of blood vessels in many organs of elderly people. However, cardiomyopathy and/or arrhythmias occur in only a few cases.

## DISORDERS OF WHITE BLOOD CELLS

## Leucopenia

Leucopenia is defined as a reduction in circulating leucocytes. The classification of leucocytes is shown in Figure 13.9.

## Neutropenia

Neutropenia, a deficiency of neutrophil granulocytes, is the most important form of leucopenia. The lower limit of normal neutrophil count is $2.5 \times 10^9$/L (except in Black people and in the Middle East, where it is $1.5 \times 10^9$/L). Levels of less than these values are classified as neutropenia.

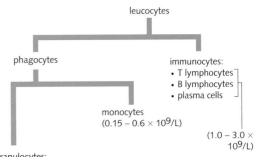

**Fig. 13.9** Classification of leucocytes.

Neutropenia may be selective or part of a general pancytopenia. The causes of both types are listed in Figure 13.10.

Clinical features depend on the degree of neutropenia:

* mild—usually asymptomatic
* moderate to severe ($< 0.5 \times 10^9$/L)—associated with a progressive increase in risk and severity of infection
* levels of $< 0.2 \times 10^9$/L are associated with a high mortality from overwhelming infection.

Severe neutropenia is termed agranulocytosis. Infections are predominantly bacterial and are usually opportunistic, most commonly Gram-positive skin organisms (e.g. *Staphylococcus* and *Streptococcus* species) or Gram-negative gut bacteria (e.g. *Pseudomonas*, *Escherichia col*, etc.).

They can be either localized (e.g. of the mouth, throat, skin or anus) or generalized (neutropenic sepsis). The latter may be rapidly fatal.

Treatment is of the underlying cause and with antimicrobial therapy.

## Leucocytosis

Leucocytosis is defined as an increase in numbers of circulating white blood cells.

## Types of leucocytosis

Each type of leucocyte (see Fig. 13.9) may be increased in number (neutrophilia, eosinophilia, etc.). Monocytosis and lymphocytosis are the terms used for increases in monocytes and lymphocytes, respectively.

Neutrophilia is the most common cause of leucocytosis, produced by common events such as acute bacterial infection or acute inflammation.

Leucocytosis can be:

* primary—caused by bone marrow disease, e.g. leukaemias, lymphomas (described later)

**Fig. 13.10** Causes of neutropenia

| Type | Cause | Clinical features |
|---|---|---|
| Selective neutropenia | Reduced granulopoiesis | Congenital: Kostmann's syndrome—autosomal recessive disease presenting in the first year of life with life-threatening infections<br>Cyclical: rare syndrome characterized by recurrent severe but temporary neutropenia with a periodicity of 3–4 weeks<br>Nutritional: vitamin $B_{12}$ or folate deficiency<br>Racial: African races |
| | Accelerated granulocyte removal | Immune:<br>• autoimmune<br>• systemic lupus erythematosus<br>• Felty's syndrome<br>• hypersensitivity and anaphylaxis<br>Infectious:<br>• viral, e.g. hepatitis, influenza, HIV<br>• fulminant bacterial, e.g. typhoid, miliary tuberculosis |
| | Drug-induced neutropenia | Drug-induced damage of either neutrophils or precursor marrow cells can occur via direct toxicity or immune-mediated mechanisms in susceptible individuals; examples of such drugs include:<br>• anticancer chemotherapy agents: chlorambucil, methotrexate<br>• anti-inflammatory: phenylbutazone, cyclophosphamide<br>• antibacterial: chloramphenicol, cotrimoxazole, sulfasalazine<br>• anticonvulsants: phenytoin<br>• antithyroid: carbimazole<br>• hypoglycaemic: tolbutamide<br>• phenothiazines: chlorpromazine, thioridazine<br>• psychotropics and antidepressants: clozapine, imipramine<br>• miscellaneous: gold, penicillamine |
| Part of general pancytopenia | Reduced granulopoiesis | Bone marrow failure, megaloblastic anaemia |
| | Accelerated granulocyte removal | Splenomegaly |

• secondary—caused by the normal response of bone marrow to abnormal conditions, e.g. infection. Also known as reactive leucocytosis (Figure 13.11).

## Malignant lymphomas

Lymphomas are clonal, neoplastic proliferations of lymphoid cells, and can be classified via cell types (B cells or T cells), tumour architecture (diffuse or follicular), and the clinical course (Hodgkin's disease or non-Hodgkin's lymphomas).

## Hodgkin's disease

Hodgkin's disease is characterized by the painless enlargement of one or more groups of lymph nodes (painless lymphadenopathy) and the presence of large binucleate cells (Reed–Sternberg cells) within them.

**Fig. 13.11** Causes of reactive leucocytosis

| Cause | Clinical features |
|---|---|
| Neutrophilia ($>7.5\times10^9$/L) | Acute infections<br>Haemorrhage/hemolysis<br>Inflammation and tissue necrosis<br>Metabolic disorders<br>Myeloproliferative diseases<br>Neoplasia<br>Steroid therapy<br>Strenuous exercise |
| Monocytosis ($>0.8\times10^9$/L) | Chronic infections, e.g. tuberculosis<br>Rickettsiosis and malaria<br>Inflammatory disorders,<br>e.g. rheumatoid disease,<br>SLE, Crohn's disease |
| Eosinophilia ($>0.44\times10^9$/L) | Allergy, e.g. asthma<br>Parasites, e.g. tapeworms<br>Skin disease, e.g. eczema, psoriasis<br>Neoplasia, especially Hodgkin's disease<br>Miscellaneous, e.g. polyarteritis nodosa, sarcoidosis |
| Basophilia ($>0.1\times10^9$/L) | Myxoedema<br>Chickenpox<br>Myeloproliferative disorders |
| Lymphocytosis ($>3.5\times10^9$/L) | Acute infections, e.g. infectious mononucleosis<br>Chronic infections, e.g. tuberculosis, brucellosis, hepatitis |

*Note: SLE, systemic lupus erythematosus*

It affects 4 per 100 000 in the UK, with a slight male excess. It can occur at any age but there are two peaks of incidence: one in young adults (15–20 years old) and the other in late middle age (40–60 years old).

The aetiology of Hodgkin's disease is obscure, as is the origin of the malignant Reed–Sternberg (RS) cells. Although no causal link has been established with Epstein–Barr virus (EBV), Hodgkin's disease sufferers are three times more likely to have had glandular fever in the past.

Hodgkin's disease often presents clinically as the enlargement of accessible nodes, most often in the upper half of the body (e.g. cervical or axillary). The disease is initially localized to a single peripheral lymph node region, but it spreads in a fairly consistent pattern to adjacent nodes via the lymphatics, and then, following splenic involvement, to other organs via the bloodstream.

One-third of patients have systemic symptoms (so-called 'B symptoms'), notably weight loss, pyrexia (Pel Epstein fevers are epsiodic fevers) and night sweats.

**Clinical Note**

The stage (extent of spread) of Hodgkin's disease is determined by the Ann Arbor staging system (Fig. 13.12). A clinical addition is the presence of 'B symptoms'—systemic features associated with poorer prognosis, namely weight loss, night sweats and unexplained fever.

Treatment depends on the stage: either localized (radiotherapy) or generalized (systemic chemotherapy). Five-year survival is approximately 75%, but long-term survivors of chemotherapy and/or radiotherapy are at increased risk of second cancers.

Diagnosis of Hodgkin's disease can only be made on examination of biopsied lymph nodes:

- Macroscopically—affected lymph nodes are enlarged, with a smooth surface and the lymph node capsule is rarely breached (cf. non-Hodgkin's lymphomas).

**Fig. 13.12** Ann Arbor staging system of Hodgkin's disease

| Stage | Comment |
|---|---|
| I | Involvement of single lymph node region (I) or of single extralymphatic organ or site (hence Ie) |
| II | Involvement of two or more lymph node regions, with all lesions confined to the same side of the diaphragm (II), or localized involvement of an extralymphatic site and one or more lymph node regions confined to one side of the diaphragm (IIe) |
| III | Involvement of lymph node regions on both sides of the diaphragm (III) which may also involve the spleen (IIIs), localized extralymphatic sites (IIIe) or both (IIIse) |
| IV | Widespread involvement of extralymphoid sites such as the liver, lung and bone marrow with or without lymph node involvement |

*Suffix A indicates the absence of systemic symptoms; suffix B indicates the presence of systemic symptoms. For example, stage IIIeB denotes involvement of lymph nodes on both sides of the diaphragm accompanied by localized involvement of an extralymphatic site with systemic symptoms.*

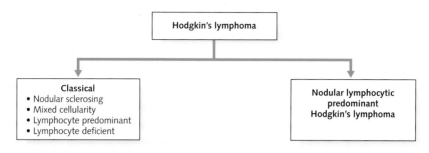

| Type | % of Classical Hodgkin's lymphoma | Lymphocytes | Reed-Sternberg | Prognosis |
|---|---|---|---|---|
| Nodular sclerosing | 60 | +++ | + | Good |
| Mixed cellularity | 30 | +++ | ++++ | Moderate |
| Lymphocyte predominant | 5 | +++ | + | Good |
| Lymphocyte deficient | 5 | + | ++ | Poor |

**Fig. 13.13**  Rye classification of Hodgkin's disease. (Adapted with permission from medicshandbook.com, 2011.)

- Microscopically—four subtypes of Hodgkin's disease are recognized and classified according to the Rye classification system (Fig. 13.13).

## Non-Hodgkin's lymphomas

Non-Hodgkin's lymphomas (NHLs) include all lymphomas other than Hodgkin's disease. They are predominantly diseases of middle and later life, with males slightly more affected than females.

The aetiology of NHLs is poorly understood but several factors have been implicated:

- Immunosuppression—increased incidence in primary immunosuppressive diseases, e.g. X-linked agammaglobulinaemia and in secondary immunosuppression, e.g. drug induced after transplantation
- Viral infection—with lymphotropic viruses, e.g. EBV, human T-lymphotropic virus (HTLV-1), HIV
- Bacterial infection—*Helicobacter pylori* infection linked to gastric lymphoma
- Radiation.

Chromosomal translocations are a feature of many types of lymphoma, for example:

- Burkitt's lymphoma—translocation 8:14
- Follicular B cell lymphoma—translocation 14:18.

These translocations cause a neoplastic transformation as a result of the transfer of an oncogene or oncogene-regulatory gene to an abnormal site. This causes the increased expression of these oncogenes, e.g *bcl-2* in follicular lymphoma, which inhibits apoptotic cell death.

The majority (70%) of NHLs are B-cell lymphomas, which are derived from follicle centre cells. These tumours have either follicular or diffuse architecture.

> **HINTS AND TIPS**
>
> Recognizing the normal development of lymphocytes (Fig. 13.14) is essential to understanding lymphomas and other neoplastic proliferations of white blood cells.

### Clinical features

The clinical manifestations of NHLs are similar to those of Hodgkin's disease but they are more varied because of their heterogeneous nature. The majority of cases present with asymmetric, painless enlargement of lymph nodes in one or more peripheral lymph node regions. However, extranodal presentation is more frequent than in Hodgkin's disease, with 20% of all NHLs originating within extranodal sites.

Systemic symptoms are often prominent in extensive disease, along with hepatosplenomegaly.

### Classification and management

The Ann Arbor staging system is used to stage NHL. However, systemic symptoms are much less common compared to Hodgkin's disease (Fig. 13.15).

Treatment is by single or combination chemotherapy with which some patients show long-term remission if not cure.

The prognosis depends on the type of lymphoma and varies widely from highly proliferative and rapidly fatal

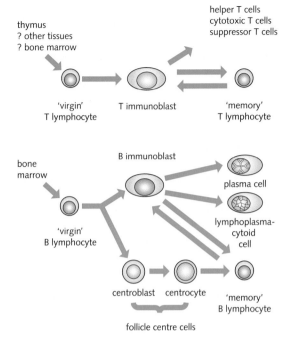

**Fig. 13.14** Normal lymphocyte development. (Adapted with permission from Essential Hematology, 5th Edition, by V Hoffbrand and J Pettit, Wiley-Blackwell, 2005.)

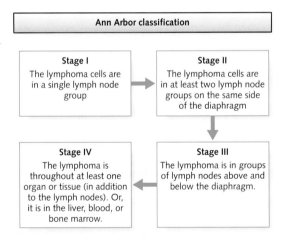

**Fig. 13.15** Ann Arbor staging system of Non-Hodgkin's disease (Adapted with permission from medicshandbook.com, 2011.)

diseases (e.g. immunoblastic lymphoma) to indolent and well-tolerated malignancies with a mean survival of about 7 years (e.g. follicular centrocytic lymphoma).

## Leukaemias

Leukaemias are neoplastic proliferations of white blood cell precursors in the bone marrow.

*Classification*—leukaemias are classified into acute or chronic based on clinical progression:

1. Acute—characterized by numerous immature 'blast' cells (leucocyte precursors) and rapid disease progression
2. Chronic—characterized by large numbers of precursor cells that are more differentiated than blast cells and associated with slower disease progression.

These groups are then further classified into two main groups depending on neoplastic cell types:

1. Myeloid leukaemia (cells of granulocytic series)
2. Lymphocytic leukaemia (cells of the lymphoid series).

*Aetiology*—in the majority of cases, the cause of leukaemia is unknown. However, certain factors are known to initiate leukaemic transformation:

- Genetics—slight familial tendency (high concordance in monozygotic twins); chromosome abnormalities (both quantitative and qualitative) are present in about 50% of patients; increased incidence in Down syndrome
- Ionizing radiation—excessive exposure in therapy, e.g. for ankylosing spondylitis, malignant disease; nuclear explosions/accidents as at Hiroshima and Chernobyl
- Drugs—prolonged chemotherapy, e.g. with alkylating agents (cause myeloid leukaemia)
- Immune status—increased incidence in immunosuppressed individuals
- Viruses—e.g. HTLV-I causes adult T cell leukaemia/ lymphoma; HTLV-II is associated with hairy cell leukaemia
- Industrial benzene exposure.

## Common features of leukaemias

The common features of leukaemias are bone marrow failure, gout and metastasis.

### Bone marrow failure

Overproduction of leucocyte precursor cells causes the suppression of normal blood cell production, thus:

- deficiency of red cell production → anaemia
- deficiency of platelet production (thrombocytopenia) → haemorrhage
- deficiency of normal leucocyte production (granulocytes and lymphocytes) → failure to control infection.

### Gout

Increased cell turnover leads to increased uric acid synthesis, which may result in gout.

### Metastasis

There is infiltration of organs such as the liver, spleen, lymph nodes, meninges and gonads by the leukaemic cells.

## Acute leukaemia

Acute leukaemia is a malignant disorder in which haemopoietic blast cells constitute > 20% of bone marrow cells.

There are two main types: acute lymphoblastic leukaemia (ALL) and acute myeloblastic leukaemia (AML). These are further subclassified according to cytological features of the blast cells. There are three subtypes for ALL ($L_1$-$L_3$) based on the degree of uniformity of cell size and vacuolation. There are eight subtypes for AML ($M_0$-$M_7$) based on the degree of cytoplasmic granularity. Figure 13.16 outlines the features of ALL and AML.

The clinical features of both AML and ALL are similar. They commonly present with symptoms of anaemia (e.g. tiredness, malaise, breathlessness, angina) and their course is typified by a series of overwhelming infections and mucosal haemorrhage.

Onset is frequently rapid and progression to death from anaemia, haemorrhage or infection occurs within weeks if no treatment is given.

The clinical course is less catastrophic in childhood ALL.

Haematological investigations reveal:

- anaemia—normocytic, normochromic
- leucocytosis—although leucopenia may be an occasional feature, despite massive marrow infiltration with blast cells
- neutropenia—susceptibility to overt infections
- thrombocytopenia—petechiae, purpura, epistaxis, bleeding gums, GI haemorrhage, cerebral haemorrhage
- blood film—this shows blast cells and can be diagnostic. If not clear from blood film, diagnosis is sought from bone marrow biopsy. This shows a hypercellular marrow with normal elements replaced by blast cells. If Auer rods are present in the cytoplasm of these cells, the pattern is AML. Cytogenetics and immunological staining can help diagnosis.

Involvement of other organs:

- Skeleton (bone pain, especially in children)—probably caused by osteolytic lesions
- Lymphadenopathy
- Symptoms and signs secondary to CNS infiltration.

Management:

- Supportive therapy—this actually increases survival and involves correction of anaemia, thrombocytopenia (i.e. blood product transfusions) and treatment of infections
- Repeated courses of combination chemotherapy to induce remission

**Fig. 13.16** Features of acute lymphoblastic and acute myeloblastic leukaemia

| Type | Acute lymphoblastic leukaemia (ALL) | Acute myeloblastic leukaemia (AML) |
|---|---|---|
| Epidemiology | Mainly (>90%) affects children of <14 years with highest incidence at 3–4 years Second increase in incidence occurs around middle-age | Occurs at all ages and is the commonest form of acute leukaemia in adults |
| Proliferating cell type | Neoplastic lymphoblasts (lymphocyte precursor cells) | Neoplastic myeloblast (granulocyte/monocyte precursor cell) |
| Degree of differentiation | Blast cells show no differentiation | Blast cells usually show some evidence of differentiation to granulocytes |
| Prognosis | Children aged 2–9 years: 50–75% cure rate Adults: 35% cure rate with chemotherapy; 50% with allogeneic bone marrow transplant | 20–25% cure rate with standard chemotherapy 50% with allogeneic bone marrow transplant |

- Bone marrow transplantation—usually reserved for those in relapsing chemotherapy-induced remission. Encouraging results in younger patients but largely depends on availability of suitable tissue-matched donor.

For the prognosis see Figure 13.16.

## Chronic leukaemias

### Chronic myeloid leukaemia

Chronic myeloid leukaemia (CML) is a disorder of proliferation, with excessive and uncontrolled neoplastic proliferation of an abnormal myeloid clone of leucocyte precursors in the bone marrow.

About 90% of cases are characterized by the presence of a specific karyotypic abnormality—the Philadelphia chromosome—within the haemopoietic stem cells. This involves reciprocal translocation of part of the long arm (q) of chromosome *22* with the long arm of chromosome 9. This creates a chimeric gene *(BCR-abl)*, which produces a tyrosine kinase thought to be involved in the pathogenesis of CML.

CML occurs in all age groups, but most frequently between the ages of 40 and 60 years. The disease has three recognized stages:

1. Chronic phase—characterized by anaemia and splenomegaly; responsive to chemotherapy
2. Accelerated phase—due to the emergence and dominance of a more malignant clone of myeloid cells. Disease becomes harder to control
3. Blast crisis phase—transformation to an acute leukaemia (usually AML), often rapidly fatal. Progression from chronic phase is unpredictable and may occur at any time.

Haematological investigation reveals leucocytosis and normocytic anaemia. Note that in contrast to acute leukaemias, neutropenia, lymphopenia and thrombocytopenia are not common in the chronic phase and that infection and bleeding are not typical.

There is sometimes massive splenomegaly (10% of cases), and often hepatomegaly.

Treatment of Philadelphia-chromosome-positive CML has recently been transformed by the drug imatinib. This novel tyrosine kinase inhibitor blocks the product of the chimeric *BCR-abl* gene and appears to offer long-term remission as long as the patient remains on the drug.

### Chronic lymphocytic leukaemia

This chronic lymphoproliferative disorder is characterized by the proliferation of an abnormal lymphoid clone of leucocyte precursors in the bone marrow.

Chronic lymphocytic leukaemia (CCL) is the most common leukaemia of adults, comprising about 30% of all leukaemias, with males affected more than females by 2:1. It is a disease predominantly of the elderly, with peak incidence at 65 years old.

This disease is much less aggressive than other leukaemias, following a predictable course over a period of years.

Haematological changes are:

- leucocytosis—small, non-functional lymphocytes of B cell origin
- anaemia and thrombocytopenia are late developments
- secondary autoimmune haemolytic anaemia develops in 10% of cases.

The lymph nodes, liver and spleen are characteristically involved and normal architecture may become completely effaced by the infiltrating cells.

### Clinical Note

The staging of CLL is summarized in Figure 13.17. Clinical features are similar to a low-grade lymphoma, but with the eventual development of bone marrow failure (anaemia, thrombocytopenia, infection).

Treatment is often reserved for the later stages, comprising combined chemotherapy and occasionally splenectomy

Survival for more than 10 years from diagnosis is common, and where CLL affects the elderly, death is often from an unrelated cause. CLL in younger individuals tends to be more aggressive.

## Myelodysplastic syndromes

This group of acquired neoplastic disorders of the bone marrow is characterized by increasing bone marrow failure with quantitative and qualitative abnormalities of all three myeloid cell lines (red cell, granulocyte/

**Fig. 13.17** Clinical features and staging of chronic lymphocytic leukaemia according to the RAI classification

| Stage | Features |
|-------|----------|
| 0 | Lymphocytosis of blood and marrow |
| I | Lymphocytosis and enlarged nodes |
| II | Lymphocytosis and enlarged liver or spleen |
| III | Haemoglobin < 11 g/dL, with features of stages 0, I or II |
| IV | Platelet count < $100 \times 10^9$/L, with features of stages, I, II or III |

monocyte and platelets) due to a defect of stem cells. They are also known as refractory anaemias.

In most cases, the disease arises *de novo* and the aetiology is likely to be as for the leukaemias. The disorders are seen as steps in the progression to leukaemia (preleukaemic) and AML develops in many instances, often after many years. However, in a significant proportion of cases, the disease is secondary to treatment with chemotherapy (with or without radiotherapy) for a previous neoplastic disease.

The hallmark of the disease is ineffective haemopoiesis resulting in pancytopenia despite a marrow of either normal or increased cellularity

Bone marrow contains morphologically abnormal cells including ring sideroblasts and hypogranular white cells, often with abnormal chromosomes.

*Clinical features*—more than half the patients are over 70 years old and more than 75% are over 50; males are affected more often than females. Symptoms are generally sequelae of the variable cytopenia, and include anaemia, infection and haemorrhage.

Diseases are subclassified depending on the presence of ring sideroblasts and the proportion of leukaemic-type blast cells in the bone marrow (Figure 13.18).

Treatment is largely supportive, by blood transfusion and treatment of infection.

Morbidity and deaths are largely attributable to the refractory cytopenias either directly (e.g. from haemorrhage) or indirectly (e.g. from transfusion-related haemosiderosis).

# Hairy cell leukaemia

This rare, B cell leukaemia is characterized by variable numbers of 'hairy' cells in the blood, bone marrow, liver and other organs. Hairy cells are so named because of their characteristic irregular outline caused by cytoplasmic projections or 'hairs'.

The disease has a peak incidence at 40–60 years old, affecting males more than females by 6:1.

It is characterized clinically by features of pancytopenia (mainly recurrent infections) and splenomegaly.

The disorder typically runs a chronic course and remission is common with chemotherapy or interferon treatment. Splenectomy is also useful in management.

# Myeloproliferative disorders

These are autonomous proliferations of one or more myeloid cells (erythroid, granulocytic, megakaryocytic) with differentiation to mature forms (Figure 13.19). Progression from one disorder to another within the group is common.

## Polycythaemia rubra vera

This idiopathic condition is characterized by an above normal increase in red cell concentration, usually with concomitant increases in haemoglobin concentration and haematocrit. Red cell mass is greatly increased.

**Fig. 13.18** Classification of myelodysplastic syndromes (MDS)

| Type of MDS | Peripheral blood | Bone marrow | Medial survival (months) |
|---|---|---|---|
| Refractory anaemia (RA) | Blasts <1% | Blasts <5% | 50 |
| RA with ring sideroblasts (RARS) | Blasts <1% | Blasts <5% Ring sideroblasts >15% of total erythroblasts | 50 |
| RA with excess blasts (RAEB) | Blasts <5% | Blasts 5–20% | 10 |
| RAEB in transformation (RAEB-t) | Blasts <5% | Blasts 20–30% or Auer rods present | 5 |
| Chronic myelomonocytic leukaemia (CMML) | Blasts <1% Monocytes >1.0 × 10$^9$/L | Blasts 5–20% Promonocytes | 10 |

**Fig. 13.19** Myeloproliferative disorders and their basic features

| Disorder | Principal proliferations | Bone marrow morphology | Clinical features |
|---|---|---|---|
| Polycythaemia rubra vera | Erythroblasts | Increased cellularity, especially erythroid | Erythrocytosis with increased Hb and PCV Often neutrophilia and thrombocytosis Pruritus (relating to basophilia) Thrombosis or haemorrhage Splenomegaly |
| Myelofibrosis | Fibroblasts | Increased deposition of collagen/reticulin; bone marrow difficult to aspirate | Leucoerythroblastic blood picture Anaemia with tear-drop poikilocytes Hepatosplenomegaly |
| Chronic granulocytic leukaemia | Myeloblasts | Increased cellularity, especially myeloid | Leucoerythroblastic blood picture Anaemia, neutrophilia, basophilia Splenomegaly |
| Essential thrombocythaemia | Megakaryoblasts | Increased megakaryocytes | Thrombocytosis Thrombosis or haemorrhage Occasional splenomegaly |

*Hb, hemoglobin; PCV, packed cell volume.*

The disorder has a prevalence of 1 per 100 000 in the UK. It typically affects the middle-aged, and males more so than females.

Progression of this disease is chronic, but about 20% of cases evolve into myelofibrosis and another 5% into acute leukaemia.

Onset is usually insidious and non-specific, e.g. malaise, fatigue, headache and dizziness. The principle symptoms are caused by vascular engorgement, increased haematocrit and thrombosis, with or without haemorrhage. Diagnosis requires raised red cell mass without another cause and palpable splenomegaly.

Treatment is by venesection or myelosuppression using chemotherapy or radioactive $^{32}$P. Treated patients have a mean survival of about 13 years, with increased morbidity and mortality from coronary and cerebral disease related to the raised haematocrit.

## Myelofibrosis

This condition is characterized by a proliferation of fibroblasts in the bone marrow and obliterative marrow fibrosis, with a corresponding massive extra-medullary haemopoiesis in the liver and spleen.

The condition is a chronic disorder of late and middle age. It may arise *de novo* (with unknown aetiology) or as an end-stage of other myeloproliferative disorders (e.g. polycythaemia rubra vera).

The disease is usually slowly progressive, with a median survival of 4 years. Acute leukaemic transformation sometimes occurs.

Clinical features are:

- blood film—typically leucoerythroblastic; erythropoiesis is ineffective leading to anaemia with marked anisocytosis (unequal sized blood cells) and teardrop poikilocytes (tear-drop shaped red cells)
- splenomegaly is invariable
- hepatomegaly is common
- increased bone density due to sclerosis (myelosclerosis is an alternative name for myelofibrosis).

Symptoms are usually caused by anaemia and massive splenomegaly. Systemic symptoms (e.g. fever, weight loss) are usually late features.

## Primary (essential/idiopathic) thrombocythaemia

This condition is characterized by increased platelet production due to a clonal proliferation of megakaryocytes without a systemic cause. It is most commonly seen in patients over 50 years of age. Its features are:

- large, atypical platelets with increased platelet count, often $> 600 \times 10^9$/L
- combined pathological haemorrhages and thromboembolic episodes
- spleen may be enlarged, but it is usually normal or reduced in size because of thromboembolic infarction.

Treatment with chemotherapy and antiplatelet drugs (e.g. aspirin) is effective and median survival with treatment is 8–10 years.

# Myeloma

This describes the malignant, monoclonal proliferation of plasma cells in the marrow. Most cases affect multiple sites (multiple myeloma), although solitary myeloma does occur (see below).

## Multiple myeloma

This typically affects the elderly, with almost all cases occurring after the age of 40. There is a male predominance.

*Pathogenesis*—normal plasma cells produce polyclonal immunoglobulins. In myeloma, only monoclonal immunoglobulins or light chains are produced; these are referred to as the 'M component' or paraprotein.

The M component is usually IgG (> 60%), but may be IgA (20%) or just the immunoglobulin light chain [κ (kappa) being more frequent than λ (lambda)]. IgM-producing plasma cells are a feature of Waldenström's macroglobulinaemia.

Serum protein electrophoresis, which shows normal levels of α- and β-globulins, but a dramatic increase in the levels of gamma-globulins (Fig. 13.20).

Diagnosis of myeloma requires two out of the following three findings:

- marrow plasmacytosis
- serum or urinary paraprotein (M component)
- skeletal lesions (see below).

distance from origin

patient with multiple myeloma IgG κ monoclonal protein 38 g/L

normal pattern

**Fig. 13.20** Serum electrophoresis showing characteristic gamma band of multiple myeloma. (Adapted with permission from Essential Hematology, 5th Edition, by V Hoffbrand and J Pettit, Wiley-Blackwell, 2006.)

### Renal impairment

In two-thirds of cases of IgG and IgA myelomas, monoclonal free light chains are also produced, which are small enough to enter the urine, where they are called Bence-Jones proteins.

During passage through the tubules, the protein precipitates as 'casts', causing damage to the tubular epithelial cells, with concomitant formation of surrounding giant cells.

Light chains that pass through capillaries are incorporated into amyloid (systemic amyloidosis); causing damage to many organs including the kidneys.

Raised blood uric acid (from increased cell turnover) worsens renal impairment (urate nephropathy), as does increased blood calcium from bone osteolysis (hypercalcaemia).

### Bone changes

These are characteristic of myeloma:

- Hypercellular marrow with a large proportion of abnormal plasma cells, especially in the skull, ribs, vertebrae and pelvis
- Osteolysis of medullary and cortical bone due to increased numbers of bone-resorbing osteoclasts: thought to be stimulated by interleukin 1 produced by the malignant plasma cells
- Osteolytic lesions are seen as 'punched out' defects in the bones, the skull showing this appearance particularly well ('pepper-pot skull')
- Generalized osteoporosis may result in pathological fractures or vertebral compression.

### Haematological findings

These are as follows:

- Anaemia—usually normochromic, normocytic
- Marked rouleaux formation—red cells pile together adhering by their rims forming cylinders
- Raised blood viscosity—depending on the type of immunoglobulin
- Reduced concentration of unaffected immunoglobulins—'immune paresis'
- Abnormal plasma cells—occasionally seen in peripheral blood, but most are in the marrow
- Neutropenia and thrombocytopenia—common features of bone marrow failure in late stages.

### Clinical Note

Clinical features of myeloma:

- Bone pain—especially backache and pathological fractures
- Anaemia—lethargy, breathlessness, tachycardia, etc.
- Repeated infections—deficient antibody levels and bone marrow failure

- Abnormal bleeding tendency—M component may interfere with platelet function and coagulation factors; thrombocytopenia in advanced disease
- Features of renal failure and/or hypercalcaemia.
  Treatment involves chemotherapy and radiotherapy but median survival is only 3 years with treatment. Allogeneic bone marrow transplant may benefit some patients.

### Solitary myeloma

This rare disease is characterized by discrete solitary tumours of proliferating monoclonal plasma cells, usually in the bone.

Proliferation does not occur in parts of the skeleton beyond the primary lesion and marrow aspirates distant from the primary tumour are usually normal.

The associated M component usually disappears following radiotherapy to the primary lesion. However, a minority of cases progress to multiple myeloma.

## DISORDERS OF THE SPLEEN AND THYMUS

## Splenomegaly

The spleen serves as the site of filtration and phagocytosis of the following:

- Effete cells and cell debris, especially red cells
- Microorganisms
- Abnormal or excess material derived from metabolic processes.

Splenomegaly (enlargement of the spleen) is a common physical sign. It can have many causes, the main types of which are summarized in Figure 13.21.

A palpable spleen is at least twice its normal size and it is vulnerable to traumatic rupture.

### Effect of splenomegaly

Irrespective of the cause, enlargement of the spleen may result in the development of hypersplenism, i.e. a decrease in the circulating numbers of

**Fig. 13.21** Causes of splenomegaly

| Cause | Comments |
|---|---|
| Infections | Bacterial, e.g. typhoid, tuberculosis, brucellosis, infective endocarditis<br>Viral: infectious mononucleosis<br>Protozoal: malaria, leishmaniasis, trypanosomiasis, toxoplasmosis |
| Congestion | Due to persistent elevation of splenic venous blood pressure,the cause of which may be:<br>• Prehepatic: thrombosis of hepatic, splenic or portal vein<br>• Hepatic: long-standing portal hypertension associated with cirrhosis<br>• Posthepatic: raised venous pressure of inferior vena cava, e.g. due to right-sided heart failure, which is transmitted to the spleen via the portal system |
| Storage disease | Heritable enzyme deficiencies, which result in storage of material in splenic macrophagic cells, e.g. Gaucher's disease, Niemann–Pick disease and Tay–Sachs disease |
| Neoplasia | Primary: rare<br>Secondary:<br>• Lymphomas: Hodgkin's disease and non-Hodgkin's lymphomas<br>• Leukaemias: especially chronic leukaemias<br>• Metastases: splenic metastases from solid tumours, e.g. carcinomas or sarcomas, are rare<br>• Extramedullary haemopoiesis, e.g. in myeloproliferative diseases and diseases with diffuse marrow replacement by tumour |
| Haematological disorders | Haematological anaemias, e.g. hereditary spherocytosis, β-thalassaemia, autoimmune haemolysis<br>Autoimmune thrombocytopenia: destruction of antibody-coated platelets in spleen results in accumulation of foamy histiocytes in sinuses |
| Immune disorders | Felty's syndrome: follicular hyperplasia in spleen associated with hypersplenism and rheumatoid disease,<br>Sarcoidosis: spleen infiltrated by granulomas<br>Amyloidosis: spleen infiltrated with amyloid |

erythrocytes, leucocytes and platelets (pancytopenia), resulting from the destruction or pooling of these cells by the enlarged spleen.

Hypersplenism is often accompanied by a compensatory response—hyperplasia of the bone marrow.

Splenectomy leads to clinical and haematological improvement.

## Congestive splenomegaly

This is enlargement of the spleen caused by any condition that leads to a persistent elevation of splenic venous blood pressure. Causes of raised splenic venous pressure are outlined in Figure 13.22.

*Morphological features*—sinusoids of the spleen are initially distended with red cells. Fibrosis of both the spleen and capsule eventually occurs and sinusoids then appear ectatic and empty.

The cut surface of the spleen has a purple-red colour with an inconspicuous white pulp and it is often flecked with firm, brown nodules (called Gamna–Gandy nodules) that represent foci of fibrosis.

Foci of extramedullary haemopoiesis are an occasional feature and are thought to be secondary to local hypoxia.

> **HINTS AND TIPS**
>
> A quick revision of splenic venous anatomy is helpful in understanding the causes of raised splenic venous

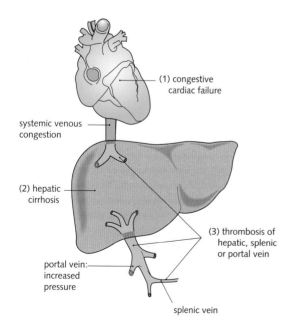

systemic venous congestion

(1) congestive cardiac failure

(2) hepatic cirrhosis

(3) thrombosis of hepatic, splenic or portal vein

portal vein: increased pressure

splenic vein

**Fig. 13.22** Causes of raised splenic venous pressure.

pressure (Fig. 13.22). These are heart failure, cirrhosis and venous thrombosis.

## Splenic infarcts

Splenic infarction follows occlusion of the splenic artery or its branches and it may be caused by:

- emboli that arise in the heart (most common). May be septic if associated with infective endocarditis.
- local thrombosis, e.g. in sickle-cell diseases, myeloproliferative disorders and malignant infiltrates.

Infarcts may be single or multiple and are generally wedge shaped and pale.

## Disorders of the thymus

The thymus is composed of lymphoid cells and specialised epithelial cells; it is known as the 'primary' lymphoid organ. It is concerned with the development and processing of the long-lived T lymphocytes prior to their distribution to lymphoid tissues and to a circulating pool of T lymphocytes.

Thymic activity is maximal in fetal and childhood stages; regression is rapid after puberty.

### Developmental disorders

#### Thymic hypoplasia and aplasia
These occur due to the developmental failure of either:

- epithelial tissue—thymus is completely absent or is represented by a fibrous streak, e.g. DiGeorge syndrome

or

- lymphoid tissue—severe combined immunodeficiency syndromes, ataxia, telangiectasia and reticular dysgenesis.

Both types of developmental disorder result in T-cell deficiency associated with a disordered, cell-mediated immune response.

### Thymic hyperplasia

This is a rare condition in which lymphoid follicles (germinal centres) composed of B cells develop in the thymic medulla. It is often accompanied by an increase in the size of the thymus and is associated with autoimmune disease, especially myasthaenia gravis. In some cases autoantibodies are thought to be produced by the lymphoid tissue.

### Thymomas

These rare tumours are derived from thymic epithelial cells; they can be benign or malignant.

Histologically thymomas are composed of uniform epithelial cells variably mixed with reactive lymphoid cells.

### Benign thymomas

The majority (80–90%) of thymomas are benign, well-circumscribed, encapsulated, lobulated tumours. Most are asymptomatic, but some present with local disease caused by the compression of adjacent mediastinal structures:

- Respiratory passages—dyspnoea and cough
- Oesophagus—dysphagia
- Great veins—cyanosis and suffusion of the face.

The remainder present with autoimmune disease. Complete surgical excision is curative.

### Malignant thymomas

Around 10–20% of thymomas are malignant and invade the local tissues. There are two types:

1. Type 1—appears cytologically benign but invades local tissues, e.g. pericardium, lungs, pleura. Rarely spread outside the thorax
2. Type 2 (thymic carcinoma)—rare malignant thymomas appearing cytologically malignant. Most are squamous cell carcinomas with a poor prognosis.

## DISORDERS OF RED BLOOD CELLS

## Abnormalities of red cell size and shape

Many haematological and systemic disorders are associated with specific abnormalities of red-cell size (anisocytosis) and/or abnormal red-cell shape (poikilocytosis) Figure 13.23.

## Anaemia classifications

Anaemia can be defined as a state in which the blood haemoglobin level is below the normal range for the patient's age and sex. The normal haemoglobin range in males is 13.0–18.0 g/dL (130–180 g/L) and in females is 11.5–16.5 g/dL (115–165 g/L). Anaemia can be classified by the underlying mechanism for reduced haemoglobin, as shown in Figure 13.24.

It is worth noting that, in clinical practice, anaemias are usually classified by the mean cell volume (MCV) of red cells—this can be increased (macrocytic anaemia), normal (normocytic) or reduced (microcytic). In general terms:

- macrocytic—megaloblastic anaemias (vitamin $B_{12}$ or folate deficiency) or haemolytic anaemias (new immature red blood cells are large in size)

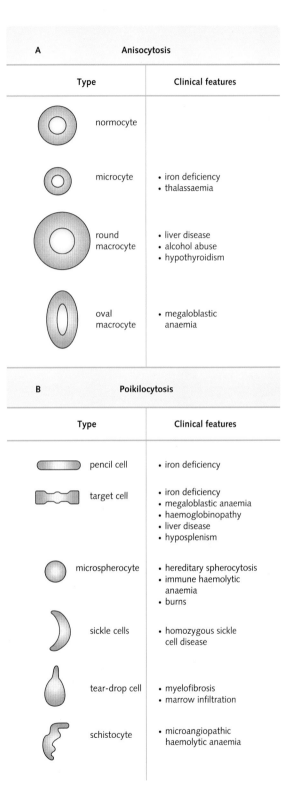

**Fig. 13.23** Diagrammatic representation of (A) abnormalities in red cell size (anisocytosis) and (B) abnormalities in red cell shape (poikilocytosis). (Adapted from Underwood, 2009.)

**Fig. 13.24** Causes of anaemia

| Cause | Clinical features |
|---|---|
| Increased red cell loss, lysis or pooling | Blood loss<br>Haemolysis:<br>• Intrinsic abnormalities of red cells: hereditary (membrane defects, enzyme defects, haemoglobinopathies) and acquired (paroxysmal nocturnal haemoglobinuria)<br>• Extrinsic abnormalities of red cells: antibody-mediated red cell destruction and mechanical trauma to red cells<br>Hypersplenism |
| Impaired red cell production | Deficiency of haematinics:<br>• Megaloblastic anaemias: lack of vitamin B$_{12}$ or folate<br>• Iron-deficiency anaemia<br>Dyserythropoiesis (production of defective cells):<br>• Anaemia of chronic disorders<br>• Myelodysplasia<br>• Sideroblastic anaemia<br>Hypoplasia of marrow (failure to produce cells):<br>• Aplastic anaemia<br>• Red cell aplasia<br>Invasion of marrow by malignant cells:<br>• Leukaemias<br>• Myeloproliferative diseases<br>• Non-haematological malignancies |

- normocytic—anaemia of chronic disease or hypoplastic anaemias (bone marrow suppression)
- microcytic—iron-deficiency anaemia (most common cause of anaemia) or thalassaemia.

The colour (quantity of haemoglobin) of a red cell is also described with the terms hypochromic (low), normochromic (normal) and hyperchromic (high).

The sections that follow describe the mechanisms that cause these anaemias.

## Anaemia from blood loss

### Acute blood loss

Following acute blood loss, a state of cardiovascular collapse may occur. On cessation of haemorrhage, the plasma volume begins to be restored from the interstitial fluid compartment; this results in haemodilution and anaemia becomes apparent.

The blood picture is:

- normocytic and normochromic anaemia
- increased reticulocytes (immature red blood cells), reflecting increased haemopoiesis
- transient leucocytosis and thrombocytosis
- plasma proteins and other biochemical constituents are restored rapidly (in 2–3 days). Full red cell restoration may take up to 6 weeks.

### Chronic blood loss

Chronic blood loss is the most common cause of iron-deficiency anaemia, causing a hypochromic microcytic blood picture. The main causes of chronic haemorrhage are:

- diseases of the gastrointestinal tract—particularly peptic ulceration, carcinoma (colorectal, stomach)
- menorrhagia.

Patients with unexplained iron-deficiency anaemia require careful screening for an occult cause of blood loss.

## Haemolytic anaemias

The basic pathological change in all haemolytic anaemias is a reduction in the lifespan of the red cells due to an increased rate of destruction; this is termed haemolysis. The effects of increased haemolysis are:

- anaemia—commonly macrocytic due to increased reticulocytes (large cells) in the blood, but may be normocytic
- erythroid hyperplasia of bone marrow
- splenomegaly
- unconjugated hyperbilirubinaemia due to red cell breakdown, which may lead to the development of pigment gall stones and jaundice (kernicterus in neonates)
- haemoglobinuria—leading to tubular damage in the kidney.

The aetiology of haemolytic anaemias can be broadly classified into:

- intrinsic abnormalities of red cells—hereditary defects, acquired defects
- extrinsic abnormalities of red cells—antibody-mediated red-cell destruction, mechanical trauma to red cells.

Hereditary defects of the red cell can be classified into:

- cell membrane defects—hereditary spherocytosis and hereditary elliptocytosis
- enzyme deficiencies—deficiency of glycolytic enzymes or hexose monophosphate shunt enzymes
- haemoglobinopathies—e.g. thalassaemias and sickle-cell disease.

## Hereditary spherocytosis and hereditary elliptocytosis

Hereditary spherocytosis is the most common cause of hereditary haemolytic anaemia in the UK. It is usually an autosomal dominant condition caused by an abnormality of spectrin, the cytoskeletal-associated membrane protein.

The cells are spherical, of reduced deformability and abnormally fragile.

Reduced deformability of the spherical red cells causes their retention in the splenic microcirculation where they undergo metabolic stress caused by a lack of glucose and acidosis. Increased fragility of metabolically stressed cells causes spontaneous lysis or premature phagocytosis by the splenic macrophages.

Blood film shows:

- increased microspherocytes, which are more deeply stained with loss of the central pallor of normal erythrocytes
- increased polychromatic cells and reticulocytes.

The general clinical features are anaemia, splenomegaly (splenectomy usually performed) and jaundice.

Hereditary elliptocytosis is similar to spherocytosis but the red cells are elliptical. This is caused by abnormalities of the cytoskeletal-associated membrane proteins ankyrin, spectrin or band 42 protein.

This condition is not as severe as hereditary spherocytosis and does not usually cause anaemia or jaundice.

## Enzyme deficiencies

In erythrocytes, 90% of glucose is metabolized anaerobically to lactate via the Embden–Meyerhof glycolytic pathway (pathway is similar to regular glycolysis except that the end product is lactate not pyruvate); 10% of glucose is used in the hexose monophosphate shunt (also known as the pentose phosphate pathway) to increase the levels of NADPH to those required for the reduction of glutathione. Reduced glutathione is essential for maintaining haemoglobin (Hb) in the reduced (ferrous) state (Fig. 13.25).

### Deficiencies of glycolytic enzymes

Pyruvate kinase deficiency is a rare, autosomal recessive defect that results in congenital chronic haemolytic anaemia. Red cells become rigid due to reduced ATP formation, and they are removed by the spleen.

This is characterized by mild anaemia, jaundice and gallstones. The blood film shows raised poikilocytosis and distorted 'prickle cells'.

Many other enzymopathies of glycolytic enzymes exist but they are extremely rare, e.g. deficiencies of hexokinase, glucose phosphate isomerase and phosphofructokinase. The effects are similar to pyruvate kinase deficiency.

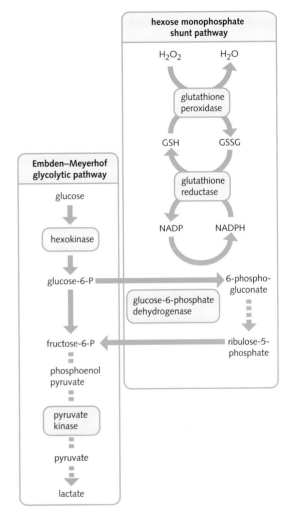

**Fig. 13.25** Metabolic pathways of the red cell. (Fructose-6-P, fructose-6-phosphate; glucose-6-P, glucose-6-phosphate; GSH, GSSG, reduced and oxidized glutathione; $H_2O_2$, hydrogen peroxide; NADP, NADPH, oxidized and reduced nicotinamide-adenine dinucleotide phosphate.)

### Deficiencies of hexose monophosphate shunt enzymes

The most common deficiencies are glucose-6-phosphate dehydrogenase (G6PD) deficiency and glutathione synthetase deficiency.

G6PD deficiency is an X-linked recessive condition that is especially common among Black races. It results in a decreased ratio of NADPH/NADP, which impairs reduction of glutathione and so increases susceptibility to oxidative stress.

Spontaneous anaemia is rare but haemolytic crises are frequently precipitated by infections, certain foods (e.g. fava (broad) beans) or certain drugs (quinine, phenacetin).

Blood film during haemolytic crises shows raised poikilocytosis with bite-shaped defects ('bite' cells) or surface blebs ('blister' cells) and Heinz bodies (red cells containing oxidized, denatured haemoglobin). The blood picture is normal between haemolytic episodes.

Female heterozygotes have the advantage of being resistant to falciparum malaria.

A deficiency of glutathione synthetase leads to defective synthesis of glutathione causing a similar syndrome to G6PD deficiency.

## Haemoglobin abnormalities (haemoglobinopathies)

Haemoglobinopathies are caused by either:

- decreased α- or β-globin synthesis—the α- and β-thalassaemias

  or

- synthesis of abnormal haemoglobin—e.g. sickle-cell disease, unstable haemoglobins.

Anaemias are usually a combined result of both dyshaemopoiesis and haemolysis.

### Thalassaemias

Normal adult haemoglobin (HbA) is composed of two α-globin chains and two β-globin chains ($\alpha_2\beta_2$). The anaemia of thalassaemias is hypochromic, with excessive production of the non-affected haemoglobin chain often producing insoluble red cell inclusions, which affect the marrow (ineffective erythropoiesis) and cause premature cell death (haemolysis).

The disease is inherited and many different causative mutations have been identified. It is common in the Mediterranean, the Middle and Far East and South-East Asia, where carrier rates of 10–15% are found.

*α-thalassaemia*—mainly caused by deletion (rather than mutation) of parts of the α-globin genes. Normal individuals have four copies of the α-globin gene, two copies on each chromosome 16. There are, therefore, four possible degrees of α-thalassaemia, depending on how many genes are abnormal (Figure 13.26). Haemolysis is less severe than in β-thalassaemia.

*β-thalassaemia*—caused by a mutation of the β-globin gene(s) leading to either reduced ($\beta^+$) or absent ($\beta 0$) synthesis of the β-globin chain. Normal individuals have two copies of each β-globin gene (one on each chromosome 11). There are, therefore, two possible degrees of β-thalassaemia:

1. Thalassaemia minor—heterozygous trait associated with mild anaemia
2. Thalassaemia major—homozygous syndrome associated with severe haemolytic anaemia.

### Sickle-cell disease

This is caused by an abnormal form of haemoglobin—HbS ($\alpha_2\beta_2^S$)—which is caused by a point mutation (resulting in the substitution of valine for glutamate) in the gene coding for the β-globin chain.

The disease is common in west and central Africa, the Mediterranean and the Middle East. In areas of Africa where malaria is endemic, up to 30% of the population is heterozygous. This is thought to be because carriage of the gene confers some protection against falciparum malaria.

HbS polymerises at low oxygen saturations, causing an abnormal rigidity and deformity of red cells, which assume a sickle shape (Fig. 13.27). As a result, deoxygenated red cells undergo aggregation (causing vascular occlusion of small vessels) and haemolysis (due to increased fragility).

### Heterozygous versus homozygous state

- Heterozygous condition—sickle-cell trait in which only 30% of the haemoglobin is HbS, resulting in no significant clinical abnormality
- Homozygous condition—sickle-cell disease in which more than 80% of the haemoglobin is HbS, the rest being HbF (fetal haemoglobin) and HbA. It is associated with serious clinicopathological features.

Figure 13.28 shows the pathogenesis and clinical features of sickle-cell disease.

### 'Crises' of sickle-cell disease

In addition to the effects of aggregation and haemolysis, sickle-cell disease is characterized by various 'crises' that occur after the age of 1 or 2 years, when HbF levels have fallen and the proportion of HbS has increased. HbF inhibits HbS polymerization, initially preventing these crises. There are three main patterns:

1. Sequestration crises—sudden pooling of red cells in the spleen and/or liver, which can lead to death from a rapid fall in haemoglobin
2. Infarctive crises—blood vessel occlusion in bone, causing the 'painful crises' (especially femoral head), spleen (leading to splenic atrophy) and skin (leg ulcers)
3. Aplastic crises—infection with parvovirus B19, which targets erythroblasts and lyses them, cause the aplastic crisis with rapid fall in blood haemoglobin.

Treatment of sickle cell disease includes the avoidance of factors known to precipitate crises, especially hypoxia. Regular blood transfusions are given to raise the haemoglobin level and reduce the proportion of HbF. Hydroxyurea chemotherapy also raises the HbF % in red cells.

Mean survival figures are variable reflecting differing standards of medical care. However, death in infancy or childhood is usual in underdeveloped countries.

**Fig. 13.26** Thalassaemia disorders

| Types of thalassaemia | | Globin chains present | Clinicopathological features |
|---|---|---|---|
| β-thalassaemia | Thalassaemia minor | Heterozygous $\beta^0\beta$ | Moderate reduction in HbA |
| | | Heterozygous $\beta^+\beta$ | Compensatory increase in $HbA_2(\alpha_2\delta_2)$ |
| | | | Mild anaemia with hypochromic cells |
| | Thalassaemia major | Heterozygous $\beta^0\beta^0$ | Hypochromic microcytic anaemia |
| | | Heterozygous $\beta^+\beta^+$ | Severe haemolysis with hepatosplenomegaly |
| | | or occasionally $\beta^+\beta^0$ | Marrow hyperplasia causing skeletal deformities |
| | | | Iron overload from repeated transfusions |
| α-thalassaemia | Silent carrier | $-\alpha/\alpha\alpha$ | Asymptomatic with normal haematology or slightly reduced MCV |
| | α-thalassaemia trait | $--/\alpha\alpha$ or $\alpha-/\alpha-$ | Asymptomatic but mild haemolytic anaemia with some microcytic cells |
| | Haemoglobin H disease | $--/\alpha-$ | Excess β-chains form tetramers: HbH |
| | | | Moderate haemolytic anaemia with hypochromia and microcytosis |
| | | | Splenomegaly |
| | Hydrops fetalis | $--/--$ | Death *in utero* |

Note: Hb, haemoglobin; MCV, mean cell volume.

## Acquired defects of the red cell

### Paroxysmal nocturnal haemoglobinuria

This rare disorder of young adults is caused by a clonal abnormality of erythrocytes, which renders them abnormally sensitive to lysis by complement. The cells lack the enzyme required for the synthesis of phosphatidyl inositol, which usually anchors several proteins to the red cell membrane. This may arise *de novo* or follow an episode of aplastic anaemia. Venous thrombosis is a frequent complication.

Haemosiderinuria is common and can cause iron deficiency. However, nocturnal haemolysis is present in only about 25% of cases. Chronic haemolysis is more usual.

## Isoimmune antibody-mediated haemolytic anaemia

### Incompatible ABO blood transfusion

This classic example of red cell haemolysis is caused by iso-antibodies (Figure 13.29).

For example, if donor blood is group A (cells contain A antigen) and recipient blood is group O (plasma contains both anti-A and anti-B antibodies), then anti-A

Fig. 13.27 Aggregation of sickle-cell haemoglobin in conditions of low oxygen.

| Fig. 13.28 Pathogenesis and clinical features of sickle-cell disease | |
| --- | --- |
| **Pathogenesis** | **Clinical features** |
| Vascular occlusion | Cerebral infarction<br>Retinopathy → blindness<br>Pulmonary infarction → acute respiratory distress<br>Cor pulmonale<br>Haematuria and polyuria<br>Splenic atrophy → hyposplenism → infections<br>Bone necrosis → osteomyelitis<br>Leg ulcers |
| Chronic haemolysis | Anaemia<br>Jaundice and gall stones<br>Haemochromatosis (due to iron overload in transfused patients) |

| Fig. 13.29 ABO blood group system | | | |
| --- | --- | --- | --- |
| **Genotype** | **Phenotype** | **Antibodies** | **Frequency of phenotype in UK** |
| OO | O | Anti-A, Anti-B | Most common |
| AA or AO | A | Anti-B | Common |
| BB or BO | B | Anti-A | Rare |
| AB | AB | None | Rarest |

antibodies of the recipient will cause agglutination and haemolysis of donor red blood cells.

**Clinical Note**

The clinical effects of an ABO incompatible transfusion:
- Massive intravascular haemolysis leading to collapse, hypotension and lumbar pain
- Haemoglobinuria is common and renal failure may ensue
- Disseminated intravascular coagulation may be triggered by red cell lysis.

The effects may be precipitated with only a few millilitres of incompatible red cells.

Transfusion-induced haemolysis due to incompatibility of the rhesus system is generally milder, since antibodies to the rhesus system are not complement fixing.

## Haemolytic disease of the newborn

This haemolysis of red blood cells in rhesus (Rh)-positive fetuses is caused by the placental passage of maternal anti-rhesus IgG antibodies from rhesus-negative mothers. It is particularly associated with D antigen of the rhesus blood group. The pathogenesis is as follows:

- First pregnancy—Rh-positive fetus in Rh-negative mother with no antibodies: healthy baby. However, if fetal red blood cells enter maternal circulation during breach of placental barrier (e.g. at birth or miscarriage), then isoimmunization of mother will occur
- Subsequent pregnancies—anti-Rh antibodies acquired by mother during previous pregnancy cause haemolytic disease of the newborn (HDN) in Rh-positive fetuses.

Incidence is now reduced by prophylactic anti-D injection in Rh-negative mothers before isoimmunization can occur.

## Autoimmune haemolytic anaemia

This is the most common type of haemolytic anaemia, caused by the immune destruction of red blood cells by the host's own antibodies. It may be idiopathic, secondary to other diseases or drug related.

It is divided into two main groups according to the temperature at which haemolytic reactions occur.

### 1. 'Warm' antibody type

The more common form, with IgG autoantibody most reactive at 37 °C leads to chronic anaemia with microspherocytes. Red cell destruction occurs in the spleen.

Clinical features are those of haemolytic anaemia: pallor, jaundice, and splenomegaly (Fig. 13.30).

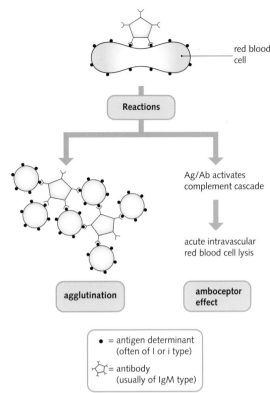

**Fig. 13.30** 'Warm' antibody-type haemolysis. The red cell membrane is modified and becomes a microspherocyte with consequences similar to hereditary spherocytosis: early sequestration in the spleen, etc. (Adapted with permission from Pathology Illustrated, 6th Edition, Churchill Livingstone, 2005.)

**Fig. 13.31** 'Cold' antibody-type haemolysis. The antibody combines with red blood cells, resulting in agglutination (clinically presenting as painful hands and feet) or the amboceptor effect (clinically presenting as paroxysmal cold haemoglobinuria-haemoglobinaemia and haemoglobinuria). (Adapted with permission from Pathology Illustrated, 6th Edition, Churchill Livingstone, 2005.)

### 2. 'Cold' antibody type

Autoantibody is IgM and is most reactive at 4 °C but it can still bind complement and agglutinate red cells at 30 °C, the temperature of peripheral tissues (hands, feet, nose and ears). There is destruction of red cells by Kupffer cells of the liver.

Clinical features are of anaemia and of blueness and coldness of the extremities, occasionally progressing to ischaemia and ulceration. Disorder is chronic and usually mild (Fig. 13.31).

Figure 13.32 summarizes the antibody-mediated haemolytic anaemias.

## Mechanical trauma to red cells

Mechanical damage to red cells may lead to reduced life-span and haemolysis.

There are several groups of mechanical haemolysis, as described below.

### Microangiopathic haemolytic anaemia

Haemolysis is caused by physical trauma to erythrocytes as they are forced through narrow areas in the vasculature. It is commonly present in:

- disseminated intravascular coagulation (see later)—red blood cells are damaged in fibrin-narrowed small blood vessels
- haemolytic uraemic syndrome
- thrombotic thrombocytopenic purpura (TTP).

Blood film shows the presence of schistocytes, helmet cells and echinocytes.

### Macroangiopathic haemolytic anaemia

This is caused by physical trauma to erythrocytes as they are forced through prosthetic (usually mechanical) heart valves.

### Malaria

Haemolysis is common in malaria. *Plasmodium* species enter the erythrocytes where they multiply and mature to form schizonts, which eventually escape by rupturing the erythrocytes. Extreme splenomegaly is often present.

**Fig. 13.32** Summary of antibody-mediated haemolytic anaemias

| Isoimmune | Autoimmune | |
| --- | --- | --- |
| | *'Warm' antibody type (auto antibody is IgG class)* | *'Cold' antibody type (auto antibody is IgM class)* |
| Transfusion reactions Haemolytic disease of the newborn | Idiopathic (50%) Secondary: <br>• chronic lymphocytic leukaemia <br>• lymphoma related <br>• systemic lupus erythematosus and other autoimmune disorders <br>• viral infections <br>• drug related, e.g. methyl-dopa, penicillin, quinidine | Idiopathic Secondary: <br>• lymphoma related <br>• infectious mononucleosis <br>• mycoplasma pneumonia |

## Megaloblastic anaemia

This type of anaemia is the result of impaired DNA synthesis in marrow precursor cells and it is caused by a deficiency of vitamin $B_{12}$ or folic acid (folate).

In the marrow, lack of vitamin $B_{12}$ or folate causes the development of abnormally large red cell precursors (megaloblasts), which develop into abnormally large red cells (macrocytes):

• Macrocytic anaemia, neutropenia and thrombocytopenia—bone marrow becomes hypercellular with megaloblasts
• Haemolytic anaemia—defective cells are prematurely destroyed.

The effects of $B_{12}$ and folate deficiency occur in most organs of the body and are prominent where cell turnover is rapid, e.g. in the marrow and mucous membranes of the alimentary tract and genitalia.

### Vitamin $B_{12}$ (cobalamin)
The source is animal products, e.g. meat and eggs.

Requirements are 1 µg per day but up to several years' supply are stored in the liver.

*Absorption*—vitamin $B_{12}$ is normally absorbed in the terminal ileum, via binding to intrinsic factor (IF), which is secreted by gastric parietal cells. The causes of vitamin $B_{12}$ deficiency are as follows:

• Pernicious anaemia—most common cause of vitamin $B_{12}$ deficiency, and in females more than males. Caused by autoimmune atrophic gastritis resulting in lack of production of IF and malabsorption of vitamin $B_{12}$. Corrected by injections of vitamin $B_{12}$
• Congenital—lack of IF
• Surgical gastrectomy—results in loss of IF

• Surgical removal of the terminal ileum—loss of vitamin $B_{12}$ absorption site
• Disease of terminal ileum (e.g. Crohn's disease)—loss of vitamin $B_{12}$ absorption site
• Bacterial overgrowth—compete for vitamin $B_{12}$
• Malnutrition—rare given liver stores but occasionally seen in veganism.

The effects of vitamin $B_{12}$ deficiency are as follows:

• megaloblastic anaemia—with associated neutropenia and thrombocytopenia
• lesions of the nervous system—myelin degeneration of posterior and lateral columns of spinal cord—subacute combined degeneration of the cord (see Chapter 5)
• malabsorption—due to mucosal changes—weight loss.

Treatment is by correction of the underlying cause (if possible), and/or injections of vitamin $B_{12}$.

### Folic acid
Sources are vegetables, cereals, meat and eggs.

Requirements are up to 200 µg per day and only 50–100 days supply is stored in the liver.

*Absorption*—folic acid is normally absorbed from the diet in the jejunum. The causes of folate deficiency are as follows:

• Malnutrition, e.g. from anorexia, alcoholism, poor diet, overcooking of food. This is the most common cause of deficiency and occurs more rapidly than vitamin $B_{12}$ deficiency because of the smaller body stores
• Malabsorption, e.g. coeliac disease, dermatitis herpetiformis, Crohn's disease

**Fig. 13.33** Comparison of vitamin $B_{12}$ and folate deficiency

|  | Vitamin $B_{12}$ deficiency | Folate deficiency |
| --- | --- | --- |
| Source | Animal produce | Most foods |
| Requirements | 1 μg/day (heat stable, body stores = several years) | Minimally 50 μg/day (heat labile, body stores = months) |
| Nutritional deficiency | Uncommon (only in vegans) | Common |
| Time of onset | Slow (years) | Over several weeks |
| Area of absorption | Absorbed in terminal ileum and requires intrinsic factor | Absorbed in jejunum (and duodenum) |
| Disease causing deficiency | Gastric or terminal ileal disease may cause deficiency | Jejunal disease may cause deficiency |
| Drug involvement | No | May be drug related (anticonvulsants or antimetabolites) |
| Neurological involvement | Neurological lesions frequent | No |

- Increased requirements, e.g. pregnancy and lactation, haemolysis, malignancy, extensive psoriasis or dermatitis
- Drugs may cause malabsorption (e.g. anticonvulsants) or may block utilization, e.g. methotrexate.

*The effects of folate deficiency*—blood and bone marrow changes are identical to those in vitamin $B_{12}$ deficiency. However, deficiency of folate is not associated with the neurological features of vitamin $B_{12}$ deficiency (Figure 13.33).

Treatment is by oral folic acid supplements, resulting in a complete reversal of the pathological features, even in malabsorption states.

## Iron-deficiency anaemia

Iron deficiency is the most common cause of anaemia.

Iron is abundant in meat, vegetables, eggs and dairy foods.

Requirements are:

- in men and postmenopausal women—1 mg per day
- in menstruating women—2 mg per day
- in pregnancy—3 mg per day
- in children—1.5 mg per day.

Absorption is via the duodenum and upper jejunum in the ferrous ($Fe^{2+}$) form.

The causes of iron deficiency are:

- chronic blood loss—most common cause (e.g. diseases of the GI tract, menorrhagia, lesions of the urinary tract)

- increased requirements, e.g. in childhood and pregnancy
- malabsorption due to gastrectomy coeliac disease
- malnutrition.

The effects of iron deficiency on the blood film are:

- hypochromic microcytic erythrocytes
- low numbers of reticulocytes for the degree of anaemia
- poikilocytosis (especially 'pencil' cells)
- anisocytosis.

Laboratory findings are as follows: reduced total serum iron, reduced serum ferritin (iron storage protein), and reduced transferrin saturation (iron carrying protein), but with a greatly increased total iron binding capacity.

Treatment is of the underlying cause and iron supplementation (ferrous sulphate).

**Clinical Note**

Clinical features of iron-deficiency anaemia are:
- anaemia—lethargy, dyspnoea, headache, palpitations
- angular cheilitis—fissures at angles of mouth
- atrophic glossitis (smooth tongue)
- oesophageal webs
- hypochlorhydria
- koilonychia (spoon-shaped nails)—seen in severe cases only
- brittle nails
- pica (indiscriminate eating of non-nutritious substances such as grass, stones or clothing).

## Dyserythropoiesis

This group of disorders is characterized by the production of defective red cells.

## Anaemia of chronic disorders

Chronic disorders are a common cause of anaemia, being second only to iron-deficiency. It may develop in patients with:

- non-organ-specific autoimmune diseases, e.g. rheumatoid disease and SLE
- chronic infective diseases, e.g. tuberculosis, malaria and schistosomiasis
- neoplasia: lymphoma and some carcinomas.

*Blood film*—mainly normocytic and normochromic but a mild degree of microcytic, hypochromic anaemia.

*Laboratory findings*—a reduced serum iron and reduced serum iron-binding capacity, but the iron stores (ferritin) are normal or increased (cf. iron-deficiency anaemia).

Erythropoietin (EPO, the hormone that stimulates erythropoiesis) is reduced, possibly due to cytokines produced by chronic disease processes. EPO injections in rheumatoid arthritis improve the anaemia.

### Sideroblastic anaemia

This anaemia, caused by defective haem synthesis, results in the accumulation of excess iron in the cytoplasm of red blood cell progenitors in the form of haemosiderin, forming cells termed ring sideroblasts.

There are two groups of the disease:

1. Primary sideroblastic anaemia—one of the myelodysplastic syndromes
2. Secondary sideroblastic anaemia—drug-, toxin-and neoplasia-related.

## Hypoplasia

This anaemia is due to the failure or suppression of red cell production in the bone marrow.

## Aplastic anaemia

A severe life-threatening disease caused by failing bone marrow stem cells, this is characterized by pancytopenia. The marrow is hypocellular, and it is replaced by fat.

It may be idiopathic or secondary to:

- whole body irradiation—therapeutically (e.g. haematological neoplasms) or in nuclear accidents (e.g. Chernobyl)
- antineoplastic chemotherapy—vincristine, busulfan
- drugs—chloramphenicol, streptomycin, chlorpromazine

- toxins—benzene
- viruses—papovavirus, HIV-1
- Fanconi's anaemia—rare autosomal recessive disorder of DNA repair.

## Red cell aplasia

This anaemia is caused by the suppression of red cell progenitor cells only. In contrast to aplastic anaemia, other blood cells are not affected. There are three main types:

1. Self-limited red cell aplasia—occurs after parvovirus infection or exposure to certain toxins
2. Chronic acquired red cell aplasia—autoimmune and it may be associated with thymomas
3. Chronic constitutional red cell aplasia—due to a hereditary defect in progenitor cells.

## Marrow infiltration

Extensive infiltration of the bone marrow may cause the obliteration of normal haemopoietic elements. It is caused by:

- leukaemias
- myelofibrosis
- disseminated carcinomas
- disseminated lymphomas.

Patients develop leucoerythroblastic anaemia characterized by circulating erythroblasts and primitive white cells. Extramedullary haemopoiesis commonly develops.

## Polycythaemia

Polycythaemia (erythrocytosis) is essentially the opposite of anaemia, defined as a sustained increase in red cell numbers, usually with a corresponding increase in haemoglobin concentration and haematocrit.

## Relative polycythaemia

This occurs when the haematocrit reading is raised due to a decrease in plasma volume, usually as a result of fluid loss (haemoconcentration). This is not 'true' (absolute) polycythaemia.

## Absolute polycythaemia

### Primary

Primary polycythaemia occurs in a rare condition termed polycythaemia rubra vera, which is one of the myeloproliferative disorders.

### Secondary

Most cases of polycythaemia are secondary to conditions resulting in:

- chronic hypoxia (common)—'appropriate' polycythaemia, e.g. high altitude, cyanotic heart disease, respiratory disease (such as chronic bronchitis, emphysema), smoking, haemoglobinopathies (resulting in defective release of $O_2$ to tissues)

- renal tumours and ischaemia (rare)—'inappropriate' polycythaemia, e.g. renal carcinomas or cysts, renal artery stenosis.

Both chronic hypoxia and renal tumours/ischaemia result in increased erythropoietin hormone production, which stimulates the bone marrow production of red cells.

Figure 13.34 compares the main features of primary and secondary polycythaemia.

## DISORDERS OF HAEMOSTASIS

## Definitions

### Purpura

This skin rash results from bleeding into the skin from capillaries. It is caused either by defects in capillaries or by defects or deficiencies of blood platelets. Individual small purple spots of the rash are called petechiae.

### Ecchymosis

This is a bruise, presenting as a bluish-black mark on the skin resulting from the release of blood into the tissues either through injury or through the spontaneous leaking of blood from the vessels.

## Abnormalities of the vessel walls

This heterogeneous group of conditions (the 'non-thrombocytopenic purpuras') is characterized by easy bruising and spontaneous bleeding from small vessels. The underlying lesions are of two main types:

1. Abnormal perivascular connective tissue which leads to inadequate vessel support
2. Intrinsically abnormal or damaged vessel wall.

Haemorrhages are mainly in the skin, causing petechiae, ecchymoses or both. In some disorders there is also bleeding from the mucous membranes. Bleeding is not usually serious.

## Infections

Some bacterial and viral infections cause purpura as a result of either vascular damage (vasculitis) by the organism or through disseminated intravascular coagulation (DIC), e.g. measles, meningococcal septicaemia.

## Scurvy and Ehlers–Danlos syndrome

Vitamin C is required for the hydroxylation of proline as a step in collagen synthesis. In both Ehlers–Danlos syndrome (an inherited disorder of collagen synthesis) and scurvy (vitamin C deficiency) capillaries are fragile because of defective collagen synthesis.

Perifollicular petechiae, bruising and mucosal haemorrhages are common.

## Steroid purpura

Long-term steroid therapy or Cushing's syndrome results in purpura caused by loss of vascular supportive tissue.

## Henoch–Schönlein purpura

This immune complex (type III) hypersensitivity reaction is usually found in children and often follows an acute infection. It is characterized by red wheals and a purple rash on the buttocks and lower legs due to bleeding into the skin from inflamed capillaries and venules.

**Fig. 13.34** Comparison of main features of primary and secondary polycythaemia

|  | Primary | Secondary |
|---|---|---|
| Prevalence | Rare | Common |
| Cause | Unknown | Hypoxia<br>Renal tumours/ischaemia |
| Erythropoietin | Normal or decreased | Increased |
| Blood film | ↑ RBCs (may be hypochromic)<br>↑ leucocytes<br>↑ megakaryocytes | ↑ RBCs (normochromic) |
| Splenomegaly | Common | None |
| *Note: RBC, red blood cell* | | |

Arthritis, acute glomerulonephritis, haematuria and GI symptoms may also occur.

It is a self-limiting condition but occasionally patients develop renal failure.

## Reduced platelet count (thrombocytopenia)

### Decreased production

This is the most common cause of thrombocytopenia (normal platelet count 150–350 × $10^9$/L).

#### Generalized disease of bone marrow
Seen in aplastic anaemia and marrow infiltration (e.g. haematological malignancies) that obliterates normal haemopoietic elements.

#### Ineffective megakaryopoiesis
- Megaloblastic anaemia (folate or vitamin $B_{12}$ deficiency)—is characterized by decreased numbers of platelets or increased numbers of megakaryocytes
- Paroxysmal nocturnal haemoglobinuria—may cause ineffective megakaryopoiesis.

### Decreased platelet survival

#### Immune destruction: autoimmune thrombocytopenic purpura
The destruction of antibody-coated platelets by the reticuloendothelial system, especially the spleen, increases the likelihood of haemorrhage:

- Skin—petechiae and ecchymoses
- Mucous membranes—e.g. epistaxis, bleeding gums, menorrhagia, haematuria, melaena
- CNS—may be fatal.

This is often associated with anaemia (secondary to blood loss).

Clinical types are:

- acute—often in children and usually self-limiting with spontaneous resolution. May be post-infective, e.g. measles
- chronic—usually in adults, mainly idiopathic but occasionally related to chronic lymphocytic leukaemia (CLL) or lymphoma. Or it may occur in association with another autoimmune disease, e.g. rheumatoid arthritis, SLE
- drug induced—e.g. quinine, heparin, sulphonamides.

#### Non-immune destruction
This is mainly through thrombotic thrombocytopenic purpura (TTP) and haemolytic-uraemic syndrome (HUS).

HUS and TTP are thought to represent the same disease process but with different distributions of thrombotic lesions.

Thrombocytopenia occurs due to abnormal platelet activation and consumption. Platelets adhere to the endothelium of capillaries and precapillary arterioles where they undergo aggregation, with fibrin deposition, which results in microvascular occlusive platelet plugs and microangiopathic haemolytic anaemia.

*Aetiology*—the underlying cause of the disorder is obscure but the following pathogenic factors have been implicated:

- Immune-mediated vessel damage
- Platelet hyperaggregation due to deficiency of an IgG inhibitor of platelet-agglutinating factor in normal plasma
- Diminished production of prostaglandin by vessel walls
- Excess of high-molecular-weight multimers of von Willebrand's factor, which interact with platelet agglutinating factor, causing platelet adhesion to vascular endothelium.

In TTP, occlusive plugs lead to widespread ischaemic organ damage, especially of the brain and kidney, resulting in neurological abnormalities and progressive renal impairment. In HUS, organ damage is limited to the kidney. Children tend to develop HUS rather than TTP.

Disseminated intravascular coagulation can also cause widespread consumption of platelets, resulting in simultaneous thrombosis and haemorrhage.

### Dilutional thrombocytopenia

Platelets are unstable at 4 °C and so blood transfusions contain few viable platelets. Therefore, transfusion with massive amounts of stored blood may cause thrombocytopenia. The effect can be minimized by replacement with specific screened products, e.g. fresh frozen plasma and platelet concentrates.

Figure 13.35 summarizes the causes of thrombocytopenia.

## Defects of platelet function

### Congenital

#### Defective adhesion (Bernard–Soulier syndrome)
This rare disease causes life-threatening haemorrhages. The platelets are deficient in glycoprotein receptors (glycoprotein Ib/IX complex), which are essential for the binding of von Willebrand's factor. The platelets are larger than normal and there is defective adherence to exposed subendothelial connective tissues and defective platelet aggregation. There is also a variable degree of thrombocytopenia.

**Fig. 13.35** Causes of thrombocytopenia

| Cause | Clinical features |
|---|---|
| Decreased platelet production | Generalized disease of bone marrow: <br> • aplastic anaemia, marrow infiltration <br> Specific impairment of platelet production: <br> • drugs: alcohol, thiazides, cytotoxics <br> • infections: measles, HIV <br> Ineffective megakaryopoiesis: <br> • megaloblastic anaemia and paroxysmal nocturnal haemoglobinuria |
| Decreased platelet survival | Immune destruction: <br> • autoimmune thrombocytopenic purpura <br> Non-immune destruction: <br> • thrombotic thrombocytopenic purpura/haemolytic-uraemic syndrome <br> • disseminated intravascular coagulation |
| Splenic sequestration | — |
| Dilutional thrombocytopenia | — |

### Defective aggregation: thromboesthaenia (Glanzmann's disease)

This failure of primary platelet aggregation is due to a deficiency of membrane receptors (glycoprotein IIb–IIIa complex) for fibrinogen binding.

### Defective secretion (storage pool disease)

A common, mild defect of platelet function. It causes easy bruising and bleeding after trauma. It is caused by a deficiency of 'dense granules' within the platelets, which normally store ADP. The decreased storage pool of ADP prevents complex platelet functions such as thromboxane release.

## Acquired

### Aspirin

Aspirin therapy is the most common cause of defective platelet function, and it produces an abnormal bleeding time.

Aspirin irreversibly inhibits cyclooxygenase, causing impairment in thromboxane $A_2$ synthesis, which is necessary for the platelet release reaction and aggregation. After a single dose the effects last 7–10 days.

Bleeding tendency is mild, with increased skin bruising and bleeding after surgery. The use of aspirin may contribute to GI haemorrhage associated with acute mucosal erosions. It can be life threatening.

### Uraemia

In uraemia, defects may be caused by an abnormal arachidonate metabolism with reduced synthesis of thromboxane. Platelet interactions with the subendothelium are abnormal and bleeding may be severe.

## Clotting factor abnormalities

## Hereditary factor abnormalities

### Von Willebrand's disease

This is the most common of the hereditary coagulation disorders. It is usually an autosomal dominant disorder of abnormal platelet adhesion associated with low factor VIII activity. The primary defect is the reduced production of von Willebrand's factor, a protein synthesized by platelets and endothelial cells which has two main functions:

1. Promotes platelet adhesion
2. Carrier molecule for factor VIII, protecting it from premature destruction.

The disease is characterized by operative and post-traumatic haemorrhage, mucous membrane bleeding (e.g. epistaxis, menorrhagia) and excessive blood loss from superficial cuts and abrasions.

Severe bleeding episodes are treated with intermediate-purity factor VIII concentrates that contain both von Willebrand's factor and factor VIII.

### Haemophilia A (factor VIII deficiency)

A common hereditary disorder of blood coagulation. It is characterized by the absence or low levels of plasma factor VIII.

Inheritance is X-linked but 33% of patients have no family history and the disorder presumably results from spontaneous mutation; it affects 1 per 10 000 in the UK.

Blood clotting time is prolonged and, in severe disease, the blood is incoagulable.

**Fig. 13.36** Classification of haemophilias

| Category | Frequency | Coagulation factor activity (% of normal) | Clinical features |
|---|---|---|---|
| Severe | 40% | <2% | Frequent spontaneous bleeding episodes from birth Degenerative joint disease |
| Moderate | 10% | 2–10% | Post-traumatic bleeding Occasional spontaneous episodes Bruising |
| Mild | 50% | 10–50% | Post-traumatic bleeding may be subclinical |

Operative and post-traumatic haemorrhage is life threatening, both in severely and mildly affected patients.

Mild, moderate and severe forms of the disease are recognized, depending on the residual clotting factor activity (Figure 13.36). Haemophilia A 'breeds true' in that the same severity of disease is seen in all affected members of a family.

*Treatment*—control can be achieved by intravenous clotting factor replacement, although antibodies against the factor VIII develop in some cases.

### Clinical Note

Haemophilia A is characterized by frequent episodes of spontaneous haemorrhage into a major joint, especially knees, hips, elbows and ankles. Without factor replacement therapy, bleeding continues until the intra-articular pressure rises sufficiently to prevent further haemorrhage (tamponade).

Resolution of acute haemarthrosis occurs slowly with recurrent bleeds producing massive synovial hypertrophy, erosion of joint cartilage and bone and changes of severe osteoarthritis.

Bleeding into muscles, retroperitoneal tissues, urinary tract and epistaxis occur.

### Haemophilia B (factor IX deficiency)

Inheritance, clinical features and treatment principles of factor IX deficiency are identical to those of haemophilia A. However, factor IX deficiency is less common, the incidence being only about one-fifth of that of haemophilia A.

The features of the most common hereditary clotting factor deficiencies are summarized in Figure 13.37.

## Acquired factor abnormalities

Acquired disorders of coagulation are far more common than the inherited disorders, and multiple clotting factor deficiencies are usual.

**Fig. 13.37** Common hereditary clotting factor abnormalities

| | Haemophilia A | Factor IX deficiency | Von Willebrand's disease |
|---|---|---|---|
| Deficiency | Factor VIII | Factor IX | Von Willebrand factor→ factor VIII deficiency |
| Inheritance | X-linked | X-linked | Dominant |
| Prevalence in the UK | 1 in 10 000 | 1 in 50 000 | 1 in 5000 |
| Main sites of haemorrhage | Muscle, joints: post trauma or post surgery | Muscle, joints: post trauma or post surgery | Mucous membranes, post trauma and operation |

## Vitamin K deficiency

Vitamin K is essential for the $\gamma$-carboxylation and hence activation of factors II, VII, IX and X, as well as proteins C and S (inhibitors). The deficiency is associated with decreased activity of these proteins, leading to coagulopathies. This may present in the newborn or in later life.

Vitamin K is obtained from green vegetables and bacterial synthesis in the gut. It is a fat-soluble vitamin and requires bile for its absorption.

Causes of vitamin K deficiency:

- inadequate diet
- malabsorption—e.g. obstructive jaundice (reduced bile), coeliac disease
- drugs—warfarin (a vitamin K antagonist). A very commonly used drug requiring regular monitoring of blood clotting (via the international normalized ratio; INR). In emergency life-threatening bleeds, vitamin K supplementation is used.

Neonates are particularly susceptible to vitamin K deficiency because of their lack of gut bacteria and low concentrations of the vitamin in breast milk. Vitamin K can be prophylactically supplemented at birth in at-risk babies.

## Liver disease

This is commonly associated with coagulation defects due to:

- impaired absorption of vitamin K caused by biliary obstruction, producing decreased activation of factors II, VII, IX and X and proteins C and S
- reduced synthesis of clotting factors and of fibrinogen, and increased amounts of plasminogen activator in severe hepatocellular disease and cirrhosis

- thrombocytopenia from hypersplenism associated with portal hypertension
- dysfibrinogenemia: functional abnormality of fibrinogen found in many patients with liver disease
- qualitative platelet disorders.

## Disseminated intravascular coagulation

Disseminated intravascular coagulation (DIC) is characterized by increased coagulation, which leads not only to widespread thrombosis but also to haemorrhage due to consumption of platelets and coagulation factors. Thus both thrombosis and haemorrhage are features of this disorder.

The disorder may cause a severe haemorrhagic syndrome with high mortality or may run a milder, more chronic course.

*Aetiology*—this is shown in Figure 13.38.

*Pathogenesis*—the causes listed in Table 13.23 activate the coagulation system in small vessels throughout the body via:

- release of procoagulant material into circulation, e.g. obstetric disorders, certain malignancies, liver disease, severe falciparum malaria and haemolytic transfusion reactions
- widespread endothelial damage, e.g. septicaemia, certain viral infections, severe burns or hypothermia
- platelet aggregation: some bacteria, viruses and immune complexes may have a direct effect on platelets.

The main effects of DIC are:

- thrombosis causes ischaemic organ damage and microangiopathic haemolysis
- consumption of platelets, clotting factors and fibrinogen causes haemorrhage

**Fig. 13.38** Causes of disseminated intravascular coagulation

| Problem | Cause |
| --- | --- |
| Infections | Septicaemia, viral infections (purpura fulminans), malaria |
| Malignancy | Carcinomas of pancreas, lung and prostate<br>Acute promyelocytic leukaemia |
| Obstetric complications | Amniotic fluid embolism, placental abruption, retained dead fetus |
| Hypersensitivity reactions | Anaphylaxis, incompatible blood transfusion |
| Widespread tissue damage | Burns, major accidental trauma, major surgery, shock, intravascular haemolysis, dissecting aortic aneurysm |
| Liver disease | Various causes |

DIC is a very important condition.

Remember that it causes both thrombosis and haemorrhage. It may be triggered by a wide variety of conditions (Table 13.23) and can be rapidly fatal if not recognized quickly.

- Activation of fibrinolytic system results in increased fibrin degradation products (e.g. D-dimer, which is measurable). These products may themselves have anticoagulant effects causing further haemorrhage.

Treatment is of the underlying cause, with clotting factor and platelet replacement.

## Thrombosis

Thrombosis is the formation of a solid mass of blood constituents—a thrombus—within the vascular system during life. It is not to be confused with a clot, which occurs in non-flowing blood.

Thrombosis can affect both arteries and veins. It is considered in detail in Chapter 6.

# Pathology of the skin  14

## TERMINOLOGY OF SKIN PATHOLOGY

### Macroscopic appearances

### Macule

This localized, flat area of altered skin colour can be hyperpigmented as in a freckle, hypopigmented as in vitiligo, or erythematous as in a capillary haemangioma.

### Papule

A small, raised, solid lesion of the skin. This is generally defined as being less than 5 mm in diameter.

### Nodule

This is similar to a papule but greater than 5 mm in diameter. It may be solid or oedematous and can involve any layer of the skin.

### Plaque

An extended papule that forms a plateau-like elevation of skin. A plaque is usually more than 20 mm in diameter, but rarely more than 5 mm in height.

### Wheal

This is similar to a papule or plaque but transitory and compressible. It is caused by dermal oedema, is red or white in colour and usually signifies urticaria.

### Blister

This fluid-filled space within the skin is caused by the separation of cells and the leakage of plasma into the space.

### Vesicle

This small blister (less than 5 mm in diameter) contains clear fluid within or below the epidermis.

### Bulla

This is similar to a vesicle but larger than 5 mm in diameter.

### Pustule

A small, pus-containing blister, a pustule commonly indicates infection, but not always (e.g. those seen in psoriasis are not infected).

### Scale

This thickened, horny layer of keratin forms readily detached fragments of skin. Scaling is caused by disturbances in the processes of keratinization and usually indicates inflammation of the epidermis (Fig. 14.1A).

### Lichenification

There is a thickening of the epidermis with exaggeration of the normal skin creases caused by abnormal scratching or rubbing of skin (Fig. 14.1B).

**Fig. 14.1** Basic lesions of the skin showing scale and lichenification.

## Excoriation

This is caused by the destruction or removal of the surface of the skin usually by scratching, but also by chemical application or other means.

## Onycholysis

This is the separation of part or all of a nail from its bed. It may occur in psoriasis and in fungal infections of the skin and nail bed, and it is more common in women.

## Microscopic appearances

Figure 14.2 is a diagrammatical representation of normal skin and normal epidermis.

## Hyperkeratosis

Thickening of the outer horny layer of the skin (stratum corneum) occurs.

## Acanthosis

This diffuse thickening of the epidermis is caused by an increased number of prickle cells in the stratum spinosum (prickle cell layer).

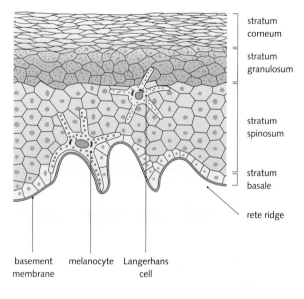

**Fig. 14.2** Normal skin and epidermis.

## Dyskeratosis

There is an abnormal premature keratinization of cells in the prickle cell layer.

## Acantholysis

The loss of cellular cohesion and separation of epidermal keratinocytes is due to the rupture of intercellular bridges. Bulla formation often results.

## Vacuolization

This is the formation of intracellular, fluid-filled spaces (vacuoles).

## Papillomatosis

In this condition, many papillomas grow on an area of skin or mucous membranes.

## Lentiginous

This describes skin whose increased pigmentation is a result of increased numbers of melanocytes.

## Erosion

This is the loss of all or part of the epidermis that does not extend into the dermis, but which heals without scarring.

## Ulceration

A full-thickness defect (epidermis and dermis) of the skin forms.

### HINTS AND TIPS

The vocabulary of dermatology is quite distinct from that of other specialties.

Learning the common dermatological terms is essential to correctly describe different skin disorders.

# INFLAMMATION AND SKIN ERUPTIONS

## Psoriasis

### Definition

Psoriasis is a chronic, non-infectious, inflammatory disease of the skin characterized by erythematous plaques covered with thick, silvery scales.

It affects about 5% of the population in the UK and it can start at any age, but the peak onset is in the second and third decades of life.

The aetiology of psoriasis is unclear; however, about 35% of patients show a family history. It is associated with HLA haplotypes Cw6, B13 and B17.

Environmental factors are thought to trigger the disease in genetically susceptible individuals.

*Pathogenesis:*

- Hyperproliferation of keratinocytes occurs
- Epidermal turnover time is greatly reduced
- Keratinocytes are normal, but the stem cell number is increased.

Thus, there is an increase in skin turnover and the granular layer is often absent. Epidermal cells are immature and there is accumulation of abnormal keratin, which results in scale. Characteristic histological features are:

- long rete ridges separated by a markedly oedematous papillary dermis in which there are large numbers of dilated capillaries
- scale—composed of flakes of thickened surface keratin, which contain remnants of nuclei (parakeratosis)
- neutrophil polymorphs migrate through the epidermis and they may be trapped beneath the thickened horny layer forming small aggregates (spongiform pustules).

*Precipitating factors*—a number of factors have been identified that can precipitate psoriasis:

- Köebner's phenomenon: trauma to skin
- Infection: β-haemolytic streptococcal throat infection may precipitate guttate psoriasis
- Drugs: β-blockers, lithium and antimalarials can precipitate or worsen psoriasis.

Psoriasis most commonly affects the extensor surfaces of the knees and elbows, the trunk and the scalp (Fig. 14.3). Nail involvement is frequent. Pitting and subungual hyperkeratosis may be followed by onycholysis.

Several types of psoriasis exist, which are of variable appearance and behaviour (Fig. 14.4).

## Complications

### Psoriatic arthropathy

About 7% of psoriasis patients develop arthropathy, which takes one of four forms:

1. Distal arthritis—the most common form. Affects the distal interphalangeal joints of the hands and feet, causing 'sausage-like' swelling of the digits
2. Rheumatoid-like arthritis—polyarthropathy similar to rheumatoid disease, but usually symmetrical and negative for rheumatoid factor (seronegative arthritis). More common in women

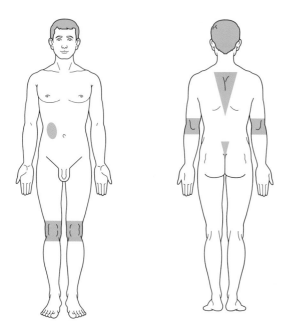

**Fig. 14.3**   Common sites of psoriasis.

3. Arthritis mutilans—progressive deformity of the hands and feet caused by erosion of the small bones. Often associated with severe psoriasis
4. Ankylosing spondylitis/sacroiliitis—in HLA-B27-positive patients.

## Management

Management of psoriasis includes topical therapy such as tar preparations, topical corticosteroids and keratolytics. Systemic therapies such as photo-chemotherapy, retinoids and cyclosporin are used in severe cases.

# Eczema and dermatitis

## Definitions

Eczema and dermatitis are synonymous terms for non-infective inflammatory conditions of the skin. They are not diseases but reactive conditions occurring in response to certain stimuli, many of which are unknown. They can be acute or chronic.

## Acute and chronic forms

### Acute eczema/dermatitis

Acute eczema/dermatitis is characterized by:

- erythema—caused by chronic inflammatory cell infiltrate (lymphocytes) around dilated vessels in the upper dermis
- fluid-filled vesicles—caused by epidermal oedema with separation of keratinocytes
- erythematous lesions—these are itchy (histamine release) and vesicles may weep and crust.

### Chronic eczema/dermatitis

Scratching of the itchy, acute-stage lesions causes secondary changes, which result in the chronic form of the condition. It is characterized by:

- thickening of the prickle cell layer (acanthosis)
- thickening of the stratum corneum (hyperkeratosis)
- elongation of the rete ridges and dermal collagenization
- dilation of dermal vessels and infiltration of the dermis with inflammatory cells.

Characteristic thickening, which occurs as a result of scratching, is termed lichenification.

## Atopic eczema

This chronic form of eczema is often associated with a strong family history of other atopic diseases such as asthma and hay fever. Uncontrollable itching is common. The condition follows a remitting/relapsing course.

| Fig. 14.4 Types of psoriasis | |
|---|---|
| **Type** | **Features** |
| Plaque | Most common type. Disc shaped, erythematous plaques covered with white silvery scale |
| Guttate | Symmetrical 'drop-like' lesions. May be associated with streptococcal infection in the young |
| Flexural | Smooth erythematous plaques, often glazed |
| Localized | Scalp, palmoplantar pustulosis, napkin (nappy area in infants), and acrodermatitis of Hallopeau (nails) types |
| Generalized | Rare, but potentially life threatening |

Although 10–15% of the population are atopic, only about 5% of these individuals will develop atopic eczema.

The aetiology of atopic eczema and other atopic diseases is not well understood. However there is a genetic predisposition.

The pathogenesis is as follows:

- Individuals prone to atopy have higher circulating levels of IgE antibodies than nonatopic individuals.
- On exposure to certain allergens, IgE-mediated, type I hypersensitivity reactions are triggered, causing mast-cell degranulation with the release of histamine and other inflammatory mediators.
- In the skin, this type of hypersensitivity reaction results in the histological changes of acute eczema, which on scratching becomes chronic eczema.

Atopic eczema presents at an early age, with 60% presenting before 1 year and 90% by 5 years.

The appearance of atopic eczema varies between different age groups (see below and Fig. 14.5):

- Infancy—babies develop the typical acute form of eczema on the face and hands, often with secondary infection
- Childhood—progression from acute to chronic condition. Usually involves flexural areas such as the antecubital and popliteal fossae, neck, wrists and ankles
- Adults—chronic condition with lichenified (and sometimes nodular) lesions. The hands are most commonly affected but a few adults also develop the chronic, severe form of generalized atopic eczema, which is often precipitated by stressful situations.

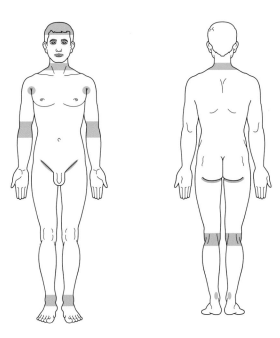

**Fig. 14.5** Distribution of atopic eczema.

**HINTS AND TIPS**

The prognosis from infantile eczema (starting before the age of 2) is actually pretty good—50% of cases will clear by 5 years and 90% will clear by 12 years of age.

The complications are:

- bacterial infection—typically with *Staphylococcus aureus*
- viral infection—increased susceptibility to the development of viral warts, molluscum contagiosum and to widespread eruption following secondary infection with herpes simplex (eczema herpeticum)
- sleep disturbance (itchiness)—potentially causing behavioural or developmental difficulties.

The treatment for atopic eczema is topical therapy (emollients, topical steroids and antibiotics), systemic therapy (antihistamines and antibiotics) and allergen avoidance (e.g. house-dust mite, rarely certain foodstuffs).

## Contact dermatitis

Contact dermatitis is a form of dermatitis precipitated by exogenous agents (Fig. 14.6). It can be classified into:

- irritant contact dermatitis—the most common form. Caused by contact of the skin with abrasives, acids, alkalis, solvents or detergents
- allergic contact dermatitis—caused by a type IV (delayed-type) hypersensitivity reaction to allergens such as nickel.

Lesions are localized to the site of contact, and they are most common on the hands and face.

Management is by identification and reduction in contact of the allergen/irritant (e.g. by protective gloves) and by topical therapy (e.g. steroids).

## Other forms

### Seborrhoeic dermatitis

This is a common, chronic inflammatory condition in which the skin is reddened and covered by thick, waxy or white scale. The eruption often occurs in the sebaceous gland areas of the scalp and face, although other areas may also be involved.

The aetiology is unknown but genetic factors and overgrowth of the yeast commensal *Pityrosporum ovale* have been implicated.

There are four common patterns in the clinical presentation (as shown in Fig. 14.7):

1. Scalp and facial involvement—affects the side of the nose, scalp margin, eyebrows and ears; excessive dandruff is usually present. Most common in young males. Causes 'cradle cap' in infants

**Fig. 14.6** Distribution and causes of contact dermatitis.

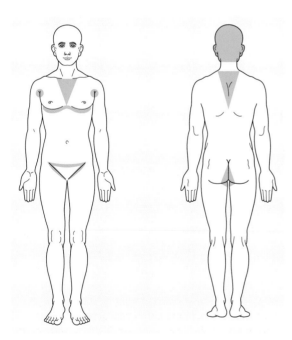

**Fig. 14.7** Distribution of seborrhoeic dermatitis.

2. Petaloid—affects the presternal area
3. *Pityrosporum folliculitis*—erythematous follicular eruption with papules or pustules, typically affecting the back

4. Flexural—involvement of the axillae, groin and sub-mammary areas, often secondarily colonized by *Candida albicans*.

The management is as follows:
- Medicated shampoos for scalp lesions
- Topical antifungals for facial, truncal and flexural involvement
- Topical hydrocortisone.

### Discoid eczema
A condition of unknown aetiology, this is characterized by 'coin-shaped', symmetrical, eczematous lesions, which typically affect the limbs of elderly men and young men who drink alcohol excessively. Secondary bacterial infection is common.

### Asteatotic eczema (eczema craquelé; winter eczema)
This dry eczema with cracking of the skin appears as a fine, 'crazy-paving' pattern of fissuring, commonly affecting the limbs and trunk of the elderly. Causes are the overwashing of patients in institutions, a dry winter climate, hypothyroidism or the use of diuretics.

**HINTS AND TIPS**

The terms 'dermatitis' and 'eczema' essentially describe the same reactive condition, i.e. they are histopathologically identical. Although the terms are often used interchangeably, eczema is sometimes used to describe the reaction that occurs in response to an endogenous stimulus, whereas dermatitis is used to describe the reaction that occurs in response to an exogenous stimulus.

## INFECTIONS AND INFESTATIONS

## Bacterial infections

### Normal skin microflora

The skin is colonized by numerous microorganisms known as microflora or commensals (see Chapter 4). Some examples are:

- *Staphylococcus epidermidis*
- *Staphylococcus aureus.*
- Streptococci.
- *Pseudomonas aeruginosa.*
- Anaerobes.
- *Candida* species.

### Overgrowth of normal flora

Some diseases are caused by an overgrowth of normal flora:

- Trichomycosis axillaris—overgrowth of coryne-bacteria, which form yellow concretions on axillary hair
- Pitted keratolysis—overgrowth of micrococci, which digest keratin causing malodorous and pitted erosions with depressed discoloured areas, often on the feet. Occurs with high humidity and hyperhidrosis (increased sweating).

### Staphylococcal infections

#### Impetigo

This highly contagious superficial skin infection is caused by either group A streptococci or *Staphylococcus aureus*. It is relatively rare in the UK, typically affecting children with poor hygiene.

#### Ecthyma

This is a full-thickness infection of epidermis by *Staphylococcus aureus.*

The clinical features of ecthyma are as follows:

- Characterized by circumscribed, ulcerated and crusted infected lesions that eventually heal with scarring

**Clincal Notes**

Impetigo is characterized by the development of large, thin-walled bullae, often on the face, which leave areas of yellow crusted exudate (classically described as honey-coloured). Satellite lesions of impetigo occur due to autoinfection from the primary site.

Common differential diagnoses are herpes simplex or fungal infections.

The management of impetigo is by the removal of crusts with saline soaks and the application of topical antibiotics (usually penicillins); widespread infection can be treated with systemic antibiotics.

- Occurs most commonly on the legs, usually as a result of an insect bite or neglected minor injury
- May also be seen in drug addicts due to the use of contaminated needles.

The management of ecthyma is by systemic and topical antibiotics.

#### Folliculitis

This infection of multiple hair follicles is usually caused by *Staphylococcus aureus*.

The clinical features of folliculitis are:

- characterized by the production of tiny pustules located in the necks of hair follicles (superficial folliculitis)
- in men, it commonly affects the beard area
- in women, it commonly affects the legs after hair removal by shaving or waxing.

A furuncle (boil) is when a deep inflammatory nodule develops within folliculitis, resulting in an expanding collection of pus that destroys the follicle and extends into the surrounding dermis.

A carbuncle is a deep abscess formed in a group of follicles with multiple drainage channels, resulting in a painful suppurating mass; it may cause systemic symptoms.

The management of folliculitis is through systemic and topical antibiotics.

Carbuncles often need surgical drainage.

#### Staphylococcal scalded skin syndrome

An acute toxic illness usually of infants, this is characterized by the shedding of sheets of skin, and it is caused by the potent exotoxin (exfoliatoxin) produced by a specific strain of *Staphylococcus aureus*.

The clinical presentation is as follows:

- Extensive disruption of the epidermis, with widespread confluent blistering and denuded erythematous areas resembling scalding of the skin

- May follow impetigo, due to the spread of localized staphylococci into the bloodstream.

*Management*—this is a serious condition treated with potent systemic antibiotics and managed like superficial burns.

## Streptococcal infections

### Erysipelas

This acute, erythematous, superficial cellulitis is caused by *Streptococcus pyogenes.*

The clinical presentation is as follows:

- Usually affects the face or the lower leg and appears as a painful red swelling
- Lesion is usually well demarcated and often oedematous and tender
- Often preceded by fever and flu-like symptoms
- Streptococci usually gain entry to the skin via a fissure.

Severe infection requires parenteral antibiotic treatment, usually penicillin. Less severe cases can be treated with oral antibiotics.

### Necrotizing fasciitis

A deep-spreading infection of the fat, fascia and muscle, this is caused by *Streptococcus pyogenes.*

The condition presents as an ill-defined erythema typically affecting the leg and associated with a high fever. Infected tissues become rapidly necrotic.

It usually occurs in otherwise healthy subjects after minor trauma. It may lead to toxaemia and multisystem organ failure.

*Management*—is by extensive emergency surgical debridement (removal of dead tissue); systemic antibiotics are essential.

## Mycobacterial infections

Tuberculosis (TB) of the skin is uncommon in the UK but is occasionally seen in the elderly and in recent immigrants from Asia.

Cutaneous manifestations of TB:

- Lupus vulgaris—the most common *Mycobacterium tuberculosis* skin infection in the UK. It usually occurs following reactivation of pre-existing disease and presents as a slowly progressive chronic skin lesion characterized by reddish-brown plaques. Typically, it affects the head or neck.
- Scrofuloderma—cutaneous involvement resulting from spread of infection from an underlying lymph node (usually cervical). Fistulae and scarring may occur.
- Warty tuberculosis—warty plaque that occurs on inoculation of the skin in an individual with immunity from a previous infection. Typically it affects the

hands, knees or buttocks. Rare in Western countries, this is the most common form of cutaneous TB in developing countries.

All types are characterized by giant cell granulomatous inflammation in the dermis leading to the destruction of dermal collagen and skin appendages. Scarring is common and sometimes destruction of deeper tissues such as cartilage occurs.

Treatment is with a 6- or 9-month course of antibiotics.

## Spirochaetal infections

### Syphilis

Syphilis is a chronic infectious disease caused by the spirochaete *Treponema pallidum,* which is usually transmitted by sexual intercourse. Skin manifestations tend to present during the secondary stage, in which there is an inflammatory response in the skin and mucous membranes.

The clinical presentation is as follows:

- Presents about 4–12 weeks after the onset of primary chancre (primary stage)
- Characterized by a non-itchy, pink or copper-coloured papular eruption on the trunk, limbs, palms and soles of the feet. It is often accompanied by lymphadenopathy and general malaise
- Other signs are moist warty papules (condylomata lata) in the anogenital area, buccal erosions and diffuse patchy alopecia
- Untreated, the eruption resolves in 1–3 months.

Management is by intramuscular penicillin. Sexual partners must be traced and they—and the patient— must be assessed for other venereal diseases.

### Lyme disease

This cutaneous and systemic infection is caused by the spirochaete *Borrelia burgdorferi* and spread by certain ticks. The majority of cases develop a slowly-extending erythematous rash at the site of the tick bite. Intermittent systemic symptoms include fever, malaise, headache, neck stiffness, and muscle and joint pain.

## Other bacterial infections

### Anthrax

This rare infection is caused by *Bacillus anthracis* associated with farm animals, particularly cattle.

A haemorrhagic bulla forms at the site of inoculation. This may be followed by vasculitis and a necrotizing, haemorrhagic inflammation of the skin.

The disease has a variable clinical course but death can occur if it is not rapidly diagnosed and treated.

Figure 14.8 provides a summary of bacterial skin infections.

**Fig. 14.8** Summary of bacterial skin infections

| Causative bacteria | Associated skin disease |
|---|---|
| Commensal overgrowth | Erythrasma, trichomycosis axillaris, pitted keratolysis |
| Staphylococci | Impetigo, ecthyma, folliculitis, scalded skin syndrome |
| Streptococci | Erysipelas, impetigo, necrotizing fasciitis |
| Mycobacteria | TB (lupus vulgaris, scrofuloderma, warty tuberculosis), leprosy |
| Spirochaetes | Secondary syphilis, yaws/bejel/pinta, Lyme disease |
| Others | Anthrax, Gram-negative infections |

*Note: TB, tuberculosis*

## Viral infections

### Viral warts (verrucae)

These common, benign, hyperkeratotic, papillomatous growths on the skin are caused by infection with human papillomavirus (HPV). The link between HPV infection of the skin and future skin cancer risk is currently unclear.

Keratinocytes in the stratum granulosum (granular layer) beneath the wart are often vacuolated due to the viral infection.

### Common warts
Firm, dome-shaped, horny papules (1–10 mm across), and usually multiple, warts are found mainly on the hands; they can also affect the feet, face and genitalia.

### Plantar warts
These occur on the soles of the feet and are often covered by callus (hyperkeratosis). Pressure causes inward growth, which results in tenderness.

### Plane warts
Flat, skin-coloured papules usually found on the face. These are usually multiple. They resist treatment but eventually resolve spontaneously.

### Genital warts
These affect the genitalia and the perianal region, and are linked to increased cervical cancer risk in women (see Chapter 11).

### Management
Hand and foot warts frequently disappear spontaneously. Resistant varieties are treated with topical 'wart paints' (salicylic acid, lactic acid, gluteraldehyde, etc.) or with cryotherapy. Genital warts generally require cryotherapy or curettage and cautery with a local anaesthetic.

## Molluscum contagiosum

This presents as discrete, multiple, pale papules with a central depression. It is caused by a DNA poxvirus.

*Clinical presentation*—mainly affects children or young adults. The most commonly affected areas are the face, neck and trunk, but it can affect the upper thighs when sexually acquired.

The virus is transmitted by contact, including sexual transmission, or on towels.

Untreated, the papules disappear in 6–9 months.

The treatment is by curettage, cryotherapy or by expressing the content of the papule under local anaesthetic.

## Herpes simplex

A common, acute vesicular eruption of the skin or mucous membranes, this is caused by infection with herpes simplex virus (HSV).

Pathologically:

- HSV blisters are highly contagious and they are transmitted through direct contact
- virus penetrates the epidermis or mucous membrane and replicates in the epithelial cells
- following primary infection, the virus enters a latent stage within infected cells or the dorsal root ganglion (e.g. cold sores—herpes labialis)
- reactivation can occur at any time, even years after initial infection
- recurrence is thought to be precipitated by respiratory infection, sunlight or local trauma.

*Clinical presentation*—there are two types of HSV:
1. HSV type 1—primary infection usually occurs in childhood and causes the common cold sore, present on or around the lips. Epithelial infection may be accompanied by fever, malaise or local lymphadenopathy. Lasts for about 2 weeks

2. HSV type 2—this is mainly associated with genital herpes and it is sexually transmitted (see Chapter 11).

However, both type 1 and 2 viruses can cause genital herpes and cold sores, depending on the site of the initial infection.

Complications are:

- secondary bacterial superinfection—usually staphylococcal
- eczema herpeticum—atopic eczema may be complicated by herpes simplex infection. Causes corneal dendritic ulceration that can threaten sight. Rarely, eczema herpeticum can be fatal
- disseminated herpes simplex—occasionally occurs in the newborn or in immunosuppressed patients. Active HSV is transmissible from mother to baby at birth and is an indication for elective caesarian section
- chronic herpes simplex—common in HIV patients
- herpes encephalitis—serious complication of HSV infection
- erythema multiforme—immune-mediated disease characterized by erythematous lesions on the hands and feet.

Management is by topical aciclovir (used for mild facial or genital herpes simplex) and oral aciclovir (prescribed for severe episodes of HSV infection).

## Herpes zoster (shingles)

This acute, vesicular eruption occurs in a dermatomal distribution. It is caused by the reactivation of latent varicella zoster virus (VZV).

Following an attack of chickenpox, the virus remains dormant in the dorsal root ganglion of the spinal cord. On reactivation (the causes of which are unknown), the virus migrates down the sensory nerve to affect one or more dermatomes on the skin.

### Clinical Note

Shingles clinical presentation:
- Densely grouped vesicles and erythema in the distribution of one dermatome
- Usually thoracic dermatomes, except in the elderly (in whom the ophthalmic division of the trigeminal nerve is more common)
- Pain, tenderness and paraesthesia may precede vesicular eruption
- Vesicles become pustular and form crusts, which separate after 2–3 weeks to leave scarring
- Vesicular blisters contain virus, which when shed may cause chickenpox in VZV-naïve contacts
- Local lymphadenopathy is common.

Complications are:

- secondary bacterial infections
- postherpetic neuralgia—occurs in one-third of those over 60 years old, but infrequently in patients under 40 years old. Pain usually subsides within 6 months
- ophthalmic scarring—corneal ulcers and scarring may occur following shingles of the ophthalmic division of the trigeminal nerve
- motor palsy—rare; viral involvement may spread from the posterior horn of the spinal cord to the anterior horn to infect motor nerves, resulting in palsies or paralysis of individual muscles or muscle groups
- disseminated herpes zoster—may occur in the immunosuppressed leading to potentially fatal varicella pneumonia or encephalitis.

Management is with oral aciclovir, which, if taken within 48 hours of onset, decreases the duration and the intensity of the disease; it may also prevent post-herpetic neuralgia. Symptomatic treatment with rest, analgesia and calamine lotion is also important.

## Fungal infections

### Dermatophyte infections

Dermatophytes are filamentous (hyphal) fungi, which reproduce by spore formation. They commonly inhabit the keratin of the skin, hair and nails producing superficial mycoses (Figure 14.9).

Dermatophytes are collectively termed 'ringworm' but they comprise three genera:

1. Microsporum, e.g. *Microsporum canis*
2. Trichophyton, e.g. *Trichophyton rubrum* and *Trichophyton interdigitale*
3. Epidermophyton, e.g. *Epidermophyton floccosum*.

Management is either topical or systemic depending on the extent of infection. Humid and sweaty conditions, including occlusive footwear, should be minimized.

### Candida albicans

*Candida albicans* is a yeast-type fungus. It is a commensal of the vagina and alimentary canal and commonly produces opportunistic infections. Predisposing factors may be humidity, obesity, diabetes and oral antibiotic therapy.

*Clinical presentation*—in infection, hyphal forms of *Candida albicans* are seen, and the infection is termed candidosis (or candidiasis), which can present in numerous patterns as discussed below.

**Fig. 14.9** Dermatophyte infections and their clinical effects

| Affected area | Most common organism | Clinical presentation |
|---|---|---|
| Tinea corporis (trunk and limbs) | *Trichophyton verrucosum, Microsporum canis, Trichophyton rubrum* | Single or multiple ring lesions with scaling and erythema, especially at the edges<br>Usually asymmetrical |
| Tinea pedis (athlete's foot) | *Trichophyton rubrum, Trichophyton interdigitale, Epidermophyton floccosum* | Redness, erosion and scaling which is often interdigital, but diffuse involvement of skin also occurs<br>Common in young men; increased predisposition by communal washing, swimming baths, occlusive footwear, and hot weather<br>Most common form of ringworm in the UK |
| Tinea capitis (scalp/hair) | *Microsporum canis, Microsporum audouinii, Trichophyton tonsurans, Trichophyton schoenleinii* | Hair loss and scaling<br>Usually affects children |
| Tinea cruris (groin) | *Trichophyton rubrum, Epidermophyton floccosum, Trichophyton interdigitale* | Red, scaly, itchy rash with brown patches; more common in men and often seen in athletes ('jock itch')<br>Starts on groin flexures and spreads to thighs |
| Tinea manuum (hand) | *Trichophyton rubrum* | Unilateral diffuse powdery scaling of the palm |
| Tinea unguium (nails) | *Trichophyton rubrum, Trichophyton interdigitale* | Thick, crumbling nails more commonly affecting toenails<br>Incidence of onychomycosis increases with age |

## Genital

This is especially common in the vagina ('thrush') where white-yellowish plaques on the inflamed mucous membranes produce itching/discomfort, and sometimes a white vaginal discharge.

## Oral

White plaques adhere on the tongue or inside the cheeks.

### Intertrigo

A superficial inflammation of two skin surfaces that are in contact (e.g. between the thighs or under the breasts) is often aggravated by *Candida albicans* infection.

## Mucocutaneous

This pattern of candidiasis occurs in individuals with T cell defects, most commonly occurring in Addison's disease and hypoparathyroidism. It causes chronic *Candida albicans* intertrigo and nail and mouth infections.

## Management

Management is by:

- topical therapy—for body folds and oral and genital *Candida*
- systemic therapy—a short course is useful for recurrent or persistent candidosis (reduces bowel carriage), also as long-term treatment for mucocutaneous candidiasis.

## Infestations

### Insect bites

These are a cutaneous inflammatory reaction to insect parts or to injected foreign substances. Common culprits include garden insects (gnats, etc.), insects of household pets (fleas, mites) and bedbugs.

Bites are usually grouped on a limb and lesions vary from itchy wheals to quite large bullae, depending on the insect and the type of immune response elicited.

Secondary bacterial infection of excoriated insect bites is common.

It can be managed by the elimination of the cause, if within the household, and with topical hydrocortisone or calamine lotion.

### Scabies

Scabies is caused by the burrowing of the female mite *Sarcoptes scabiei* through the stratum corneum where she lays her eggs. After a few days the eggs hatch into larvae, which moult and mature in the epidermis. The new mites mate in the stratum corneum. The male dies and the fertilized female burrows into the skin and continues the cycle.

*Clinical presentation*—very itchy, raised lesions, often red and scaling, typically arise on the sides of fingers, palms, nipples and genitalia.

**Fig. 14.10** Skin involvement in lepromatous and tuberculoid forms of leprosy

| Lepromatous form | Tuberculoid form |
|---|---|
| Minimal immune response (occurs in patients with low cellular immunity) | Vigorous T-cell-mediated (delayed) hypersensitivity |
| Bacteraemia occurs to peripheral sites | Bacteraemia rare |
| Many skin lesions with symmetrical distribution | Few skin lesions with asymmetrical distribution |
| Macules, papules, plaques and nodules | Raised, red plaques with hypopigmented centre. Sensation is often impaired within the plaque |
| Typically involves arms, legs, buttocks and face | Often affects the face |
| Progression causes a thickened, furrowed appearance of face (leonine facies) with eyebrow loss | Progression is slow; combined effect of extensive destruction of tissue by immune response and repeated trauma to desensitised areas results in severe disfigurement, especially to hands and feet |
| Untreated, this form is lethal due to the impaired immune response | Eventually heals spontaneously |

Linear tracks (the burrows), about 1 cm long, are often seen, and the mite can sometimes be removed by blunt needle to confirm the diagnosis.

Itching causes excoriation that frequently results in secondary bacterial infection. Untreated, the condition becomes chronic.

*Management*—scabies is transmitted by direct transfer and, therefore, all contacts require treatment.

*Treatment*—is with topical scabicides applied to the whole body.

## Tropical skin infections and infestations

### Leprosy (Hansen's disease)

This chronic granulomatous disease is caused by *Mycobacterium leprae*.

Leprosy is rare in the UK but is common in tropical and subtropical areas. There are about 10 million patients worldwide.

Transmission is by the inhalation of nasal droplets, after which the incubation period may be many years.

The clinicopathological features of leprosy depend on the degree of cell-mediated immunity instigated against the infection by the host. This may vary in a spectrum from strong (tuberculoid leprosy) to weak (lepromatous leprosy).

*Clinical presentation*—*Mycobacterium leprae* has a predilection for nerves (causing peripheral neuritis—see Chapter 5) and the skin. Figure 14.10 shows the skin involvement in the lepromatous and tuberculoid forms of leprosy.

*Management*—is by antibiotic treatment (usually multiple) for at least 2 years.

### Leishmaniasis

A common disease in the tropics and subtropics caused by the protozoan *Leishmania*, this is transmitted by sand flies. Three forms of the disease exist, caused by different species of *Leishmania* (Figure 14.11)

*Management*—cutaneous leishmaniasis often heals spontaneously over several months. However, other forms require pentavalent antimonials intravenously for 10–21 days.

### Larva migrans

Also known as 'creeping eruption', this is caused by the larvae of dog hookworms. Larvae burrow through the skin (most commonly the feet), leaving intensely itchy tracks in their wake. Treatment is with topical tiabendazole, although the larvae die spontaneously after a few weeks, as they cannot complete their life cycle in humans.

### Deep mycoses

These systemic diseases are caused by fungal invasion. They include:

• blastomycosis—wart-like ulcers on the face, neck and limbs, plus lung disease

**Fig. 14.11** Different types of leishmaniasis

| Type of leishmaniasis | Endemic areas | Protozoan | Clinical presentation |
|---|---|---|---|
| Visceral (kala azar) | Asia, Africa and South America | *Leishmania donovani* | Affects lymphatic system, spleen and bone marrow, causing splenomegaly, hepatomegaly, anaemia and disability; patchy pigmentation may occur on face, hands and abdomen |
| Cutaneous | Mediterranean coast, Middle East and Asia | *Leishmania tropica* | Characterized by 'oriental sore', a red–brown nodule that appears at site of inoculation and which either ulcerates or spreads slowly to form crusty plaque |
| Mucocutaneous | Central and South America | *Leishmania braziliensis* | Characterized by a skin lesion similar to that of oriental sore but is followed by necrotic ulcers which cause deformity of nose, lips and palate |

- histoplasmosis—lung disease plus granulomata of the skin (pathologically similar to tuberculosis)
- mycetoma—chronic granulomatous sinuses on the foot or hand
- Sporotrichosis—chronic granulomatous skin infection.

### Onchocerciasis

This endemic disease of Africa and Central America is caused by the nematode worm *Onchocerca volvulus*, which is transmitted to humans by a gnat. The worms cause an itchy papular eruption on the skin, which progresses to form fibrous nodules with lichenification and pigmentary change. Microfilariae also invade the eye, resulting in total or partial blindness (called 'river blindness' in Africa).

## DISORDERS OF SPECIFIC SKIN STRUCTURES

## Sweat and the sebaceous structures

### Acne vulgaris

This inflammatory disorder of the pilosebaceous apparatus is characterized by comedones (blackheads and whiteheads), papules, pustules, nodules, cysts and scars. It is extremely common in adolescents, the peak age for clinical acne being 18 years.

*Aetiopathogenesis*—the cause of acne is uncertain but the androgen-sensitive sebaceous glands show a hyper-responsiveness to testosterone that results in the following sequence of events:

- Increased sebum excretion
- Hyperkeratosis of pilosebaceous ducts

- Blockage of pilosebaceous units with excess keratin and sebum, causing comedo formation
- Colonization of ducts with *Propionibacterium acnes*
- Release of inflammatory mediators.

Figure 14.12 illustrates the pathogenesis of acne.

*Clinical presentation*—comedones (singular comedo) tend to be limited to the face, shoulders, upper chest and back. They are of two types:

1. Open as in blackheads—dilated pores with dark plugs of keratin and sebum
2. Closed as in whiteheads—small, cream-coloured, dome-shaped papules formed through sebum and keratin accumulations deeper in the ducts.

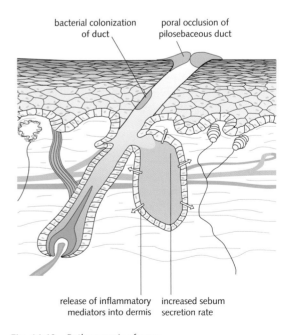

bacterial colonization of duct

poral occlusion of pilosebaceous duct

release of inflammatory mediators into dermis

increased sebum secretion rate

**Fig. 14.12** Pathogenesis of acne.

**Fig. 14.13** Management of acne vulgaris

| Type | Treatment | Comment |
| --- | --- | --- |
| Topical treatment (mild acne) | Benzoyl peroxide | Reduced numbers of *Propionibacterium acnes* but may cause irritation |
| | Tretinoin | Reduces number of non-inflamed lesions but may cause irritation |
| | Antibiotics | Used in treatment of mild or moderate acne |
| Systemic treatment (moderate or severe acne) | Antibiotics | e.g. tetracyclines or erythromycin for a minimum of 4 months |
| | Antiandrogens | Usually combined with an oestrogen and prescribed to females over a period of 6–12 months; suppresses sebum production and is also a contraceptive |
| | Retinoids | Isotretinoin: reduces sebum excretion, inhibits *Propionibacterium acnes* and is anti-inflammatory; 4- to 6-month course; very effective but side effects common |

The colonization of ducts with *Propionibacterium acnes* causes the evolution of comedones into inflammatory papules, nodules or cysts, which often form scars on healing. This may persist until the early twenties and even into the fifth decade of life in a few patients, especially in women.

Management of acne is shown in Figure 14.13.

## Rosacea

This chronic inflammatory disease of the face is characterized by erythema, telangiectasia and pustules.

The aetiology of rosacea is unknown.

Telangiectatic dilatation of the upper dermal vessels is common, and it causes erythema. Fragments of the mite *Demodex folliculorum* are commonly found in follicles but its role in the pathogenesis is unclear.

Follicular pustules often develop in the markedly dilated hair follicles.

Rupture of the follicles stimulates a granulomatous reaction that leads to a florid, lumpy form of rosacea.

### Clinical Note

Rosacea typically affects the middle-aged or elderly. There is intermittent facial flushing on top of persistent erythema. Rosacea is often complicated by:
• rhinophyma—hyperplasia of sebaceous glands and connective tissue of the nose
• eye involvement—blepharitis (inflammation of the eyelids) and conjunctivitis
• the condition is exacerbated by sunlight and topical steroids.

Management is by oral tetracycline but this will not reverse telangiectasia or prevent erythema. Plastic surgery may be required for rhinophyma.

# Hair disorders

## Alopecia

This describes the loss of hair. It is commonly classified into three main types: diffuse non-scarring, localized non-scarring and scarring (cicatricial).

### Diffuse non-scarring

There is a diffuse reduction in hair density. The patient usually notices excessive numbers of hairs on the pillow, brush or comb.

The causes of diffuse non-scarring alopecia are:
• male pattern/androgenic alopecia—inherited, androgen-dependent hair loss. Extremely common in men but it also occurs in women, becoming more pronounced after the menopause
• endocrine related—hypo- and hyperthyroidism, pituitary or adrenal hypoactivity. Androgen-secreting tumours in women can produce male pattern baldness

- nutrition related—iron or zinc deficiency, malnutrition especially kwashiorkor (protein deficiency)
- telogen effluvium—hair follicles, which are usually out of phase, can, under certain circumstances, become synchronized into the resting phase (telogen) and then shed in unison 3 months later. The causes of synchronization are high fever, childbirth, surgery, drugs or stress
- drug induced—e.g. cytotoxics, heparin, warfarin, carbimazole, colchicine and vitamin A.

### Localized non-scarring
There is patchy hair loss. The causes are:

- alopecia areata—common condition associated with autoimmune disorders, atopy and Down syndrome. The growth phase of hair is prematurely arrested
- infections, e.g. with scalp ringworm (tinea capitis) or secondary syphilis
- trauma/traction.

It typically presents in the second or third decade of life with bald patches on the scalp, but the eyebrows and beard can also be affected. The nails may show pitting.

The course is unpredictable, varying from the progressive enlargement of bald patches to the regrowth of hair (more common).

A poor prognosis is indicated if the onset is prepubertal, associated with atopy or shows extensive involvement.

Rarely, complete scalp alopecia (totalis) or loss of all bodily hair (universalis) occurs.

### Scarring (cicatricial) alopecia
This is caused by scarring of the scalp with the destruction of hair follicles.

The causes of scarring are:

- irradiation/burns (chemical or thermal)
- infection, e.g. shingles of the ophthalmic division of the trigeminal nerve, tinea capitis or tertiary syphilis
- lichen planus/lupus erythematosus—erythema, scaling and follicular changes may result in scarring
- pseudopelade—end stage of an idiopathic or unidentified destructive inflammatory process in the scalp.

## Excess hair

### Hirsutism
This is the growth of coarse, pigmented hair with an androgenic distribution in a female.

Figure 14.14 shows the aetiology of hirsutism.

### Hypertrichosis
This is excessive growth of hair in a non-androgenic distribution. It is less common than hirsutism and can be:

**Fig. 14.14** Aetiology of hirsutism

| | |
|---|---|
| Idiopathic | Most common form; probably due to increased hypersensitivity of end-organ to androgens |
| Iatrogenic | e.g. androgens, progestogens |
| Virilising tumours | e.g. ovarian or adrenal tumours |
| Endocrine disorders | Congenital adrenal hyperplasia, Cushing's syndrome, acromegaly |

- localized, e.g. on melanocytic naevi or following topical steroid usage
- generalized—fine terminal hair appears on the face, limbs and trunk. Mostly drug induced but it can also be caused by anorexia nervosa (or malnutrition), porphyria, cutanea tarda or underlying malignancy.

## Nail disorders

## Congenital disease

Congenital conditions are as follows:

- Racket nails—most common congenital nail defect characterized by broad, short, thumb nails
- Nail-patella syndrome—nails (and patellae) are absent or rudimentary
- Pachyonychia congenita—rare autosomal dominant condition causing thickened, discolored nails present from birth.

## Trauma

Traumatic conditions are as follows:

- Subungual haematoma—bleeding under the nail following trapping of a finger- or toenail
- Splinter haemorrhages—almost always occur with infective endocarditis, but they may also be trauma or psoriasis induced
- Onychogryphosis—big toenails become thickened and horn-like, usually in response to trauma
- Brittle nails—usually due to repeated exposure to detergents and water.

## Nail involvement in the dermatoses

These are:

- alopecia areata—pitting and roughness of nail surface
- psoriasis—pitting, nail thickening, onycholysis, brown patches, subungual hyperkeratosis, splinter haemorrhages
- eczema—pitting and transverse ridging. Often shiny from repeated scratching.

## Infections

Infections are:

- tinea unguium—fungal infection of the nails (Figure 14.15)
- chronic paronychia—*Candida albicans* infection of the nails, common in wet-workers (see p. 292)
- acute paronychia—typically, a bacterial infection of the nails usually caused by staphylococci.

## Tumours of the nails

The tumours are:

- viral warts—common around the nail-fold
- periungual fibroma—associated with tuberous sclerosis
- malignant melanoma—subungual malignant melanoma, which produces a pigmented longitudinal streak in a nail and may cause its destruction.

## Nail changes in systemic disease

Systemic disorders can often cause specific nail changes, which can help in the diagnosis of these conditions. Figure 14.15 gives examples of nail changes and their possible causes.

## DISORDERS OF PIGMENTATION

## Hypopigmentation

### Vitiligo

This common disorder (1% of the population) is characterized by the appearance of symmetrical white or pale macules on the skin, which are caused by focal melanocyte loss.

*Aetiopathogenesis*—it has been suggested that vitiligo is an autoimmune disease of melanocytes, as it is often associated with other autoimmune diseases, such as pernicious anaemia, thyroid disease and Addison's disease.

The exact aetiology is unknown but about 30% of patients have a family history.

*Clinical presentation*—vitiligo affects all races, but is more conspicuous in dark-skinned individuals.

Onset is usually between 10 and 30 years of age. It commonly affects the hands, wrists, knees, neck and areas around orifices (e.g. mouth). It has an unpredictable course, ranging from progression to repigmentation (rarely).

Vitiligo is managed with camouflage cosmetics and sunscreens (for both cosmetic reasons and to reduce risk of burning and skin cancer). Topical steroids occasionally induce repigmentation in darker skins. PUVA (psoralen and UV-A) is occasionally beneficial.

## Albinism

This is a rare (1 in 20 000) autosomal recessive disease characterized by the lack of pigmentation in the skin, hair and eyes. Melanocyte numbers are normal but melanin production fails because of a deficiency or defect in the enzyme tyrosinase.

The skin is white or pink, the hair is white and pigmentation is lacking in the eye. It is associated with poor sight, photophobia and nystagmus. Albinos have an increased risk of skin tumours on exposure to UV light.

Prenatal diagnosis is possible.

## Phenylketonuria

This autosomal recessive inborn error of metabolism is caused by a deficiency of phenylalanine hydroxylase, which normally converts phenylalanine to tyrosine.

Patients also have fair hair and skin because of impaired melanin synthesis (tyrosine is a precursor of melanin). The concentration of phenylalanine and its metabolites is increased and damages the neonatal brain. Untreated, mental retardation and choreoathetosis develop, although a low phenylalanine diet can prevent neurological damage.

The prevalence is 1 per 25 000 and it is detected by routine screening tests (heel-prick or Guthrie test performed around day 5 of life).

A summary of the causes of hypopigmentation is given in Figure 14.16.

## Hyperpigmentation

### Freckles and lentigines

#### Freckles (ephelides)

Freckles are small, light-brown, well-demarcated macules that darken on exposure to sunlight. They contain normal numbers of melanocytes but melanin production is increased. They are common in childhood, especially in fair-skinned children. No treatment is required.

#### Lentigines

Lentigines (also known as lentigos) are similar in appearance to freckles but they are more scattered and they do not darken in the sun. Their outline may be more irregular than freckles. They contain increased numbers of melanocytes and may develop in childhood, but they are more common in a sun-exposed, elderly skin. They respond to cryotherapy.

### Drug-induced pigmentation

This can be caused by stimulation of melanogenesis or by drug deposition in the skin. Drugs commonly responsible include amiodarone, bleomycin, psoralens, chlorpromazine and minocycline.

**Fig. 14.15** Nail changes and their possible causes

| Nail change | Description | Possible causes |
|---|---|---|
| Beau's lines | Transverse ridges | Severe illnesses that affect nail growth, e.g. pneumonia or myocardial infarction |
| Brittle nails | Easily broken nails | Repeated exposure to water/detergent, iron deficiency, hypothyroidism, ischaemia of digits |
| Colour change | Black transverse bands | Cytotoxic drugs |
| | Blue | Haematoma, cyanosis, antimalarials |
| | Blue–green | *Pseudomonas* infection |
| | Brown | Fungal infection, cigarette stains, chlorpromazine, gold, Addison's disease |
| | Brown patches | Psoriasis |
| | Brown longitudinal streak | Melanocytic naevus, malignant melanoma, Addison's disease |
| | Red–brown streaks (splinter haemorrhages) | Infective endocarditis, trauma |
| | White spots | Trauma to nail matrix (not calcium deficiency) |
| | White (leuconychia) | Hypoalbuminaemia |
| | Yellow | Psoriasis, tinea unguium, jaundice, tetracycline |
| | Yellow nail syndrome | Defective lymphatic drainage |
| Clubbing | Swelling of nail with loss of angle between nail-fold and nail plate | Respiratory: pulmonary tuberculosis, bronchiectasis, empyema, lung cancer, fibrosing alveolitis. Cardiovascular: infective endocarditis, congenital heart disease. Other less common diseases, e.g. asbestosis, Crohn's disease, ulcerative colitis, cirrhosis |
| Koilonychia | Concave (spoon-shaped) nails | Iron deficiency anaemia. Repeated exposure to detergents |
| Nail-fold telangiectasia | Reddened nail-folds caused by dilated capillaries | Inflammatory connective tissue disorders including systemic sclerosis and dermatomyositis |
| Onycholysis | Separation of part or all of nail from its bed | Psoriasis, tinea unguium, trauma, thyrotoxicosis, tetracyclines |
| Pitting | Small holes in nail-bed | Psoriasis, eczema, alopecia areata, lichen planus |
| Ridging | Transverse | Beau's lines, eczema, psoriasis, chronic paronychia |
| | Longitudinal | Secondary to trauma |

**Fig. 14.16** Summary of causes of hypopigmentation

|  | Cause | Example |
|---|---|---|
| Generalized hypopigmentation | Genetic | Albinism and phenylketonuria |
| Patchy hypopigmentation | Endocrine | Hypopituitarism (↓ACTH and ↓MSH) |
|  | Infective | Leprosy, yaws, pityriasis versicolor |
|  | Postinflammatory | Cyrotherapy, eczema, psoriasis, morphoea, pityriasis alba |
|  | Chemical | Substituted phenols, hydroquinone |
|  | Other | Vitiligo, lichen sclerosus, halo naevus |

Note: ACTH, adrenocorticotrophic hormone; MSH, melanin-stimulating hormone

**Fig. 14.17** Summary of causes of hyperpigmentation

| Cause | Problem |
|---|---|
| Genetic | Inherited: freckles, neurofibromatosis (café-au-lait spots), Peutz–Jeghers syndrome<br>Acquired: lentigines |
| Endocrine | Chloasma, Addison's disease, Cushing's syndrome, hyperthyroidism and acromegaly |
| Metabolic | Biliary cirrhosis (jaundice), haemochromatosis (iron deposition), porphyria |
| Nutritional | Carotenemia (orange discoloration), malnutrition/malabsorption, pellagra |
| Postinflammatory | Eczema, lichen planus, systemic sclerosis |
| Drugs | e.g. oestrogens, amiodarone, bleomycin, psoralens, chlorpromazine and minocycline |
| Other | Acanthosis nigricans, malignant melanoma, naevi, argyria (deposition of silver), chronic renal failure |

## Other causes

### Addison's disease

This is characterized by hypoadrenalism, with overproduction of adrenocorticotrophic hormone (ACTH) by the pituitary gland. ACTH stimulates melanogenesis, resulting in hyperpigmentation of mucosae and skin creases.

Addisonian-like pigmentation is also seen in Cushing's syndrome, hyperthyroidism and acromegaly.

### Peutz–Jeghers syndrome

This rare, autosomal dominant disorder is characterized by perioral lentigines and intestinal polyps.

Figure 14.17 provides a summary of the causes of hyperpigmentation.

## BLISTERING DISORDERS

Blisters are fluid-filled spaces within the skin caused by the separation of two layers of tissue and the leakage of plasma into the space. The type of blister formed (Fig. 14.18) depends on the level of separation. It can be:

- subcorneal—bullous impetigo or pustular psoriasis
- intraepidermal—acute eczema, herpes simplex/zoster, pemphigus, friction blisters
- subepidermal—pemphigoid, dermatitis herpetiformis, cold and thermal injury.

## Pemphigus

This rare but potentially fatal group of autoimmune disorders is marked by successive outbreaks of blisters on the skin and in the mouth.

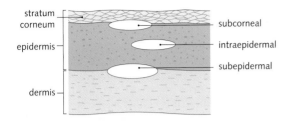

stratum corneum — subcorneal
epidermis — intraepidermal
— subepidermal
dermis —

**Fig. 14.18** Location of blisters within the skin.

*Aetiopathogenesis*—patients have circulating IgG autoantibodies that bind to intercellular junctions in the epidermis. Binding of IgG activates complement and adjacent keratinocytes are induced to release proteolytic enzymes. Cellular adhesion is lost (acantholysis), and an intraepidermal separation occurs.

This is also associated with other organ-specific autoimmune disorders, such as myasthenia gravis.

*Clinical presentation*—the most common form is pemphigus vulgaris, which typically affects middle-aged people. Oral erosions precede cutaneous blistering in 50% of cases. Flaccid, superficial blisters develop over the scalp, face, back, chest and flexures.

If left untreated, the blistering is progressive and ultimately fatal (due to the loss of electrolytes and protein). Pemphigus is associated with a 15% mortality rate. It is managed with systemic steroids and other immunosuppressive agents.

## Bullous pemphigoid

This is a chronic, itchy blistering disorder of the elderly.

*Aetiopathogenesis*—an autoimmune disorder, in which IgG antibodies are deposited at the basement membrane.

Inflammatory cells attracted by complement activation release proteolytic enzymes resulting in subepidermal bullae formation, which tend to remain intact.

*Clinical presentation*—large, tense blisters commonly appear on the limbs, trunk and flexures, but are occasionally localized to one site, often the lower leg. Oral lesions occur in only 10% of cases. An urticarial eruption may precede the onset of blistering.

The disease is self-limiting in about 50% of cases and is managed with systemic steroids and other immunosuppressants.

## Dermatitis herpetiformis

This presents as a rare eruption of symmetrical itchy blisters on the extensor surfaces.

*Aetiopathogenesis*—the aetiology is unknown but associated with coeliac disease (see Chapter 8). It is characterized by granular IgA at the dermal papillae of normal-looking skin and villus atrophy of the small intestine.

It usually presents in the third or fourth decade of life, with males more often affected than females by 2:1. There are groups of small, intensely itchy vesicles on the knees, elbows, scalp, buttocks and shoulders.

Despite villus atrophy in most patients, symptoms of gastrointestinal (GI) disturbances are uncommon. It should be managed with a gluten-free diet with or without dapsone.

A summary of blistering disorders is given in Figure 14.19.

### HINTS AND TIPS

Blistering diseases are rare but important because they can be severe and are potentially fatal. Pemphigus vulgaris is the most life-threatening type of blistering disorder.

**Fig. 14.19** Summary of blistering disorders

| Disorder | Type of bullae | Autoimmunity | Clinical features |
| --- | --- | --- | --- |
| Pemphigus vulgaris | Intraepidermal | IgG deposited on intercellular junctions | Flaccid, superficial bullae<br>More common in middle-aged<br>High mortality |
| Bullous pemphigoid | Subepidermal | IgG deposited on basement membrane | Large, tense bullae<br>More common in elderly<br>Self-limiting in about 50% of cases |
| Dermatitis herpetiformis | Subepidermal | IgA deposited on dermal papillae | Small, itchy vesicles<br>Usually presents in 3rd or 4th decade; males > females<br>Associated with coeliac disease |

# TUMOURS OF THE SKIN

## Benign tumours of the skin

### Epidermal tumours

#### Seborrhoeic wart

This common, benign tumour of basal keratinocytes typically occurs on the trunk, face and arms of the elderly. The aetiology of these tumours is unknown. They are also known as basal cell papilloma:

- Warts are often greasy looking (hence seborrhoeic), but they are not associated with seborrhoea nor with sebaceous glands
- Rare before 35 years old, then usually multiple, varying in size from a few millimetres to several centimetres
- Progress from lightly pigmented, small papules to darkly pigmented, warty nodules
- Often have a 'pasted on' appearance with well-defined edges.

Microscopically, all lesions show basal cell proliferation, hyperkeratosis and a variable degree of pigmentation.

#### Actinic keratosis

This presents as roughened, scaly brownish-to-red lesions, usually less than 1 cm across, which bleed when rubbed. They typically arise on sun-exposed areas (also known as solar keratosis), especially the face, scalp and hands of the middle-aged and elderly.

Histologically, they show hyperkeratosis and parakeratosis, abnormal keratinocytes with loss of maturation, and a mild to moderate degree of pleomorphism and mitotic figures.

The lesions are considered as premalignant, with 20% of them evolving into squamous cell carcinoma.

#### Cysts

These benign, keratin-filled, firm, skin-coloured cysts are normally 1–3 cm in diameter.

Common types are epidermal cysts (derived from the epidermis) and pilar cysts (derived from the outer root sheath of the hair follicle). These are often incorrectly grouped together as sebaceous cysts.

### Dermal tumours

#### Dermatofibroma (histiocytoma)

These firm, reddish-brown papules are common in young adults, females more than males, and usually appear on the lower legs.

Histologically, they consist of intertwining bands of collagen fibres formed by proliferating fibroblasts, with reactive hyperplasia and hyperpigmentation of overlying epidermis. Dermatofibroma can be mistaken for a melanocytic naevus or malignant melanoma.

#### Pyogenic granuloma

A benign, rapidly growing, bright-red nodule arising mainly on the fingers or face, typically at a site of trauma (e.g. a thorn prick) and more commonly in young adults and children. It is neither pyogenic nor granulomatous but is a well-circumscribed dermal lesion of proliferating capillaries and inflammation that closely resembles a haemangioma.

Excision and histological examination are required to rule out malignant melanoma.

#### Keloid

This is an excessive proliferation of connective tissue occurring in previously injured skin (a form of scar), but extending beyond the margin of the original injury. Commonly seen in the healing of acne vulgaris. Characteristics are:

- firm, smooth, erythematous nodules of irregular shapes, occurring mainly over the upper back, chest or ear lobes
- more common in Black people
- highest incidence in second to fourth decades of life.

Treatment is by steroid injection into the keloid.

#### Campbell de Morgan's spot (cherry angioma)

Small, bright-red papules (1–2 mm diameter) composed of benign capillary proliferations commonly arise on the trunk in elderly or middle-aged patients.

#### Lipoma

A soft, subcutaneous tumour of mature adipocytes. This is often multiple and mostly found on the trunk, neck and upper extremities.

Figure 14.20 provides a summary of benign skin tumours.

## Naevi

### Definition

Naevi are benign, coloured lesions on the skin formed from a proliferation of one or more of the normal constituent cells of the skin. Although often congenital (birthmarks), they may be acquired.

### Melanocytic naevi

These consist of localized benign proliferations of melanocytic cells and are the most common type of naevus (also known as 'moles'). They present in most Caucasians but they are less prevalent in those with Down syndrome; they are also less common in Black people.

The aetiology of naevi development is unknown but it seems to be an inherited trait in many families:

| Tumour type | Example |
|---|---|
| Benign epidermal tumours | Viral wart<br>Actinic keratosis<br>Seborrhoeic wart<br>Milia<br>Cysts<br>Skin tags |
| Benign dermal tumours | Dermatofibroma<br>Melanocytic naevus<br>Cherry angioma<br>Pyogenic granuloma<br>Keloid<br>Lipoma<br>Chondrodermatitis nodularis |

**Fig. 14.20** Summary of benign skin tumours

- About 1% of naevi are congenital
- Majority develops during childhood or adolescence; numbers reach a peak at puberty and they have a tendency to decline during adult life
- A few new naevi develop during the third and fourth decade of life, especially if provoked by excessive sun exposure or pregnancy.

Naevi can be classified according to the position of the naevus cells within the skin as follows:

- Junctional naevi—flat circular macules consisting of rounded nests of melanocytes in the lower epidermis at the dermoepidermal junction
- Compound naevi—papules or nodules with an irregular surface, which consist of junctional nests of melanocytes combined with an intradermal mass of melanocytic cells
- Intradermal naevi—dome-shaped papules/nodules composed entirely of melanocytic cell clusters within the upper dermis (no junctional component present).

These different types of naevi are thought to arise by progression from junctional to intradermal (Fig. 14.21).

Other variants are:

- congenital naevi—usually over 1 cm in diameter; they may be protuberant or hairy and have a risk of malignant change, which is believed to be proportional to the size of the lesion
- blue naevi—steely blue intradermal naevus, usually solitary and most commonly found on the extremities
- halo naevi—white halo of depigmentation surrounds naevi. Represents involution of naevus following immune response against naevus cells. Mainly seen in children and adolescents
- familial dysplastic naevus syndrome—familial condition characterized by large numbers of atypical and 'dysplastic' naevi. Affected individuals have a greatly increased risk of developing malignant melanoma.

The majority of naevi are entirely benign but malignant changes can occur. Junctional components of junctional or compound naevi carry the highest risk for malignancy. Invasion is preceded by nuclear pleomorphism with increased mitoses and cellular atypia. Clinically, malignant naevi appear larger than normal and have an irregular edge, surface and pigmentation. They are also more likely to be itchy and to bleed.

The management is as follows:

- Increase public awareness about significance of change in pigmented lesions
- Excision and histological examination of suspicious naevi.

## Vascular naevi

These common naevi are usually congenital or developed soon after birth. They are composed of small dermal blood vessels. There are four main types:

1. Salmon patch—most common type (present in about 50% of neonates), typically on neck or eyelids. Usually fades quickly
2. Port wine stain naevus—irregular red/purple macule, which often affects one side of the face

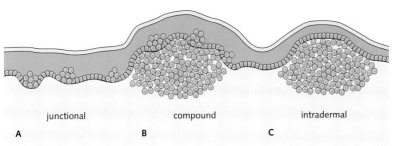

junctional     compound     intradermal
A              B            C

**Fig. 14.21** Types of melanocytic naevi.

3. Capillary haemangioma (strawberry naevus)—common, red, nodular lesion, which develops during the first few weeks of life, reaches its maximum size in the first 12 months and then involutes. Most cases have regressed by 5–7 years of age

4. Cavernous haemangioma—similar to strawberry naevus but composed of larger and deeper channels and presents as a nodular swelling. Regression is not as complete.

The treatment is by camouflage cosmetics or laser treatment for port wine stains. Strawberry naevi are usually left to involute but cavernous haemangiomas may require surgery.

## Epidermal naevi

These warty, pigmented and often elongated naevi are usually congenital or develop in early childhood. Most are a few centimetres long but they can be extensive. Treatment is by excision but recurrence is common.

## Connective tissue naevi

Rare, skin-coloured papules composed of coarse collagen bundles in the dermis. Common in tuberous sclerosis.

Figure 14.22 provides a summary of naevi.

## Malignant melanoma (melanocarcinoma)

This malignant tumour of melanocytes usually arises in the skin. Incidence in the UK is 10 per 100 000 per year but it is rising steadily. Five-year survival is nearly 80% in males and over 90% in females, although women are more often affected than men by 2:1.

It occurs in all races but it is more common in Caucasian races. Incidence is proportional to geographical latitude, which suggests an effect of UV radiation. The most common site in males is on the back but in females it is the lower leg.

The aetiology is unknown but repeated exposure to UV radiation is thought to play an important role.

Major risk factors for the development of malignant melanoma (with decreasing risk) are:

- familial dysplastic naevus syndrome—rare but lifetime risk of melanoma is over 50%
- multiple melanocytic naevi—50 naevi over 2 mm in diameter
- congenital naevus
- previous malignant melanoma
- immunosuppression
- fair skin—melanin pigmentation appears protective.

## Classification

Four main types of malignant melanoma are recognized.

### 1. Superficial spreading malignant melanoma
A flat tumour with variable pigmentation and irregular edges. This is the most common type, accounting for 50% of all UK cases. There is a female preponderance and it is most common on the lower leg.

### 2. Lentigo malignant melanoma
A nodular lesion arising in a pre-existing lentigo maligna. This typically occurs in sun-damaged skin of the face in elderly patients. It comprises about 15% of UK cases.

Lentigo maligna is similar to a benign lentigine but it is generally larger, at over 2 cm, and it has atypical melanocytes.

### 3. Acral lentiginous malignant melanoma
This resembles the lentigo malignant melanoma but it affects the palms, soles and nail-beds (subungual melanoma). It comprises 10% of UK cases but it is the

| Fig. 14.22 Summary of naevi | |
| --- | --- |
| **Type of naevus** | **Comments** |
| Melanocytic | Very common, usually multiple, pigmented and benign<br>Consists of nests of melanocytic cells<br>Classified into junctional, compound and intradermal<br>Types are congenital, blue, halo, Becker's and dysplastic |
| Vascular | Common, usually congenital, composed of small dermal blood vessels<br>Types are salmon patch, port wine stain, capillary haemangioma ('strawberry'), cavernous haemangioma |
| Epidermal | Warty, pigmented and often linear |
| Connective tissue | Rare, skin-coloured, collagenous naevi |

most common form of malignant melanoma in oriental people, suggesting it develops independently of UV radiation exposure. It is often diagnosed late and consequently has poor survival figures.

### 4. Nodular malignant melanoma

A pigmented nodule that may grow rapidly and ulcerate, this accounts for 25% of UK melanomas. It is more common in males, typically arising on the trunk. The preceding in-situ phase of growth is very difficult to identify in nodular melanoma.

## Staging and prognosis of malignant melanoma

Local invasion of the malignant melanoma is assessed using the Breslow method (Fig. 14.23). The Breslow thickness is the measured thickness in millimetres (on a histological section) from the granular layer of the epidermis to the deepest identifiable melanoma cell.

The Breslow thickness is directly related to the risk of metastasis (Fig. 14.24). Tumours are divided into one of three prognostic groups—good, intermediate or poor—depending on their Breslow thickness.

**Fig. 14.23** Staging of malignant melanomas using the Breslow thickness technique.

| | Breslow thickness (mm) | 5-year survival rate (%) |
|---|---|---|
| Prognosis | | |
| Good | <1.0 | 93 |
| Intermediate | 1–3.5 | 67 |
| Poor | >3.5 | 31 |

**Fig. 14.24** Five-year survival rates for malignant melanomas of different Breslow thickness

*Diagnosis*—one or more of the following changes observed or reported in a naevus or pigmented lesion may suggest malignant melanoma:

- Size—usually increased
- Shape—irregular outline
- Colour—irregular pigmentation
- Inflammation—at the edge of lesion
- Crusting—oozing or bleeding lesion
- Itchiness—a common symptom.

## Malignant epidermal tumours

### Basal cell carcinoma (rodent ulcer)

A malignant tumour that arises from the basal keratinocytes of the epidermis, this is the most common form of human cancer, typically seen on the face in elderly or middle-aged subjects. It is five times more common than squamous cell carcinoma (see below).

Tumours are locally very invasive, but they almost never metastasize.

Risk factors for the development of basal cell carcinoma include:

- repeated UV exposure—tumours are more common in light-skinned races, with increasing incidence towards the Equator
- X-ray irradiation
- chronic scarring
- genetic predisposition.

### Clinical Note

The differential diagnosis of malignant melanoma includes:
- benign lentigine
- benign melanocytic naevi
- dermatofibroma
- haemangioma
- pigmented basal cell carcinoma
- seborrhoeic wart.

Management is by surgical excision (rarely plus radiotherapy) with regular follow-up to detect recurrence, which may be:
- local—at edge of excised site
- lymphatic—in regional lymph nodes or in lymphatics between tumour and nodes
- at distant sites—due to haematogenous spread.

Tumours are typically composed of basophilic cells that invade the dermis. They appear as well-defined lobules and islands of cells.

*Clinical presentation*—they typically occur on sun-exposed sites, commonly around the nose, inner canthus of the eyelids and the temple.

Tumours grow slowly but relentlessly and they may destroy underlying cartilage, bone and soft-tissue structures.

There are three main types of basal cell carcinoma:

1. Nodular—most common form. Skin-coloured nodule, which may show numerous telangiectatic vessels and a glistening pearly edge. Often has central ulceration with an adherent crust
2. Superficial (or multifocal)—flat, red plaque often with an irregular rim-like edge and light pigmentation. Often multiple and most commonly seen on the trunk
3. Morpheic—flat, thickened, whitish-yellowish waxy plaque with indistinct edges. These may have focal areas of ulceration.

*Management*—complete excision is usually the best treatment but is not always possible. Radiotherapy or cryotherapy is often used for non-excisable tumours. Recurrence is about 5% at 5 years for most methods of treatment.

## Squamous cell carcinoma

This malignant tumour is derived from keratinocytes of the upper layers of the epidermis. Typically seen on the face in elderly or middle-aged subjects, with a male preponderance. Tumours are locally invasive and they may also metastasize.

Its aetiology is related to:

- chronic sunlight exposure
- chemical carcinogens (e.g. tar, arsenic and machine oil)
- X-ray radiation
- chronic ulceration and scarring
- smoking (lip lesions—aggressive, frequently metastasizes)
- common wart virus (HPV) in immunosuppressed individuals
- genetic (e.g. xeroderma pigmentosum).

Histologically, tumours consist of disorganized keratinocytes with typical malignant cytology, which destroy the dermoepidermal junction and form invading strands into the dermis. Foci of keratinization are seen within the tumour.

The clinical presentation is:

- dome-shaped nodules, which usually arise in sun-exposed sites such as the face, neck, forearm or hand
- nodules typically develop into roughened keratotic areas, ulcers or horns
- often difficult to distinguish from keratoacanthomas (see below)
- less aggressive form may arise within actinic keratosis as a small papule, which progresses to ulcerate and then crust over
- more aggressive forms may arise at the edge of chronic skin ulcers (rare).

*Management*—the treatment of choice is surgical excision. Radiotherapy can be used in some cases.

## Intraepidermal carcinoma (Bowen's disease)

This carcinoma in situ typically occurs on the lower leg in elderly women. Its predisposition is associated with previous exposure to arsenicals. It is characterized by:

- slowly extending, pink or lightly pigmented, scaly plaques up to several centimetres in size. Can look like psoriatic plaques
- full-thickness dysplasia with prominent nuclear pleomorphism and large numbers of mitoses.

Carcinomas usually remain in situ for many years but have the capacity to transform into squamous cell carcinomas.

## Other tumours of the skin

### Keratoacanthoma

This benign, self-limiting tumour typically arises on the face of elderly white males. It grows very rapidly, changing from a small, red papule to a large, domed nodule with raised edges and a central mass of keratin within a few weeks. It resembles a squamous cell carcinoma but does not invade deeply and never metastasizes.

The majority spontaneously regress within a few months.

### Mycosis fungoides (cutaneous T cell lymphoma)

This rare, slowly progressive (years) tumour of CD4 + (T helper) lymphocytes evolves in the skin. There are four stages:

1. Premycotic phase—erythematous eczematous lesions. May persist for 10 or more years
2. Infiltrative phase—erythematous plaques develop, typically affecting the trunk. This stage may last for years
3. Fungoid phase—tumour nodules or ulcers develop within the plaques suggesting systemic spread. Has a mean survival time of 2.5 years
4. Systemic disease—involvement of lymph nodes or internal organs.

## Dermatofibrosarcoma

This is a locally invasive dermal tumour of proliferating myofibroblasts with low-grade malignancy. It is similar in appearance to dermatofibromas but tends to be more invasive and is characterized by protuberant nodules on the epidermis. It does not metastasize but often recurs following excision.

## Kaposi's sarcoma

This malignant disorder is characterized by bluish-brown plaques or nodules formed from a proliferation of small blood vessels and spindle cells in the dermis. It is caused by infection with the Kaposi sarcoma virus (human herpes virus 8 (HHV8)).

Intradermal haemorrhage with haemosiderin deposition occurs within the nodules.

It commonly occurs in association with acquired immunodeficiency syndrome (AIDS) but is also endemic with cytomegalovirus in certain African regions. The lesions may be single or multiple, often beginning on the feet and with a tendency to metastasize.

# SELF-ASSESSMENT

# Single best answer questions (SBAs)

## Chapter 2 Inflammation, repair and cell death

1. A 12-year old boy with a 1-day history of sore throat was seen by his GP. On physical examination, the most prominent finding was a purulent pharyngeal exudate. He most likely has an acute inflammation. In acute inflammation which of the following is true?
   a. The predominant cell type is the neutrophil polymorph
   b. The inflammation is usually initiated by cell-mediated immunity
   c. The duration may be for months
   d. Plasma cells are frequently present
   e. Lymphocytes are present at the start of the process

2. The histopathology report for a tissue biopsy shows that it is acute inflammation. Which of the following features is seen in a tissue undergoing acute inflammation?
   a. Vasoconstriction
   b. Increased blood flow
   c. Histamine sequestration
   d. Diuresis
   e. Nitrate release

3. Which of the following statements about necrosis is correct?
   a. Is a physiological response to injury
   b. Maintains plasma membrane integrity
   c. May be stimulated by oxygen free radicals
   d. Does not result in an inflammatory response
   e. Is an energy-dependent process

4. Apototic cells usually exhibit distinctive morphological features. Which of the following is true of pure apoptosis?
   a. Is only a pathological process
   b. Occurs in groups of cells
   c. Results in cell shrinkage and fragmentation
   d. DNA is cleaved by proteases
   e. Results in an inflammatory response

5. The histopathology report for a tissue biopsy shows that it is fat necrosis. Which of the following situation is most likely to exhibit fat necrosis?
   a. Brain aneurysm
   b. Muscle injury
   c. Trauma to bowel
   d. Trauma to breast
   e. Myocardial infarction

## Chapter 3 Cancer

6. During an oncology department MDT meeting, the oncologist mentions some medical terminology. Which of the following definition is correct?
   a. Dysplasia is a change from one type of differentiated tissue to another
   b. Anaplasia is an almost complete lack of differentiation
   c. Carcinoma is a benign tumour of epithelial derivation
   d. Metaplasia is the disordered development of cells with loss of organization
   e. Carcinoma in situ is a carcinoma with stromal invasion

7. Which of the following statement regarding cancers is correct?
   a. Tumours arise from single cells
   b. Lymphomas are benign lymphoid cell tumours
   c. Cells in a tumour are always genetically identical
   d. Transcoelomic spread occurs through the lymphatic system
   e. Sound waves may cause cancer

8. You are reading a histopathology report which describes the excised tumour as malignant. Which of the following are common features of malignant tumours?
   a. Decreased density of nuclear chromatin
   b. Exophytic growth
   c. Nuclear pleomorphism
   d. Few mitotic figures
   e. Metastatic spread

9. Which of the following statement about tumour suppressor genes is correct?
   a. Tumour suppressor genes encode proteins that positvely regulate cell growth
   b. *p53* and *RB1* are oncogenes
   c. Gain of function of tumour suppressor genes results in neoplastic growth
   d. Viral proteins cannot deregulate tumour suppressor function
   e. *p53* triggers apoptosis and cell cycle arrest

## Chapter 4 Infectious disease

10. Which of the following is true of viruses?
    a. Are prokaryotes
    b. Always possess RNA nucleic acid

c. If of the non-enveloped type, may release new particles by budding
d. Are obligate extracellular parasites
e. May cause cell lysis

11. A 34-year-old man who presented with infection with a resistant species of enterobacteria was commenced on oral ciprofloxacin. Which of the following is true of bacterial antibiotic resistance?

a. Is uncommon
b. Is conferred via extrachromosomal RNA
c. Cannot be directly transferred between bacteria
d. May occur through the alteration of the target site for an antibiotic
e. MRSA is virtually impossible to treat

# Chapter 5 Pathology of the nervous system

12. A 65-year-old woman presented with headache, vomiting, nausea, papilloedma. Upon admission to hospital, the patient was noticed to have gait instability, urinary incontinence and focal neurological signs. A diagnosis of hydrocephalus was made. Which of the following is true of hydrocephalus?
a. Is a decrease in the volume of CSF within the brain
b. It results in the constriction of the cerebral ventricles.
c. Increased absorption of CSF at the arachnoid villi is the commonest form
d. A ventricular shunt can be used in the management
e. All causes of hydrocephalus are acquired

13. A 34-year-old woman was hit in the head by a cricket ball. After she was hit, she managed to walk off the field without any symptoms. By the time she reached hospital, she had died. Upon autoposy a diagnosis of extradural haemorrhage was made. Which of the following is true of extradural haemhorrages?
a. Occurs between the dura and outer surface of the arachnoid membrane
b. Is not usually associated with a skull fracture
c. Is due to bleeding from the cortical bridging veins
d. May be associated with a post-traumatic lucid period
e. Is not a surgical emergency

14. Upon autopsy an incidental finding of Alzheimer's dieases was made. Which of the following is true of Alzheimer's disease?
a. Is usually familial
b. Is caused by senile plaques of amyloid protein
c. Neurofibrillary tangles occur within neurones
d. Affects half of all people over the age of 80 years
e. Is not usually associated with memory disturbance

15. A patient with an intracranial neoplasm was informed by the neurosurgeon that he had a tumour.

Which of the following is true about the neoplasms of the CNS?
a. Gliomas are the least common primary CNS tumour
b. Astrocytomas rarely affect children
c. Oligodendrogliomas are slow-growing tumours
d. Meningiomas commonly invade deep CNS tissue
e. Prostatic carcinoma often causes brain metastases

# Chapter 6 Pathology of the cardiovascular system

16. A 24-year-old man was found to have a ventricular septal defect upon echocardiogram. Which of the following is true of ventricular septal defect:
a. Usually produces a right-to-left shunt of blood
b. Produces respiratory depression
c. Produces a diastolic murmur
d. May be of a membranous or muscular location
e. Is the least common congenital cardiac abnormality

17. Coarctation of the aorta was diagnosed in a 4-year-old child. Which of the following is true of coarctation of the aorta?
a. Is more common in females
b. Causes hypotension distal to the narrowing
c. Is often associated with a bicuspid mitral valve
d. Rarely causes serious complications
e. Is associated with weak and delayed femoral pulsations

18. Upon autoposy an incidental finding of atherosclerosis was made. Which of the following is true of atherosclerosis?
a. It is characterized by the accumulation of protein rich material in the intima of arteries
b. It is common in the pulmonary arteries
c. It is associated with hypocholesterolaemia
d. It may be seen as a pathological response to endothelial injury
e. It is characterized by neutrophil lipid uptake to form foam cells

19. During a routine checkup in the GP, a 34-year-old man had consistently high blood pressure of 149 mmHg systolic. Benign hypertension is characterized by:
a. Fibrinoid necrosis of arterioles
b. Hypotrophy of the muscular media of the arteries
c. Fibroelastic thinning of the intima
d. Hyaline deposition in arteriole walls
e. Sudden and severe increase in blood pressure

20. A 56-year-old man has arrived in hospital complaining of chest pains which radiated to his left hand, and upon investigation had ECG changes concurrent with acute myocardial infarction. Which of the following is true of myocardial infarction?
a. Results in necrosis of the myocardium following severe ischaemia

b. Induces chronic inflammatory changes
c. The infarct tissue is replaced by new cardiac muscle
d. Occlusion of the left anterior descending coronary artery results in an inferior MI
e. Management includes thrombolysis regardless of ECG changes

21. A 67-year-old man presents to the GP with breathlessness upon exertion, orthopnea and oedema of legs, feet and ankles. Which of the following of heart failure is true?
    a. Is when the heart is unable to maintain cardiac output or can do so only by increasing filling pressure
    b. Right-sided heart failure is more common than left-sided failure
    c. Left-sided heart failure may commonly develop as a result of right-sided failure
    d. Is not a complication of myocardial infarction
    e. Is not associated with valve disease

22. After a 12-hour plane flight, a 53-year-old female flight attendant noticed a heavy ache over the right calf, with associated swelling and tenderness. Which of the following is true of thrombosis?
    a. A thrombus is the pathological term for a clot
    b. Is predisposed by both blood stasis and turbulence
    c. Antiphospholipid antibody decreases risk of arterial and venous thrombosis
    d. The most common site of venous thrombosis is the portal vein
    e. Malignancy sometimes decrease the risk of venous thrombosis

# Chapter 7 Pathology of the respiratory system

23. A 45-year-old man presented to his GP due to a slow growing lump in his neck and hoarseness of voice. Upon biopsy carcinoma of the larynx was diagnosed. Which of the following is true of carcinoma of the larynx?
    a. Is usually sited in the subglottic region
    b. Has a negative association with cigarette smoking
    c. Commonly spreads by the haematogenous route
    d. Is usually of squamous cell differentiation
    e. Usually presents before the age of 35 years

24. A 56-year-old man who is a chronic smoker presented to hospital with an acute exacerbation of chonic obstructive pulmonary disease. Which of the following is true of chronic obstructive pulmonary disease?
    a. Is characterized by chronic bronchitis, emphysema and bronchiolitis
    b. The obstructive lung disease can be completely reversed with bronchodilators
    c. Causes hypoinflated lungs
    d. Is exclusively a disease of smokers
    e. Lung fibrosis is a feature of emphysema

25. Which of the following is true of chronic bronchitis?
    a. Defined as a productive cough on most days for 1 month of the year for at least 2 successive years
    b. Most cases are due to cigarette smoking
    c. Hypersecretion of mucus is associated with hypotrophy of the bronchial mucus-secreting glands
    d. Is characterized by an acute inflammation of the bronchioles
    e. Lung function tests show a restrictive pattern

26. A 12-year-old boy presents to his GP with coughing, wheezing and shortness of breath. The GP subsequently diagnosed him with asthma. Which of the following is true of asthma?
    a. Causes irreversible airway narrowing
    b. May be caused by a type II hypersensitivity reaction
    c. Bronchospasm, oedema and mucus plugging are commonly seen
    d. Is sometimes associated with $\alpha$-1-antitrypsin deficiency
    e. Hypotrophy of bronchial smooth muscle may occur

27. Which of the following is true of cystic fibrosis?
    a. Is associated with infections with *Pseudomonas*
    b. Is the most common autosomal dominant condition in Europe
    c. Is due to defective transport of potassium ions
    d. Is not associated with malabsorption
    e. Is due to a mutation in a gene on chromosome 9

28. A 67-year-old man has come into hospital with bronchial breathing in the right lung base, and associated crackles. A clinical diagnosis of pneumonia was made. Which of he following is true of pneumonia?
    a. Pneumonia is most commonly caused by viral infectons
    b. Most cases of bacterial community-acquired pneumonia are due to Gram-negative organisms
    c. Lung fibrosis, abscess and empyema may complicate pneumonia
    d. Red hepatization describes a pathological stage in bronchopneumonia
    e. Is less likely to occur if there is pre-existing pulmonary oedema

29. A 29-year-old woman with cervical lymphadenopathy is seen in a surgical outpatient clinic. An excision biopsy was performed and sent for histopathology. Which of the following is true of pulmonary tuberculosis?
    a. Is most commonly due to *Mycobacterium avium intracellulare*
    b. Is caused by direct cytopathic effects of the infecting organism
    c. Does not have an association with silicosis
    d. Is a common cause of death in AIDS
    e. Is not characterized histologically by granulomas

30. A 78-year-old smoker complaining of a persistent dry cough had a chest X-ray which showed a 2 cm mass lesion in the right upper zone. Biopsies was sent for

histological examination. Which of the following is true of lung carcinoma:
a. Is most commonly of adenomatous differentiation
b. Is not associated with cigarette smoking
c. Is not associated with asbestos exposure
d. Has rarely metastasized at the time of presentation
e. Is the most common cause of death from neoplasia in the UK

31. Which of the following is true of idiopathic pulmonary fibrosis?
a. Is an infectious condition
b. Causes interstitial atrophy
c. Is an obstructive lung disease
d. Causes peripheral lung honeycombing
e. Is not a cause of finger clubbing

32. A 48-year-old man has suddenly developed sudden onset of chest pain, cough, dyspnoea, tachypnoea and marked anxiety. Two days ago he had just underwent an operation. Which of the following is true of a pulmonary embolism?
a. May cause pulmonary hypotension and infarction
b. May be precipitated by mural thrombus in left ventricle
c. Can cause pulseless electrical activity (electromechanical dissociation) of the heart
d. Is always thromboembolic
e. Is usually caused by thromboembolism from arm veins

33. Which of the following is true of malignant mesothelioma?
a. Develops rapidly after exposure to asbestos
b. Mainly spreads via the bloodstream
c. Is slowly progressive with a long life-expectancy
d. Has been decreasing in incidence
e. Is associated with recurrent pleural effusions

# Chapter 8 Pathology of the gastrointestinal tract

34. Which of the following is true of squamous cell carcinoma of the oral cavity?
a. Occurs least commonly on the lips
b. Is more common in women than men
c. Has a positive association with cigarette smoking
d. Has a positive association with moderate alcohol intake
e. Has a 5-year survival of about 10%

35. Which of the following is true of oesophageal carcinoma?
a. Is most commonly adenocarcinoma
b. May develop into Barrett's metaplasia
c. Adenocarcinoma is the most likely pattern in heavy smokers or drinkers
d. Has a 5-year survival of about 50%
e. Causes dysphagia

36. Which of the following is true of oesophageal varices?
a. Are dilated submucosal veins in the oesophagus
b. They are not associated with cirrhosis of the liver
c. Rupture causes slight bleeding
d. Are associated with portal vein hypotension
e. Sclerotherapy is not used in the management

37. Which of the following is true of *Helicobacter pylori* associated gastritis?
a. Is an example of an acute gastritis
b. *Helicobacter pylori* colonizes the epithelium above a layer of mucus
c. Epithelial damage is caused by the immune response against *Helicobacter pylori*
d. Is most commonly seen at the pyloric fundus
e. Is almost always a transient infection

38. Which of the following is true of gastric carcinoma?
a. Is usually of squamous cell type
b. Is more common in females than males
c. Occurs most commonly in the body of the stomach
d. Is commoner in Europe than Japan
e. Has a positive association with *Helicobacter pylori* infection

39. Which of the following is true of portal hypertension?
a. May be classified as prehepatic, hepatic or posthepatic
b. Is most commonly caused by portal vein thrombosis
c. Is not a cause of ascites
d. May cause Budd-Chiari syndrome
e. Causes the regression of portosystemic shunts

40. Which of the following is true of liver cirrhosis?
a. A reversible condition in which the liver's normal architecture is diffusely replaced by nodules
b. A rare cause of cirrhosis is alcohol liver disease
c. A common cause of cirrhosis is autoimmune chronic hepatitis
d. Nodules are formed from regenerated hepatocytes separated by bands of collagenous fibrosis
e. Prothrombin time is reduced

41. A 65-year-old has noticed that he has a full distended abdomen and has complained of shortness of breath. Which of the following is true of ascites?
a. Is the accumulation of free fluid in the peritoneal cavity
b. Cirrhosis is associated with exudative ascites
c. Signifies liver disease
d. Grey Turner's sign is seen
e. Sodium-containing drugs are useful in the management of ascites

42. Which of he following is true of Wilson's disease?
a. Is an autosomal dominant condition
b. It results from a mutation in a gene for a copper transporter protein
c. Free copper overspills into the blood and deposits in the cornea and the brain
d. There are no psychiatric symptoms
e. The liver is not affected

43. Which of the following is true of Hepatitis B?
    a. Is a RNA virus
    b. May be transmitted by drinking infected water
    c. Initial infection is chronic in the majority of cases
    d. Vaccination utilizes the hepatitis B surface antigen (HbsAg)
    e. Cirrhosis and hepatocellular carcinoma are not complications of chronic infection

44. A 54-year-old woman presented with increasing abdominal distension. Physical examination revealed an enlarged liver. Her serum alpha-fetoprotein is 40 times the upper limit of normal. Which of the following is true of hepatocellular carcinoma (HCC)?
    a. Is the most common malignant tumour of the liver
    b. Has a positive association with hepatitis A
    c. Is more common in males than females
    d. Has a median survival of 3 years following diagnosis
    e. Arises from bile duct epithelium

45. A 43-year-old woman is noted to have mild jaundice and some weight loss. Her alkaline phosphatase level is elevated and she has a positive anti-mitochondrial antibody. She was subsequently diagnosed with primary biliary cirrhosis. Which of the following is true of primary biliary cirrhosis?
    a. Is more common in males
    b. Is not associated with autoimmune diseases
    c. Is relatively easy to treat
    d. Is strongly associated with ulcerative colitis
    e. Causes scar formation by bridging fibrosis

46. Which of the following is true of carcinoma of the pancreas?
    a. Is not associated with excess alcohol ingestion
    b. Is more common in women than men
    c. Is not surgically resectable
    d. Is normally squamous in origin
    e. Usually occurs in subjects older than 60 years of age

47. A 25-year-old woman presented with a 1-week history of right lower-quadrant pain and fever. She has also noticed an increase in the frequency of stools and occasional bloody diarrhoea. Following endoscopic biopsy, a diagnosis of Crohn's disease was made. Which of the following is true of Crohn's disease?
    a. Is not associated with erythema nodosum
    b. Has a negative association with cigarette smoking
    c. May occur only in the colon
    d. Is characterized histologically by non-caseating granulomas
    e. Never causes uveitis

48. A 45-year-old man has developed iron deficiency anaemia secondary to chronic bloody diarrhoea. A colonic biopsy showed the presence of ulcerative colitis. Which of the following is true of ulcerative colitis?
    a. Is characterized by transmural inflammation
    b. Has a positive association with cigarette smoking
    c. Is characterized by granulomatous inflammation

d. Is commonly complicated by fistulae
e. Is characterized by continuous disease distribution in the colon

49. Which of the following is true of coeliac disease?
    a. Is caused by a normal immune response to gluten
    b. Is associated with intestinal villous hypertrophy
    c. Most commonly affects the large intestine
    d. Anti-endomyseal antibodies are a useful blood test to aid diagnosis
    e. A gluten-free diet improves symptoms but the intestinal changes are irreversible

50. Which of the following is true of colorectal carcinoma?
    a. Is often a progression from adenoma
    b. Familial adenomatous polyposis patients rarely develop colorectal cancer if untreated
    c. Is staged by the Breslow system
    d. Usually presents earlier if affecting the right (ascending) colon
    e. Most commonly develops in the caecum

## Chapter 9 Pathology of the kidney and urinary tract

51. Which of the following is true of adult polycystic kidney disease?
    a. Only one kidney is affected
    b. It is an inherited autosomal recessive disease
    c. There are no vascular associations
    d. Enlarging cysts replace and compress functioning renal parenchyma
    e. Hypertension is important for the management

52. Which of the following is true in glomerular disease?
    a. Nephrotic syndrome in an adult is strongly suggestive of minimal change nephropathy
    b. Most cases of membranous nephropathy have an identifiable cause
    c. Minimal change disease rapidly progresses to renal failure in children
    d. A focal proliferative glomerulonephritis with autoantibodies against type III collagen is indicative of Goodpasture's syndrome
    e. Streptococcal sore throat may be a cause of proliferative glomerulonephritis

53. Which of the following is true of renal cell carcinoma?
    a. Is more common in males
    b. Usually develops at the lower pole of the kidney
    c. Proteinuria is a common presenting feature
    d. Cigarette smoking is protective
    e. All cases are sporadic as no genetic association has been identified

54. A 67-year-old man with haematuria was diagnosed with bladder cancer. Which of the following is true of bladder cancers?

a. Is largely a disease of women
b. Is usually a squamous cell carcinoma
c. Does not cause urinary obstruction
d. Most commonly arises at the base of trigone and around the ureteric orifices
e. Is not linked to exposure to environmental carcinogens

## Chapter 10 Pathology of the endocrine system

55. Which of the following is true of Graves' disease?
   a. Is equally common in males and females
   b. A minority of individuals are positive for thyroid-stimulating hormone (TSH)-receptor antibodies in their serum
   c. Causes no change in the thyroid gland
   d. Only a minority of individuals show signs of exophthalmos
   e. Causes the same change in thyroid hormone levels as Hashimoto's thyroiditis

56. Which of the following is true of malignant thyroid tumours?
   a. Include toxic adenomas
   b. May be caused by childhood radiation exposure
   c. Papillary adenocarcinomas tend to be found in elderly patients
   d. Medullary carcinoma is derived from thyroxine-secreting cells
   e. Anaplastic carcinoma is not associated with a history of multinodular goitre

57. The following are causes of Cushing's syndrome:
   a. Addison's disease
   b. Adrenocorticotrophic hormone (ACTH) administration
   c. Saline fluid adminstration
   d. Phaeochromocytomas
   e. Waterhouse-Friderichsen syndrome

58. Which of the following is true of Type I diabetes mellitus?
   a. Is not an autoimmune-induced disorder
   b. Has no genetic predisposition
   c. Is a disease of middle-aged/elderly onset
   d. Shows destruction of insulin secreting cells of the islets of Langerhans
   e. Shows plasma insulin levels that are raised or normal

59. Which of the following is true of Type II diabetes mellitus?
   a. Is a disease most commonly of children
   b. Is thought to develop from tissue insulin resistance
   c. Is commonly treated with insulin in the first instance
   d. May be complicated by diabetic ketoacidosis
   e. Is not associated with vascular complications

## Chapter 11 Pathology of the reproductive system

60. Which of the folowing is true of carcinoma of the uterine cervix?
   a. Is usually of adenomatous differentiation
   b. Is preceded by cervical intraepithelial neoplasia (CIN)
   c. Has no association with some serotypes of human papilloma virus (HPV)
   d. Has no association with cigarette smoking
   e. Has no association with HIV infection

61. A 26-year-old woman is diagnosed with endometrosis. Which of the following statements regarding endometriosis is correct?
   a. Is defined as endometrial glands or stroma occurring outside of the uterus
   b. Rarely affects the ovaries
   c. Not caused by retrograde menstruation
   d. Worsens after the menopause
   e. Invariably causes infertility

62. Which of the following is true of pelvic inflammatory disease?
   a. Is a combined inflammatory disorder of the fallopian tubes, ovaries and peritoneum
   b. Intrauterine contraceptive device is not a predisposing factor
   c. *Pseudomonas* is a common aetiological agent
   d. Is characterized by chronic inflammation
   e. Pelvic inflammatory disease is an autoimmune disorder

63. A 30-year-old woman is diagnosed with ectopic pregnancy, which of the following statements about ectopic pregnancy is true?
   a. A fertilized ovum implants inside the uterine cavity
   b. The most common site is the uterus
   c. Aetiology may be due to previous episodes of salpingitis
   d. Proliferation of the ectoblast causes erosion of the submucosa and bleeding
   e. The embryo typically survives to term

64. Which of the following is true of pre-eclampsia?
   a. Is defined as high blood pressure during pregnancy where it was previously normal
   b. Is more common in a first pregnancy or with multiple pregnancies
   c. Is thought to be the result of placental hyperperfusion
   d. The main risks are to the mother rather than the fetus
   e. May persist for several months after delivery

65. Which of the following is true of breast carcinoma?
   a. Most common cause of death in women aged over 60 years of age

b. Predisposing factors include mutation of *BRCA1* and *BRCA2* genes
c. Screening is not carried out in the UK
d. Tamoxifen can be used if oestrogen-receptor negative
e. Ductal carcinoma is the rarest type

66. A 76-year-old man presents with urinary retention had a digital rectal examination which suggested that he had an enlarged prostate with a craggy nodular feel. Biopsy of the lesion suggested malignancy. Which of the following is true of prostate carcinoma?

a. Is a squamous cell carcinoma
b. Affects the central zone of prostate
c. Is more likely to cause urinary symptoms than benign prostatic hyperplasia
d. Rarely extends outside of the prostatic capsule
e. The majority have a well-differentiated glandular pattern

---

# Chapter 12  Pathology of the musculoskeletal system

67. Which of the following is true of osteoporosis?
a. Is an uncommon bone disorder
b. Is not a cause of pathological fractures
c. Microscopically, bone trabeculae are thickened
d. Diagnosis is by X-ray of the affected bones
e. Bones appear less dense on X-ray and lumbar vertebral bodies often appear more biconcave than normal

68. A 56-year-old woman is on long-term corticosteroid therapy for severe rheumatoid arthritis. Which of the following is true of rheumatoid arthritis?

a. Affects 10% of the population
b. The likelihood of onset increases with age, therefore peaking in the elderly
c. All patients have circulating rheumatoid factor
d. Causes the development of a pannus and inflammatory joint destruction
e. There are no extra-articular features

---

# Chapter 13  Pathology of the blood and immune systems

69. Which of the following is true of the human immunodeficiency virus (HIV)-1.
a. Is a DNA virus
b. Contains its own reverse transcriptase for replication
c. Binds to B cell lymphocytes
d. Is not associated with *Pneumocytis carinii* infection
e. Is associated with *Mycobaderium avium intracellulare* infection

70. Which of the following is ture of amyloidosis?
a. Amyloid is a well characterized polypeptide
b. Amyloid does not take up Congo red stain
c. Has no systemic effects
d. The most common amyloid in reactive systemic amyloidosis is the AL type
e. May follow long-term haemodialysis

71. Which of the following is true of leucopenia and leucocytosis?
a. Agranulocytosis is used to describe severe thrombocytopenia
b. Neutropenia forms part of Kostmann's syndrome
c. Leucocytosis is most commonly caused by an increase in lymphocytes
d. Leucocytosis always indicates infection
e. Basophilia is commonly seen in allergic reactions

72. A lymph node biopsy was performed on a 45-year-old man who presented with a low-grade fevers, night sweats and generalized malaise for a couple of months. He was found to have cervical lymphadenomapthy. A diagnosis of Hodgkin's disease was confirmed upon biopsy. Which of the following is true of Hodgkin's disease?
a. Is characterized histologically by Reed-Sternberg cells
b. Is more common in females than males
c. Is staged using the Rye classification
d. Has a better prognosis if B symptoms are present
e. Of the mixed cellularity type has the most favourable prognosis

73. Which of the following is true of non-Hodgkin's lymphoma?
a. Is not linked to immunosuppression
b. Gastric lymphoma has been linked to *Escherichia coli* gastroenteritis
c. The majority of cases are derived from T cells
d. Point mutations of susceptibility genes are commonly associated
e. Extranodal presentation is more common than in Hodgkin's disease

74. A 67-year-old man was found to have numerous small, mature lymphocytes. A diagnosis of chronic lymphocytic leukaemia was made. Which of the following statements is correct regarding chronic lymphocytic leukaemia?
a. Is characterized cytogenetically by the Philadelphia chromosome
b. Is the least common leukaemia in adults
c. Has a median survival of 9 months
d. Is more common in females than males
e. May affect lymph nodes

75. Which of the following is true of sickle-cell disease?
a. Is caused by a point mutation in the DNA coding for the a-globin chain
b. Is more common in Europe than Africa
c. Is associated with gallstones
d. Is associated with hypersplenism
e. Does not confer resistance to malarial infection

**76.** Which of the following is true of haemolytic anaemia?
   a.  Is not commonly isoimmune
   b.  Does not cause brain damage in neonates
   c.  When autoimmune, 'warm' type results in macrospherocytosis
   d.  When autoimmune, 'cold' type results in red cell agglutination
   e.  Is not associated with lymphoma

---

## Chapter 14 Pathology of the skin

**77.** Which of the following definitions are correct regarding skin pathology?
   a.  Nodule is a raised lesion less than 5 mm across
   b.  Vesicle is a blister greater than 5 mm across
   c.  Macular describes a raised lesion of altered skin colour
   d.  Pustule is a blister containing clear fluid
   e.  Spongiosis means epidermal oedema

**78.** Which of the following is true of psoriasis?
   a.  Is an infective condition
   b.  Is characterized by a reduced turnover of epithelial cells
   c.  May be precipitated by lithium administration
   d.  Commonly affects skin at the antecubital fossa
   e.  Is not associated with pitting of the nails

**79.** Which of the following is true of atopic eczema?
   a.  Is decreasing in incidence
   b.  Is less common where there is a strong family history
   c.  Is a type II hypersensitivity reaction
   d.  Increases in incidence with increasing age through childhood
   e.  Increases the likelihood of skin infection

**80.** Which of the following is true of blistering disorders?
   a.  Pemphigoid describes subcorneal separation of skin tissue
   b.  Pemphigus is associated with erosions
   c.  Pemphigoid has a higher untreated mortality than pemphigus
   d.  Pemphigus is associated with coeliac disease
   e.  Dermatitis herpetiformis involves granular IgG deposition at the dermal papillae of normal looking skin

**81.** Which of the following is true of malignant melanoma?
   a.  Arises from epidermal keratinocytes
   b.  Is associated with intermittent intense UV light exposure
   c.  Has no increase in incidence with familial dysplastic naevus syndrome
   d.  With a depth of invasion of 3.5 mm has a good prognosis
   e.  Never arises within lentigo maligna

# Extended-matching questions (EMQs)

In each of the following questions, select the condition listed that is most likely to fit the given description.

## 1. Nervous system:

A. Acute bacterial meningitis
B. Viral meningitis
C. Multiple sclerosis
D. Subarachnoid haemorrhage
E. Meningioma
F. Extradural haemorrhage
G. Guillain-Barré syndrome
H. Alzheimer's disease
I. Hydrocephalus
J. HSV encephalitis

1. The diagnosis in a patient with diffuse ventricular dilatation on CT scanning of the brain, who has had ventriculopertioneal shunt surgery.
2. A possible diagnosis in a 70-year-old woman whose husband complains that she has been getting increasingly forgetful over a period of months.
3. The diagnosis in a 23-year-old man presenting with rapidly developing focal neurological signs several hours after he sustained a head injury in a motorbike accident.
4. A condition that causes episodes of acute CNS demyelination separated in time and space.
5. The diagnosis in a patient with an infection of the leptomeninges that has caused brain abscess. Lumbar puncture revealed a cloudy CSF with increased protein and decreased glucose.

## 2. Cardiovascular system:

A. Ventricular septal defect
B. Angina pectoris
C. Infective endocarditis
D. Polyarteritis nodosa
E. Coarctation of the aorta
F. Myocardial infarction
G. Dissecting aortic aneurysm
H. Tetralogy of Fallot
I. Giant cell arteritis
J. Aortic stenosis

1. A condition that causes headache, dizziness, intercostal bruits and radiofemoral pulse delay.
2. The diagnosis in a patient with sudden onset chest pain, radiating to between the scapulae, who develops asymmetry of pulses in his arms and legs. Chest X-ray reveals mediastinal widening.
3. The diagnosis in an elderly patient who has an ejection systolic murmur and a propensity for syncope. A narrow pulse pressure and slow-rising carotid pulse are also detected.
4. A condition that has the potential to cause scalp tenderness, headache and blindness. Erythrocyte sedimentation rate is significantly raised.
5. A condition that causes a left-to-right shunt with pansystolic murmur.

## 3. Respiratory system:

A. Squamous cell carcinoma of the lung
B. Small cell lung cancer
C. Extrinsic (atopic) asthma
D. Chronic obstructive pulmonary disease
E. Pulmonary tuberculosis
F. Cystic fibrosis
G. Malignant mesothelioma
H. Intrinsic (non-atopic) asthma
I. Adenocarcinoma of lung
J. Sarcoidosis

1. A response to noxious agents causing reduced $FEV_1$, reduced $FEV_1/FVC$ ratio and characterized by a CD8+ T-cell infiltration.
2. The likely diagnosis in a 45-year-old non-smoker, with no past history of respiratory illness, who presents with shortness of breath and wheezing. Salbutamol inhaler completely resolves the breathing difficulties.
3. The cause of abnormally thickened mucus affecting both the lung and pancreas.
4. A lung condition that may cause cough, haemoptysis, shortness of breath and chest pain, and which is exquisitely sensitive to chemotherapy and radiotherapy in its early stages.
5. The likely diagnosis in a patient with a granulomatous condition affecting the lung and other organs. Blood tests reveal hypercalcaemia and a raised serum angiotensin converting enzyme.

## 4. Gastrointestinal system:

A. Barrett's oesophagus
B. Wilson's disease

315

C. Colorectal carcinoma

D. Crohn's disease

E. Coeliac disease

F. Haemochromatosis

G. Whipple's disease

H. Oesophageal varices

I. Hepatocellular carcinoma

J. Gallstones

1. The most likely diagnosis in a 25-year-old woman complaining of a 3-month history of diarrhoea, who has recently developed a blistering rash on her elbows.
2. The diagnosis in a 27-year-old female who presents with intermittent diarrhoea and weight loss. Endoscopy reveals multiple small bowel strictures occurring between areas of normal looking bowel.
3. A condition of metaplastic change.
4. A complication of portal hypertension.
5. The diagnosis in a 50-year-old male with leaden grey pigmentation of his groins and axillae. A liver biopsy shows increased iron deposition and some hepatic fibrosis.

## 5. Renal and urinary systems:

A. Membranous nephropathy

B. Alport's disease

C. Benign nephrosclerosis

D. Minimal change disease

E. Goodpasture's syndrome

F. Focal segmental glomerulosclerosis

G. Acute tubular necrosis

H. Amyloidosis

I. Hydronephrosis

J. Medullary sponge kidney

1. The likely diagnosis in a 5-year-old boy who develops facial swelling. Urinalysis reveals heavy proteinuria, but no blood. A kidney biopsy shows no abnormality on light microscopy.
2. The likely diagnosis in a 25-year-old man who is being investigated for renal failure. He is complaining that he is having to change the prescription for his glasses every few weeks to see clearly and that he is struggling to hear some sounds.
3. Describes a form of acute renal failure that is normally reversible and may be caused by an ischaemic or toxic insult.
4. Describes a complication of urinary tract obstruction.
5. The diagnosis in a 55-year-old man presenting with haemoptysis and haematuria. A renal biopsy shows crescentic change and IgG deposits in the basement membrane.

## 6. Endocrine system:

A. Type I diabetes mellitus

B. Hypoparathyroidism

C. Cushing's syndrome

D. Hypothyroidism

E. Addison's disease

F. Cranial diabetes insipidus

G. Hyperthyroidism

H. Type II diabetes mellitus

I. Hyperparathyroidism

J. Adrenal crisis

1. The most likely diagnosis in a patient who presents with diarrhoea, vomiting, abdominal pain and profound hypotension. She has been on regular prednisolone to treat her temporal arteritis for over a year, but recently suddenly stopped taking it because she was worried about the side effects.
2. Is primarily a disorder of insulin production.
3. Is the most likely diagnosis in a patient who has recently had mumps infection, with persisting fatigue in recovery. She has now developed a painful lump in her neck, and has noticed that she has cold hands and is 'really suffering the cold weather'.
4. Is characterized by central obesity, moon face, hypertension, osteoporosis, menstrual irregularity and hirsutism.
5. Is a disorder of polyuria and polydipsia that is caused by a failure of hormone production from the posterior pituitary.

## 7. Reproductive system:

A. Pre-eclampsia

B. Cervical cancer

C. Fibroids

D. Choriocarcinoma

E. Ectopic pregnancy

F. Adenomyosis

G. Breast cancer

H. Benign ovarian cyst

I. Endometriosis

J. Endometrial cancer

1. Is a potential cause of abnormal ovarian tissue that undergoes cyclical bleeding and commonly predisposes to infertility.
2. Is subject to 'triple assessment' in suspicious lesions.
3. A condition that has risk factors for development including HPV infection, combined oral contraceptive use, multiple sexual partners and smoking.
4. Is a tumour of trophoblastic tissue.

5. Is the most likely diagnosis in a 24-year-old female complaining of severe lower abdominal pain that came on very suddenly, and who has signs of cardiovascular collapse and shock.

## 8. Musculoskeletal system:

A. Osteogenesis imperfecta

B. Osteoid osteoma

C. Paget's disease

D. Dermatomyositis

E. Osteoarthritis

F. Osteoporosis

G. Osteosarcoma

H. Metastatic disease

I. Osteopetrosis

J. Duchenne muscular dystrophy

1. The most common tumour found in bones.
2. Is the likely diagnosis in a 60-year-old man presenting with bone pain of the femur. On X-ray of the affected bone, alternating areas of increased and decreased bone density are seen. Blood tests are normal with the exception of a highly elevated alkaline phosphatase.
3. Is a degenerative disease of articular cartilage.
4. Is the term given for a group of hereditary disorders that result in abnormal type I collagen formation.
5. An X-linked inherited condition that results in failure to produce dystrophin protein.

## 9. Haematological and immunological systems:

A. Chronic lymphocytic leukaemia

B. Hodgkin's disease

C. Vitiligo

D. Non-Hodgkin's lymphoma

E. Chronic myeloid leukaemia

F. Myeloma

G. Myasthenia gravis

H. Thalassaemia

I. Acute myeloid leukaemia

J. Megaloblastic anaemia

1. Is a disorder in which the Philadelphia chromosome abnormality is detected within affected cells.
2. Is a disease characterized by the development of Reed-Sternberg cells.
3. Is the likely diagnosis in a 50-year-old male who presents with worsening back pain and persistent tiredness. Bone imaging show lytic bone lesions and serum electrophoresis reveals an intense gamma-globulin band.
4. Is an autoimmune disease characterized by a raised serum titre of antiacetylcholine receptor antibodies.
5. Is an example of a haemoglobinopathy.

## 10. Dermatological system:

A. Acantholysis

B. Dermatitis

C. Plaque

D. Parakeratosis

E. Acne vulgaris

F. Ulceration

G. Macule

H. Bullous pemphigoid

I. Blister

J. Pemphigus vulgaris

1. A localized, flat area of altered skin colour that may be hyperpigmented, hypopigmented or erythematous.
2. A disorder that causes increased sebum excretion and blockage of pilosebaceous ducts.
3. A disorder characterized by the development of intraepidermal bullae.
4. Is a microscopic appearance in psoriasis.
5. The loss of cellular cohesion and separation of epidermal keratinocytes due to the rupture of intercellular bridges.

# SBA answers

1. **A.** The neutrophil polymorph is the predominant cell type in acute inflammation. Acute inflammation is mediated by chemical factors. The duration of acute inflammation is a few hours to a few weeks. Plasma cells are not present. They are involved in humoral antibody-mediated immunity. Lymphocytes are involved in chronic inflammation.

2. **B.** Vasodilatation is a feature of acute inflammation, not vasoconstriction. Increased blood flow (hyperaemia) is seen. Histamine is one of the chemical inflammatory mediators and is released. Oedema occurs due to increased hydrostatic and decreased oncotic pressures. Nitric oxide is another inflammatory mediator that increases vascular permeability.

3. **C.** Necrosis is a pathological response to injury. Necrosis does not maintain plasma membrane integrity. Oxygen free radicals may stimulate necrosis. Necrosis is associated with a local inflammatory response. Necrosis is an energy-independent process.

4. **C.** Apoptosis can be either a pathological or physiological process. Single cells are usually involved. Cells appear fragmented and shrunk (apoptotic bodies). DNA fragmentation occurs in an energy-dependent process, and is cleaved by endonucleases. There is no inflammatory response.

5. **D.** Fat necrosis can be seen after trauma to breast, usually presenting as a painless palpable mass. The lesion usually consist of haemhorrage in the early stages and later central liquefactive necrosis of fat.

6. **B.** Dysplasia is the disordered development of cells resulting in an alteration in their size, shape and organization. True – anaplasia is the almost complete lack of differentiation. Carcinomas are derived from epithelial cells. Metaplasia is an adaptive response resulting in the replacement of one differentiated cell type with another. Carcinoma in situ is an epithelial tumour with features of malignancy but it has not invaded through the basement membrane.

7. **A.** Tumours originally arise from single cells that proliferate to form a clone of cells. Lymphoma is a malignant lymphoreticular tumour. Tumours pick up additional mutations as they develop (tumour heterogeneity). Transcoelomic spread occurs via the pleural, pericardial and peritoneal cavities. Ultraviolet radiation is an important cause of many skin cancers, sound has no part to play.

8. **C.** Variation in nuclear size and shape (pleomorphism) is characteristic of malignant tumours. Malignant tumour cells show increased chromatin density. Malignant tumours tend to show endophytic growth. Malignant tumours tend to have lots of mitotic figures. The ability of malignant tumours to invade tissue allows metastatic spread.

9. **E.** Tumour suppressor genes encode proteins that negatively regulate cell growth. P53 and RB1 are tumour suppressor genes located on chromosomes 17 and 13, respectively. Loss of the protective functional role of tumour suppressor genes results in neoplastic growth. Viral proteins such as HPV E6 can deregulate tumour suppressor function. The so-called guardian of the genome triggers apoptosis and cell cycle arrest.

10. **E.** Host cell lysis is a method of release of new viral particles. Viruses are neither prokaryotes nor eukaryotes. Both RNA and DNA viruses exist. Budding occurs in enveloped viruses, e.g. HIV. Viruses are obligate intracellular parasites.

11. **D.** Altering the antibiotic target site is one mechanism for antibiotic resistance. Bacterial antibiotic resistance is very common. Resistance is conferred through extrachromosomal DNA called plamids. Resistance can be transferred by bacterial conjugation, transduction or transformation. Although resistant to many common antibiotics, MRSA is still treatable (e.g. vancomycin).

12. **D.** Hydrocephalus is an increase in the volume of CSF. Cerebral ventricles become expanded and dilated. Obstruction to the flow of CSF is the commonest form of hydrocephalus. A ventricular shunt with one-way valve can be used in the management. Congenital hydrocephalus may be diagnosed antenatally via ultrasound.

13. **D.** It is associated with a post-traumatic lucid interval that can last for several hours. Extradural haemorrhage occurs between the skull and the dura. Extradural haemorrhage is nearly always associated with a linear skull fracture, usually of the temporal bone. The artery usually involved is the middle meningeal artery. Prompt neurosurgery results in a good outlook.

14. **C.** Neurofibrillary tangles occur within neurons of patients with Alzheimer's disease. Only 5% of Alzheimer's disease is familial, 95% is sporadic. Senile plaques of amyloid protein are seen in Alzheimer's disease. Alzheimer's disease affects 15% of those aged above 80 years old. Memory disturbance is a common early presentation in Alzheimer's disease.

15. **C.** Oligodendrocytomas are slow-growing tumours. Gliomas are the most common primary CNS tumour, accounting for 50% of cases.

Astrocytomas are more common in children than adults. Meningiomas commonly compress rather than invade deeper CNS tissue. Prostatic carcinoma metastases to the brain are extremely rare.

16. **D.** Small defects often involve membranous areas, larger defects also involve the muscular wall. Ventricular septal defects cause a left-to-right shunt because of the higher pressure of the left side. Ventricular septal defects cause tachypnoea. The pansystolic murmur is caused by high pressure blood on the left side flowing to the right side. Ventricular septal defects are the most common of all congenital heart disease (25–30%).

17. **E.** Coarctation of aorta causes weak femoral pulses with radiofemoral delay. Coarctation of the aorta is more common in males by 2:1. Coarctation of the aorta causes hypertension distal to the stenosis. It is associated with a bicuspid aortic valve in 50% of cases. Serious complications in severe cases include heart failure and aortic dissection. Coarctation of aorta causes weak femoral pulses with radiofemoral delay.

18. **D.** It may be seen as a pathological response to endothelial injury. Atherosclerosis is the accumulation of lipid rich material in the intima of arteries. It is rare in pulmonary arteries, being seen more commonly in, for example, the aorta. Atherosclerosis is associated with both hypercholesterolaemia and diabetes mellitus. Macrophages take up lipid within a plaque to produce foam cells.

19. **D.** Hyaline is deposited in the arterial walls resulting in hyaline arteriosclerosis. Fibrinoid deposition occurs in malignant hypertension. In benign hypertension thickening and hypertrophy of the muscular media are seen histologically. Thickening of the elastic intima is seen histologically. Benign hypertension is characterized by stable elevation of blood pressure over many years.

20. **A.** Myocardial infarction results in necrosis of the myocardium following severe ischaemia. MI induces acute inflammatory changes. The infarct tissue is replaced by a collagenous scar. Occlusion of the right coronary artery results in an inferior MI. Management includes analgesics, thrombolysis and anticoagulants. However only STEMI (ST elevated MI) should have thrombolysis.

21. **A.** Heart failure is where the heart cannot maintain adequate cardiac output, or can only do so by increasing filling pressure. Left-sided failure is more common than right-sided. The progression of left-sided heart failure is the most common cause of right-sided failure. Heart failure may be a complication of myocardial infarction due to ventricular remodelling. Heart failure commonly follows severe aortic, mitral or pulmonary valve disease.

22. **B.** Both stasis and turbulence predispose to thrombosis (one of Virchow's triad). Thrombus occurs in flowing blood, a clot occurs in non-flowing blood. Antiphospholipid antibody promotes thrombosis, as seen in systemic lupus erythematosus. The most common site is the deep veins of the leg (deep vein thrombosis). Malignancy increases the risk of thrombosis, especially cancers of the breast, lung, prostate, pancreas and bowel.

23. **D.** The majority are of well-differentiated keratinizing squamous epithelium. The most common affected site for carcinoma of the larynx is the glottic region (60%). Cigarette smoking is a major risk factor in the aetiology. The tumour spreads mainly through local invasion to adjacent laryngeal structures. Carcinoma of the larynx usually occurs over the age of 40 years, affecting men more than women.

24. **A.** COPD is characterized by chronic bronchitis, emphysema and bronchiolitis. COPD is incompletely reversible by bronchodilators. Lungs are hyperinflated in COPD. Commonly smokers, but may occur without smoking in those occupationally exposed to dust or with $\alpha$-1-antitrypsin deficiency. Emphysema causes permanent airways dilatation and tissue destruction without fibrosis.

25. **B.** Cigarette smoking is very important in the aetiology. Chronic bronchitis is defined as a productive cough on most days for 3 months of the year for at least 2 successive years. Hypersecretion is associated with hypertrophy and hyperplasia of the bronchial mucus-secreting cells. Is characterized by chronic inflammation. Lung function tests show an obstructive pattern.

26. **C.** Bronchospasm, oedema and mucus plugging are commonly seen. Asthma reverses spontaneously or with bronchodilators. Asthma may be caused by a type I hypersensitivity reaction. $\alpha$-1-antitrypsin deficiency is associated with COPD development. Bronchial smooth muscle hypertrophy may occur.

27. **A.** Repeat infections occur in the stagnated secretions with organisms such as *Pseudomonas*. CF is the most common autosomal recessive condition in Europe (chromosome 7). Mutation results in a defective cystic fibrosis transmembrane regulator, impaired transport of Cl$^-$ ions. Malabsorption occurs due to reduced pancreatic secretions (mucus plugs in exocrine glands). The most common mutation is the deletion of phenylalanine 508 on chromosome 7.

28. **C.** Lung fibrosis, abscess and empyema may complicate pneumonia. Bacterial origin in 80–90% of cases. Gram-negative bacteria are associated with hospital-acquired pneumonia, Gram-positives with community-acquired. Lung fibrosis, abscess and empyema may complicate pneumonia. Red hepatization occurs in lobar pneumonia. Pulmonary oedema does increase the risk of pneumonia.

29. **D.** Immunocompromised patients are very susceptible to tuberculosis. Tuberculosis is caused by the organism *Mycobacterium tuberculosis*. Pathogenesis is due to host hypersensitivity reaction to constituents of the bacteria cell wall. Predisposing factors include chronic lung diseases such as silicosis. Immunocompromized patients are very susceptible to tuberculosis. Tuberculous granulomas are called tubercles.

30. **E.** Lung cancer is the most common cause of neoplasia in the UK. Squamous cell carcinoma is the most common form of lung cancer. Cigarette smoking is a major aetiological factor in the formation of lung cancer. Occupational exposure to asbestos increases risk of lung cancer and mesotheliomas. Metastatic spread is seen in 70% of patients at presentation.

31. **D.** Peripheral honeycombing describes the appearance on a cut lung surface (or CT scan). Idiopathic pulmonary fibrosis is not an infectious condition. It causes interstitial thickening with fibrosis. It is a restrictive airways disease. Idiopathic pulmonary fibrosis is one of the causes of finger clubbing.

32. **C.** Pulmonary embolism is a potential cause of pulseless electrical activity of the heart. Causes pulmonary hypertension and infarction. This would cause arterial embolism. Usually thromboembolic, but can involve fat, amniotic fluid, air, foreign bodies or tumour. Thromboembolism from deep leg veins is the most common cause of pulmonary embolism.

33. **E.** Mesothelioma is associated with recurrent pleural effusions. There is a long latency between asbestos exposure and mesothelioma. Haematogenous spread is rare in mesothelioma. Rapidly progressive with death usually occurring within 10 months of diagnosis. The incidence has been increasing per year.

34. **C.** There is a direct relationship between the number of cigarettes smoked and oral cancer risk. The lips are the most common site for squamous cell carcinoma of the oral cavity. The incidence is twice as high in males as in females. Moderate alcohol intake has been shown to decrease the risk of oral cancer. Oral cancer has a 5-year survival rate of about 50%.

35. **E.** Dysphagia is seen especially where the middle and upper oesophagus is affected. Squamous cell carcinoma is more common. Oesophageal adenocarcinoma may develop from Barrett's metaplasia. Heavy smoking and drinking are associated with squamous-cell carcinoma. Five-year survival from oesophageal carcinoma is less than 10%.

36. **A.** Oesophageal varices are dilated submucosal veins in the oesophagus. They are commonly associated with cirrhosis of the liver. Rupture causes torrential bleeding and haematemesis. Are associated with portal vein hypertension. Sclerotherapy can be used in the management by the injection of an irritant that causes thrombophlebitis.

37. **C.** Epithelial damage is mediated by the immune response against *Helicobacter pylori*. The gastritis is initially acute, but then becomes chronic. *Helicobacter pylori colonizes* the epithelium below a layer of mucus. Gastritis is most commonly found at the antrum. Infection often persists for many years.

38. **E.** Patients with antibodies to *Helicobacter pylori* have a higher risk of gastric cancer. The vast majority of gastric tumours are adenocarcinomas. Males are more affected than females. Sixty per cent of tumours are found at the pylorus. Interesting geographical pattern with incidence higher in East Asia than Europe.

39. **A.** The prehepatic, hepatic, posthepatic classification system is useful. Portal hypertension is most commonly caused by cirrhosis. Portal hypertension may cause ascites and splenomegaly. Budd-Chiari syndrome (hepatic vein thrombosis) is a cause of portal hypertension. Portosystemic shunts become enlarged.

40. **D.** Nodules are formed from regenerated hepatocytes separated by bands of collagenous fibrosis. Cirrhosis is an irreversible condition. A common cause of cirrhosis is alcohol liver disease (also hepatitis B and C). An uncommon cause of cirrhosis is autoimmune chronic hepatitis (also cystic fibrosis). Prothrombin time is increased due to reduced synthesis of anticoagulation factors.

41. **A.** Ascites is the accumulation of free fluid in the peritoneal cavity. Cirrhosis causes transudative (low protein) ascites. Non-hepatic causes of ascites include malignancy, nephrotic syndrome and heart failure. Shifting dullness on percussion of the abdomen signifies ascites, Grey Turner's sign is a sign of retroperitoneal bleeding. The treatment of ascites involves sodium restriction.

42. **C.** Free copper overspills into the blood and deposits in the cornea and the brain. Wilson's disease is an autosomal recessive condition. It results from a mutation in a gene for a calcium transporter protein. Psychiatric disorders occur. Chronic hepatitis and cirrhosis are common.

43. **D.** Vaccination for hepatitis B utilizes the surface antigen, HBsAg. Hepatitis B is a DNA virus. Transmission routes are blood-borne, sexual contact and vertical. Initial infection is subclinical and transient in 65% of cases. Cirrhosis and hepatocellular carcinoma are potential complications of chronic infection.

44. **C.** Males are affected more than females (8:1 ratio). The majority of malignant liver tumours are metastatic (lung, breast, colon, stomach). Predisposing factors include hepatitis B. Prognosis

is very poor with a median survival rate of less than 6 months post diagnosis. It is cholangiocarcinoma that arises from the bile duct epithelium, not HCC.

**45. E.** The scar formation in primary biliary cirrhosis is by bridging fibrosis. Primary biliary cirrhosis is much more common in females than males (10:1). Associations with several autoimmune diseases are seen, e.g. rheumatoid arthritis, SLE. Drugs are ineffective and affected individuals eventually need a liver transplant. Ulcerative colitis is strongly associated with primary sclerosing cholangitis.

**46. E.** Patients are usually over the age of 60 at presentation. Pancreatic cancer has a positive association with excess alcohol consumption. It is more common in males than females. Curative surgical resection is rarely possible with a Whipple's prodecure. Lesions are typically moderately differentiated adenocarcinomas.

**47. D.** Non-caseating granulomas present in the bowel wall and mesenteric lymph nodes. Systemic complications which develop in a minority of patients with Crohn's include skin disease. There is an increased incidence of Crohn's in cigarette smokers. Granulomatous inflammation can occur anywhere from the mouth to the anus. There is an association between Crohn's and eye disease.

**48. E.** The disease is continuous, spreading to the whole of the large bowel. Ulcerative colitis is characterized by superficial inflammation. Interestingly, smoking is associated with a decreased risk for UC. Inflammation is diffuse and limited to the mucosa. Features include infiltration of inflammatory cells, crypt abscesses and atrophy (Crohn's is complicated by fistulae).

**49. D.** Serum screening for anti-endomyseal antibodies is a useful aid to diagnosis. Coeliac disease is due to an abnormal immune response to gluten. Villous atrophy and crypt hyperplasia are seen. A disease of the small intestine. There is a slow but partial or total recovery in villous structure.

**50. A.** Colorectal carcinoma is thought to develop from adenomas. By the age of 45, 90% of individuals with FAP will have developed carcinoma. Staged by the modified Dukes system (A-D). Left-sided carcinomas cause early mechanical obstruction to faeces and so present earlier. The rectosigmoid is the most common area affected.

**51. D.** Enlarging cysts replace and compress functioning renal parenchyma. Both kidneys are progressively replaced by cyst. It is an inherited autosomal dominant disease. Associations are with berry aneurysms of the cerebral arteries. Uncontrolled hypertension accelerates the development of renal failure.

**52. E.** Streptococcal glomerulonephritis may follow throat infection. Membranous nephropathy is the most common cause of adult nephrotic syndrome. Eighty to ninety per cent of membranous nephropathy cases are idiopathic. Children with minimal change disease have a good prognosis with corticosteroids. Goodpasture's syndrome is indicated by anti-collagen IV antibodies and glomerulonephritis.

**53. A.** Renal cell carcinoma is more common in males than females (3:1). Carcinoma usually occurs at the upper kidney pole. Haematuria, loin pain and a loin mass are more typical features. Smoking increases the risk of renal cell carcinoma. Renal cell carcinoma may rarely be linked to von Hippel-Lindau syndrome.

**54. D.** The most commonly affected sites are the base of trigone and ureteric orifaces. Men are affected more often than women (3:1). Almost all cases are transitional cell carcinoma. Bladder cancer may obstruct urinary flow. Known environmental carcinogens include certain dyes, rubbers and cigarette components.

**55. D.** Only about 5% of patients show exophthalmos. Graves' disease is much more common in women than men (8:1). Ninety-five per cent of Graves' individuals are serum positive for TSH-receptor antibodies. Diffuse hypertrophy and hyperplasia of the acinar epithelium are seen. Graves' disease causes thyrotoxicosis, Hashimoto's thyroiditis causes hypothyroidism.

**56. B.** There is a link between childhood radiation exposure (e.g. Chernobyl) and thyroid cancer. Toxic adenomas are benign tumours that secrete thyroid hormones. Papillary carcinomas tend to develop in younger patients. Medullary carcinoma is derived from parafollicular C cells that secrete substances like calcitonin and serotonin. In about half of anaplastic carcinoma cases there is a history of multinodular goitre.

**57. B.** Iatrogenic administration of ACTH can cause Cushing's syndrome. Addison's disease results in a hypofunction of the adrenal cortex. Iatrogenic administration of prednisolone can cause Cushing's syndrome, but saline fludis do not. Phaeochromocytoma is a tumour of the chromaffin cells that results in the secretion of catecholamines. Waterhouse-Friderichsen syndrome is caused by adrenal gland haemhorrage due to Neisseria infections.

**58. D.** Histologically destruction of insulin secreting cells of the islets of Langerhans is observed. Type 1 diabetes mellitus is an autoimmuneinduced disorder, which may be triggered by a viral infection. Genetic predisposition association with HLA-DR genotype. Type 1 diabetes mellitus is a disease of childhood/adolescent onset. Plasma insulin absent or low.

**59. C.** Insulin resistance is an important first step in the development. Type II diabetes is almost exclusively a disease of adults. Commonly treated by diet and oral hypoglycaemic agents, although insulin may eventually be required. Diabetic ketoacidosis is a complication of type I diabetes. Macrovascular and microvascular complications occur in diabetes.

60. **B.** Cervical intra-epithelial neoplasia is a dysplastic preneoplastic proliferative state. The majority of cervical tumours are squamous cell carcinomas. HPV 16, 18 and 33 have been identified in cervical carcinoma. Cigarette smoking has a positive association with cervical cancer. HIV infection has a positive association with cervical cancer due to its immunosuppressive action.

61. **A.** Endometriosis is defined as endometrial glands or stroma occurring outside of the uterus. The ovaries are a commonly affected site. Retrograde menstruation is a common theory of aetiology. Endometriosis is oestrogen dependent and therefore improves after the menopause. It is a common cause of infertility but only 30% of those with endometriosis are infertile.

62. **A.** Pelvic inflammatory disease is a disorder of the fallopian tubes, ovaries and peritoneum. Predisposing factors include intrauterine contraceptive devices. *Neisseria gonorrhoeae* is a common aetiological agent. Initially inflammation is acute; untreated PID may progress to chronic inflammation. Pelvic inflammatory disease is a disease of infection.

63. **C.** Aetiology may be due to previous episodes of salpingitis (inflammation of the fallopian tube). Ectopic pregnancy results when a fertilized ovum implants outside the uterine cavity. The most common site is the fallopian tube, especially the ampulla. Proliferation of the trophoblast causes erosion of the submucosa, which precipitates severe bleeding. Tubal pregnancy invariably results in rupture of the fallopian tube and death of the fertilized ovum.

64. **B.** First and multiple pregnancies are more commonly affected. Pre-eclampsia also requires proteinuria, otherwise it is just gestational hypertension. It is thought pre-eclampsia develops from placental ischaemia. Pre-eclampsia is associated with fetal growth retardation and low birth weight. It resolves within 24 hours of delivery.

65. **B.** Mutation of tumour suppressor genes *BRCA1/2* are implicated in some inherited cancers. Carcinoma of the breast is the most common cause of death in women aged 35–55 years. Screening by mammography is available for all women over the age of 50. The antioestrogen tamoxifen can be used in oestrogen-receptor-positive tumours. Ductal carcinoma is the most common histological subtype.

66. **C.** The majority of prostate carcinomas have a well differentiated glandular pattern. It is an adenocarcinoma. Prostate carcinoma affects the peripheral zone. Benign prostatic hyperplasia is more likely to cause urinary symptoms as it affects the central zone. Commonly extends outside of the prostatic capsule.

67. **E.** X-ray changes include decreased bone density and 'fish' lumbar vertebrae. Osteoporosis is very common, especially in elderly women. Osteoporosis may cause pathological fractures. Bone trabeculae are thinned and reduced in number. Diagnosis is by bone densitometry.

68. **D.** Associated with the development of a pannus and inflammatory destruction of joints. Rheumatoid arthritis affects 1% of the UK population. Onset is normally distributed with a peak between 35 and 45 years old. Many, but not all, are positive for rheumatoid factor. Rheumatoid disease has widespread extraarticular manifestations.

69. **E.** HIV infection is characterized by atypical mycobacterium infection. HIV is an enveloped RNA retrovirus. Host reverse transcriptase is required for viral replication. HIV binds CD4 positive cells via its gp120 cell surface glycoprotein. Opportunistic infections include *Pneumocystis carinii*.

70. **E.** Amyloidosis may complicate long-term haemodialyis. Numerous potential proteins can fold abnormally to produce amyloid. Amyloid takes up the Congo red stain. Abnormal macrophage control systems appear to aid amyloid aggregation, and has systemic effects in the liver, kidneys and the tongue. The AA type is seen in reactive systemic amyloidosis.

71. **B.** Neutropenia is part of the autosomal recessive Kostmann's syndrome. Agranulocytosis describes severe neutropenia. Neutrophil increase is the most common cause of leucocytosis. Primary leucocytosis occurs in bone marrow disease, e.g. leukaemia, lymphoma. Eosinophilia is commonly seen in allergic reactions.

72. **A.** Reed-Sternberg cells are seen in Hodgkin's lymphoma. Males are affected more than females. The staging system used for Hodgkin's lymphoma is the Ann Arbor system. Suffix B indicates the presence of systemic symptoms and a worse prognosis. Mixed cellularity with numerous RS cells has a poor prognosis.

73. **E.** Extranodal involvement is more common in non-Hodgkin's lymphoma. Non-Hodgkin's lymphoma has been linked to immunosuppression. *Helicobacter pylori* infection has been linked to gastric lymphoma. Seventy per cent of non-Hodgkin's lymphomas are derived from B cells. Chromosomal translocations are a common feature of many lymphomas.

74. **E.** Lymph nodes can be affected with normal architecture becoming effaced by infiltrating cells. The Philadelphia chromosome occurs in chronic myeloid leukaemia. Chronic lymphocytic leukaemia is the commonest leukaemia in adults. Survival of more than 10 years postdiagnosis is common. True – males are affected more than females.

75. **C.** Chronic haemolysis may result in gall stones and jaundice. Sickle-cell anaemia is caused by a mutation in the gene encoding the β-globin chain.

It is common in West and East Africa, the
Mediterranean and the Middle East. Hyposplenism
is seen (autosplenectomy). HbS confers protection
against malaria by creating a hostile environment
for the plasmodium parasite in the RBC.

76.  'Cold' type autoimmune haemolytic anaemia
results in red cell agglutination. Autoimmune
haemolytic anaemia may be associated with
lymphoma. Haemolytic anaemia is most
commonly autoimmune. Causes brain damage in
neonates (kernicterus). 'Warm' type autoimmune
haemolytic anaemia results in microspherocytosis.

77.  E.  Spongiosis means epidermal oedema. A nodule is a
raised lesion greater than 5 mm across. A vesicle is
a blister less than 5 mm across. A macule is a
localized flattened lesion of pigmented skin. A
pustule is a small pus-containing blister, often
indicating infection.

78.  C.  Lithium may precipiate or worsen psoriasis.
Psoriasis is a chronic, non-infective inflammatory
disease. The epidermal proliferation rate is
increased 20-fold. Psoriasis commonly affects the
elbows, knees, trunk and scalp. Nail involvement is
common, with pitting and thickening of the nail.

79.  E.  Bacterial and viral infections complicate atopic
eczema. The incidence of atopic eczema is
increasing. Family history is a strong risk factor for
the development of atopic eczema. Atopic eczema
is caused by a type I hypersensitivity reaction.
Atopic eczema decreases in incidence with
increasing age through childhood.

80.  B.  Pemphigus is associated with erosions.
Pemphigoid is subepidermal separation of tissue.
Pemphigus has a higher untreated mortality than
pemphigoid. Dermatitis herpetiformis is a
blistering condition associated with coeliac disease.
Dermatitis herpetiformis involves granular IgA
deposition at the dermal papillae in normal-
looking skin.

81.  B.  Repeated exposure to UV radiation may play an
aetiological role. Malignant melanoma is a tumour
of melanocytes. Familial dysplastic naevus
syndrome is a major risk factor. A Breslow thickness
(staging of malignant melanoma) of > 3.5 mm has
a poor prognosis. Malignant melanoma may arise in
a preexisting lentigo maligna.

# EMQ answers

## 1. Nervous system:

1. I. Hydrocephalus. An increase in CSF within the brain that may be congenital or acquired. Often treated with ventriculoperitoneal shunt surgery.
2. H. Alzheimer's disease. Memory disturbance is a common initial presentation of disease.
3. F. Extradural haemorrhage. Almost always the result of skull fracture, with decline in neurological function occurring after several hours of a post-traumatic lucid interval.
4. C. Multiple sclerosis. Diagnosis requires at least two episodes of CNS demyelination separated in time (i.e. recovery between episodes) and space (i.e. affecting different CNS areas).
5. A. Acute bacterial meningitis. Often presents with fever, headache, petechial rash and neck stiffness. CSF is cloudy because of increased neutrophils.

## 2. Cardiovascular system:

1. E. Coarctation of the aorta. Causes headache, dizziness, interstitial bruits and radiofemoral pulse delay.
2. G. Dissecting aortic aneurysm. Classically causes central chest pain radiating to the back between the scapulae with pulse asymmetry. Chest X-ray changes include mediastinal widening, aortic knuckle distortion and left-sided pleural effusion.
3. J. Aortic stenosis. Syncope, angina and even sudden death are potential consequences of reduced cardiac output.
4. I. Giant cell arteritis. Affects the temporal arteries to cause scalp tenderness. Also often associated with polymyalgia rheumatica.
5. A. Ventricular septal defect. Other congenital causes of a left-to-right shunt include atrial septal defect and patent ductus arteriosus.

## 3. Respiratory system:

1. D. Chronic obstructive pulmonary disease. Obstructive lung pattern with chronic inflammation in response to noxious stimuli (most commonly cigarette smoking) that is only partially reversible with bronchodilators.
2. H. Intrinsic (nonatopic) asthma. This is late-onset asthma that is often triggered by upper respiratory tract infection. IgE levels are normal (unlike atopic asthma).
3. F. Cystic fibrosis. A hereditary, multisystem disease that causes abnormally thick mucus. Affects several organs, but effects on the lung and pancreas are most marked.
4. B. Small cell lung cancer. Unique amongst lung cancers for its response to radiotherapy and chemotherapy, but prognosis remains very poor.
5. J. Sarcoidosis. Multisystem granulomatous disease of unknown aetiology that commonly causes lung disease. Raised serum angiotensin converting enzyme levels aid diagnosis.

## 4. Gastrointestinal system:

1. E. Coeliac disease. A disease of malabsorption causing villous atrophy in the small intestine. The rash is that of dermatitis herpetiformis, which is strongly associated with coeliac disease.
2. D. Crohn's disease. Usually presents early in adult life causing full thickness granulomatous inflammation of any site in the GI tract. This commonly leads to strictures, but in a 'skip lesion' pattern, hence the normal areas of bowel on endoscopy.
3. A. Barrett's oesophagus. Metaplastic replacement of normal squamous epithelium with glandular columnar epithelium. Predisposes to adenocarcinoma of the oesophagus.
4. H. Oesophageal varices. Dilatation of oesophageal veins as a complication of portal hypertension.
5. F. Haemochromatosis. Caused by excessive iron deposition in the liver and elsewhere. This leads to cirrhosis if untreated. Excess melanin causes leaden grey pigmentation of skin.

## 5. Renal and urinary systems:

1. D. Minimal change disease. Most common cause of nephrotic syndrome in children. Changes only seen on renal biopsy if examined by electron microscopy.
2. B. Alport's syndrome. A hereditary glomerulonephritis that commonly causes renal failure in the second decade of life in males affected by the X-linked

form. Ocular disease and deafness to high-pitched sounds are associated features.

3. G. Acute tubular necrosis. Usually reversible renal failure caused by ischaemia or toxins.

4. I. Hydronephrosis. Dilatation of the renal pelvis and calyces in response to increased pressure from distal obstruction.

5. E. Goodpasture's syndrome. Autoimmune disease targeting type IV collagen in both the kidney and the lung.

## 6. Endocrine system:

1. J. Adrenal crisis. A medical emergency caused by abrupt cessation of prolonged high-dose corticosteroids.

2. A. Type I diabetes mellitus. Autoimmune destruction of β-cells in the pancreas result in the failure of insulin production.

3. DHypothyroidism. Secondary to De Quervain's thyroiditis that may follow mumps infection. Causes a painfully enlarged thyroid gland with classical hypothyroid features of cold extremities and cold intolerance.

4. C. Cushing's syndrome. Caused by inappropriately elevated free glucocorticoid levels.

5. F. Cranial diabetes insipidus. Caused by failure of the posterior pituitary to produce antidiuretic hormone.

## 7. Reproductive system:

1. I. Endometriosis. Ectopic growth of endometrial tissue outside of the uterus.

2. G. Breast cancer. A breast lump is investigated by history/examination, imaging (mammography or ultrasound) and tissue sampling (fine-needle aspiration or core biopsy).

3. B. Cervical cancer. The same risk factors exist for development of the premalignant state, cervical intraepithelial neoplasia.

4. D. Choriocarcinoma. A malignant tumour of trophoblastic tissue, most commonly occurring from a hydatiform (molar) pregnancy.

5. E. Ectopic pregnancy. The implantation of a fertilized ovum outside the uterus. May cause severe haemorrhage from tubal rupture.

## 8. Musculoskeletal system:

1. H. Metastatic disease. The most common tumours in bone are blood-borne metastases from other primary sites.

2. C. Paget's disease. Uncontrolled bone resorption and deposition. Most common in men over the age of 40 years.

3. E. Osteoarthritis. A very common disease of articular cartilage degeneration.

4. A. Osteogenesis imperfecta. A group of disorders characterized by the development of abnormal type I collagen. Also known as 'brittle bone disease'.

5. J. Duchenne muscular dystrophy. An inherited myopathy. The lack of dystrophin protein results in tears to muscle fibres on repeated contraction.

## 9. Haematological and immunological systems:

1. E. Chronic myeloid leukaemia. Philadelphia chromosome is seen in 90% of cases.

2. B. Hodgkin's disease. A lymphoma characterized by painless lymphadenopathy and the presence of Reed-Sternberg cells (large binucleate cells).

3. F. Myeloma. Diagnosis here is based on skeletal lesions and characteristic serum electrophoresis.

4. G. Myasthenia gravis. Autoimmune disease of the post-synaptic acetylcholine receptor causing fatigability.

5. H. Thalassaemia. Caused by decreased α- or β-globin synthesis.

## 10. Dermatological system:

1. G. Macule. A localized, flat area of altered skin colour that may be hyperpigmented (e.g. freckle), hypopigmented (e.g. vitiligo) or erythematous (e.g. capillary haemangioma).

2. E. Acne vulgaris. An inflammatory disorder of the pilosebaceous apparatus, characterized by comedones, pustules, papules, nodules, cysts and scars.

3. J. Pemphigus vulgaris. Causes intraepidermal bullae, which are flaccid and superficial. Erosions commonly develop.

4. D. Parakeratosis. A histological sign of increased epidermal growth, with excessive keratin and nuclear remnants persisting in the stratum corneum.

5. A. Acantholysis. Describes the loss of cellular cohesion between epidermal keratinocytes due to the rupture of intercellular bridges.

# Glossary

**Abscess** A localized collection of pus in a tissue, cavity or confined area. Usually associated with infection.

**Aetiology** The cause of a disease.

**Anaplastic** A lack of cellular differentiation which is characteristic of some cancer cells.

**Anhidrosis** The absence of sweating.

**Atrophy** Describes the decrease in size (or wasting) of a cell, tissue or organ.

**Autocrine** Describes the process whereby a cell secretes a substance whose target for action is the secreting cell itself.

**Bursa** A small fluid-filled sac that reduces friction on movement between a tendon and bone, or between bone and skin.

**Colic** Describes a pain that gradually increases, reaches a peak and then subsides slowly. This pattern may then be repeated.

**Contralateral** On the opposite side (to a lesion).

**Crypt** A deep pit-like structure found in the wall of the small intestine.

**Dysphagia** Difficulty in swallowing.

**Dyspnoea** Shortness of breath.

**Empyema** The accumulation of pus in a cavity of the body.

**Endophytic** Used to describe a tumour that grows inwards and is thus invasive.

**Epistaxis** A nosebleed.

**Erythrocyte sedimentation rate (ESR)** A nonspecific marker of inflammation, based on the rate at which red blood cells settle in a column of liquid.

**Exophytic** Used to describe a tumour that grows outwards from an epithelial surface.

**Fistula** An abnormal communication between two epithelial lined cavities.

**Giant cell** A multinucleated cell formed from the fusion of many cells.

**Glossitis** Inflammation of the tongue.

**Histiocyte** A resident tissue macrophage which has a long lifespan.

**Hyperhidrosis** Excessive sweating.

**Hypoxia** A condition where insufficient oxygen reaches the tissues of the body.

**Iatrogenic** An inadvertent effect of medical treatment or actions.

**Idiopathic** Where the cause is unknown.

**Ipsilateral** On the same side (as a lesion).

**Paracrine** Describes the process whereby a cell secretes a substance that has an action on nearby cells.

**Parenchyma** The functional component of a gland or organ (distinct from support or connective tissue).

**Paroxysmal** Describes sudden attacks of a given effect.

**Pathogenic** Capable of causing disease.

**Petechiae** Small red spots on the skin.

**Pruritus** Itchiness.

**Ptosis** Drooping of the upper eyelid.

**Stroma** Supporting connective tissue of an organ.

**Suppurative** Any reaction that produces pus.

**Venesection** The removal of blood from a vein.

**Xanthoma** A benign yellow-coloured lesion common on the eyelid and usually indicating elevated serum cholesterol levels.

# Index